Neonatal Pulmonary Hypertension

Editors

SATYAN LAKSHMINRUSIMHA
STEVEN H. ABMAN

CLINICS IN PERINATOLOGY

www.perinatology.theclinics.com

Consulting Editor
LUCKY JAIN

March 2024 • Volume 51 • Number 1

ELSEVIER

1600 John F. Kennedy Boulevard • Suite 1800 • Philadelphia, Pennsylvania, 19103-2899

http://www.theclinics.com

CLINICS IN PERINATOLOGY Volume 51, Number 1
March 2024 ISSN 0095-5108, ISBN-13: 978-0-443-18405-5

Editor: Kerry Holland
Developmental Editor: Nitesh Barthwal

Clinics in Perinatology (ISSN 0095-5108) is published quarterly by Elsevier Inc., 360 Park Avenue South, New York, NY 10010-1710. Months of issue are March, June, September, and December. Business and Editorial Offices: 1600 John F. Kennedy Blvd., Ste. 1800, Philadelphia, PA 19103-2899. Customer Service Office: 3251 Riverport Lane, Maryland Heights, MO 63043. Periodicals postage paid at New York, NY and additional mailing offices. Subscription prices are $351.00 per year (US individuals), $398.00 per year (Canadian individuals), $475.00 per year (international individuals), $100.00 per year (US and Canadian students), and $195.00 per year (International students). For institutional access pricing please contact Customer Service via the contact information below. International air speed delivery is included in all Clinics subscription prices. All prices are subject to change without notice. **POSTMASTER:** Send address changes to *Clinics in Perinatology*, Elsevier Health Sciences Division, Subscription Customer Service, 3251 Riverport Lane, Maryland Heights, MO 63043. **Customer Service: Telephone: 1-800-654-2452** (U.S. and Canada); **1-314-447-8871** (outside U.S. and Canada). **Fax: 1-314-447-8029. E-mail: journalscustomerservice-u-sa@elsevier.com** (for print support); **journalsonlinesupport-usa@elsevier.com** (for online support).

Reprints. For copies of 100 or more, of articles in this publication, please contact the Commercial Reprints Department, Elsevier Inc., 360 Park Avenue South, New York, NY 10010-1710. Tel. 212-633-3874; Fax: 212-633-3820; E-mail: reprints@elsevier.com.

Clinics in Perinatology is also published in Spanish by McGraw-Hill Interamericana Editores S.A., P.O. Box 5-237, 06500 Mexico D.F., Mexico.

Clinics in Perinatology is covered in *MEDLINE/PubMed (Index Medicus) Current Contents, Excepta Medica, BIOSIS and ISI/BIOMED.*

Contributors

CONSULTING EDITOR

LUCKY JAIN, MD, MBA
Pediatrician-in-Chief, Children's Healthcare of Atlanta, George W. Brumley Jr. Professor and Chair, Emory University School of Medicine, Department of Pediatrics, Executive Director, Emory+Children's Pediatric Institute, Atlanta, Georgia, USA

EDITORS

SATYAN LAKSHMINRUSIMHA, MD, MBBS, FAAP
Professor and Dennis and Nancy Marks Chair, Division of Neonatology, Department of Pediatrics, University of California, Davis; Pediatrician-in-Chief, UC Davis Children's Hospital, Sacramento, California, USA

STEVEN H. ABMAN, MD
Professor, Department of Pediatrics, Director, Pediatric Heart Lung Center, University of Colorado Denver Anschutz Medical Campus, School of Medicine, Children's Hospital Colorado, Aurora, Colorado, USA

AUTHORS

STEVEN H. ABMAN, MD
Professor, Department of Pediatrics, Director, Pediatric Heart Lung Center, University of Colorado Denver Anschutz Medical Campus, School of Medicine, Children's Hospital Colorado, Aurora, Colorado, USA

GABRIEL ALTIT, MD
Neonatologist, Neonatology, McGill University Health Centre, Montreal Children's Hospital, Department of Pediatrics, McGill University, Montreal, Quebec, Canada

PRATHIK BANDIYA, MD, DM
Associate Professor, Department of Neonatology, Indira Gandhi Institute of Child Health, Bangalore, India

STEPHANIE M. BOYD, MBBS (Hons), BSc (Med), MPHTM, FRACP, CCPU
Neonatologist, Grace Centre for Newborn Intensive Care, The Children's Hospital at Westmead, Faculty of Medicine and Health, The University of Sydney, Sydney, Australia

JEANNE CARROLL, MD
Associate Professor and Medical Director, Division of Neonatology, Department of Pediatrics, University of California, San Diego, Rady Children's Hospital-San Diego, San Diego, California, USA

PRAVEEN CHANDRASEKHARAN, MD, MS
Associate Professor of Pediatrics, Division of Neonatology, Department of Pediatrics, Jacobs School of Medicine and Biomedical Sciences, State University of New York, Attending Neonatologist, Oishei Children's Hospital, Buffalo, New York, USA

MICHAEL W. COOKSON, MD
Neonatal and Perinatal Medicine Fellow, Section of Neonatology, Department of Pediatrics, University of Colorado Anschutz School of Medicine, Children's Hospital Colorado, Department of Pediatrics, Pediatric Heart Lung Center, Aurora, Colorado, USA

KRISTEN COLETTI, MD
Fellow, Division of Neonatology, Department of Pediatrics, The Children's Hospital of Philadelphia, Philadelphia, Pennsylvania, USA

OLIVIER DANHAIVE, MD
Professor and Chief, Division of Neonatology, Saint-Luc University Hospital, UCLouvain, Brussels, Belgium; Professor, Department of Pediatrics, University of California, San Francisco, San Francisco, California, USA

JACK R.T. DARBY, PhD
Early Career Researcher, Early Origins of Adult Health Research Group, University of South Australia, Adelaide, South Australia, Australia

AHMED ELSAIE, MD
Assistant Professor of Pediatrics, Section of Neonatology, Department of Pediatrics, Children's Mercy Hospital, Kansas City, Missouri, USA; Department of Pediatrics, Cairo University, Cairo, Egypt

ELIZABETH E. FOGLIA, MD, MSCE
Attending Neonatologist, Division of Neonatology, Department of Pediatrics, The Children's Hospital of Philadelphia, Perelman School of Medicine, University of Pennsylvania, Philadelphia, Pennsylvania, USA

CSABA GALAMBOS, MD, PhD
Professor, Department of Pathology and Laboratory Medicine, University of Colorado Anschutz School of Medicine, Aurora, Colorado, USA

REGAN GEISINGER, MD
Division of Neonatology, Department of Pediatrics, University of Iowa, Iowa City, Iowa, USA

HANNAH HOLMES
Division of Cardiology, Department of Pediatrics, The Hospital for Sick Children, University of Toronto, Toronto, Ontario, Canada

AJAY RAGHAV JOSHI, MBBS, DCH, DNB (Pead)
Consultant Pediatrician, Department of Pediatrics, SIGMA Hospital, Mysore, Karnataka, India

ROBERTA L. KELLER, MD
Neonatology, UCSF Benioff Children's Hospital, Department of Pediatrics, University of California, San Francisco, San Francisco, California, USA

JOHN P. KINSELLA, MD
Professor of Pediatrics, Section of Neonatology, Department of Pediatrics, University of Colorado Anschutz School of Medicine, Children's Hospital Colorado, Department of Pediatrics, Pediatric Heart Lung Center, Aurora, Colorado, USA

HARESH KIRPALANI, BM, MSc
Emeritus, Perelman School of Medicine, University of Pennsylvania, Philadelphia, Pennsylvania, USA; Emeritus, Pediatrics, McMaster University, Hamilton, Ontario, Canada

MARTIN KLUCKOW, MBBS, FRACP, PhD, CCPU
Faculty of Medicine and Health, The University of Sydney, Department of Neonatology, Royal North Shore Hospital, Sydney, Australia

SATYAN LAKSHMINRUSIMHA, MD, MBBS, FAAP
Professor and Dennis and Nancy Marks Chair, Division of Neonatology, Department of Pediatrics, University of California, Davis; Pediatrician-in-Chief, UC Davis Children's Hospital, Sacramento, California, USA

PHILIP T. LEVY, MD
Assistant Professor, Division of Newborn Medicine, Department of Pediatrics, Boston Children's Hospital, Harvard Medical School, Boston, Massachusetts, USA

RAJESHWARI MADAPPA, MBBS, DCH, DNB (Pead)
Director and Head, Department of Pediatrics, SIGMA Hospital, Mysore, Karnataka, India

SRINIVASAN MANI, MD
Clinical Assistant Professor, Section of Neonatology, Department of Pediatrics, The University of Toledo, ProMedica Russell J. Ebeid Children's Hospital, Toledo, Ohio, USA

PATRICK J. McNAMARA, MB, BCh, BAO, DCH, MSc, MRCP, MRCPCH
Professor, Division of Neonatology, Department of Pediatrics, University of Iowa, Iowa City, Iowa, USA

HUSSNAIN MIRZA, MD
Associate Professor, Section of Neonatology, Department of Pediatrics, Advent Health for Children, University of Central Florida, College of Medicine, Orlando, Florida, USA

OLIVIA J. MOIR, MSc
Division of Cardiology, Department of Pediatrics, The Hospital for Sick Children, University of Toronto, Toronto, Ontario, Canada

SHIRAN S. MOORE, MD
Neonatology, Dana Dwek Children's Hospital, Tel Aviv Sourasky Medical Center, Tel Aviv-Jaffa, Israel; Tel Aviv University, Tel Aviv, Israel

JANNA L. MORRISON, PhD
Early Origins of Adult Health Research Group, University of South Australia, Adelaide, South Australia, Australia

SUZAN COCHIUS-DEN OTTER, MD, PhD
Head of Pediatric Intensive Care, Division of Pediatric Intensive Care, Department of Neonatal and Pediatric Intensive Care, Erasmus MC University Medical Center, Rotterdam, the Netherlands

ROHIT RAO, MD, MBA
Clinical Professor of Pediatrics and Medical Director, Division of Cardiothoracic Critical Care, Department of Pediatrics, University of California, San Diego, Rady Children's Hospital-San Diego, San Diego, California, USA

DANIELLE R. RIOS, MD, MS
Associate Professor, Division of Neonatology, Department of Pediatrics, University of Iowa, Iowa City, Iowa, USA

CATHERINE A. ROTTKAMP, MD, PhD
Neonatologist, Division of Neonatology, Department of Pediatrics, University of California, Davis, Davis, California, USA

BRAHMDEEP S. SAINI, PhD
Postdoctoral Fellow, Division of Cardiology, Department of Pediatrics, The Hospital for Sick Children, University of Toronto, Toronto, Ontario, Canada

DEEPIKA SANKARAN, MD
Assistant Professor, Division of Neonatology, Department of Pediatrics, University of California, Davis, Davis, California, USA

LOURENCO SBRAGIA, MD, PhD
Professor of Surgery, Division of Pediatric Surgery, Department of Surgery and Anatomy, University of São Paulo, Ribeirão Preto, São Paulo, Brazil

AUGUSTO F. SCHMIDT, MD, PhD
Associate Professor of Pediatrics, Division of Neonatology, Department of Pediatrics, University of Miami Miller School of Medicine, Batchelor Children's Research Institute, Miami, Florida, USA

MIKE SEED, MD
Head, Division of Cardiology, Department of Pediatrics, The Hospital for Sick Children, University of Toronto, Toronto, Ontario, Canada

BINOY SHIVANNA, MD, DM, PhD
Associate Professor of Pediatrics, Division of Neonatology, Department of Pediatrics, Baylor College of Medicine, Texas Children's Hospital, Houston, Texas, USA

ROBIN H. STEINHORN, MD
Professor and Vice Dean, Department of Pediatrics, University of California, San Diego, Rady Children's Hospital-San Diego, San Diego, California, USA

EMILY S. STIEREN, MD, PhD
Neonatologist, Division of Neonatology, Department of Pediatrics, University of California, Davis, Davis, California, USA

LIQUN SUN, MD, PhD
Division of Cardiology, Department of Pediatrics, The Hospital for Sick Children, University of Toronto, Toronto, Ontario, Canada

APRIL W. TAN, MD
Assistant Professor of Pediatrics, Division of Neonatology, Department of Pediatrics, University of Miami Miller School of Medicine, Batchelor Children's Research Institute, Miami, Florida, USA

K. TAYLOR WILD, MD
Assistant Professor, Division of Neonatology, Department of Pediatrics, The Children's Hospital of Philadelphia, Philadelphia, Pennsylvania, USA

KAREN C. YOUNG, MD, MS
Professor of Pediatrics, Director, Newborn Intensive Care Unit, Division of Neonatology, Department of Pediatrics, University of Miami Miller School of Medicine, Batchelor Children's Research Institute, Miami, Florida, USA

JAMES ZIEGLER, MD
Pediatric Cardiologist, Division of Cardiovascular Diseases, Department of Pediatrics, Hasbro Children's Hospital, Brown University, Providence, Rhode Island, USA

Contents

Fetal lungs have fewer and smaller arteries with higher pulmonary vascular resistance (PVR) than a newborn. As gestation advances, the pulmonary circulation becomes more sensitive to changes in pulmonary arterial oxygen tension, which prepares them for the dramatic drop in PVR and increase in pulmonary blood flow (PBF) that occur when the baby takes its first few breaths of air, thus driving the transition from fetal to postnatal circulation. Dynamic and intricate regulatory mechanisms control PBF throughout development and are essential in supporting gas exchange after birth. Understanding these concepts is crucial given the role the pulmonary vasculature plays in the development of complications with transition, such as in the setting of persistent pulmonary hypertension of the newborn and congenital heart disease. An improved understanding of pulmonary vascular regulation may reveal opportunities for better clinical management.

Neonatal pulmonary hypertension (PH) is a devastating disorder of the pulmonary vasculature characterized by elevated pulmonary vascular resistance and mean pulmonary arterial pressure. Occurring predominantly because of maldevelopment or maladaptation of the pulmonary vasculature, PH in neonates is associated with suboptimal short-term and long-term outcomes because its pathobiology is unclear in most circumstances, and it responds poorly to conventional pulmonary vasodilators. Understanding the pathogenesis and pathophysiology of neonatal PH can lead to novel strategies and precise therapies. The review is designed to achieve this goal by summarizing pulmonary vascular development and the pathogenesis and pathophysiology of PH associated with maladaptation, bronchopulmonary dysplasia, and congenital diaphragmatic hernia based on evidence predominantly from preclinical studies. We also discuss the pros and cons of and provide future directions for preclinical studies in neonatal PH.

Pulmonary hypertension (PH) in neonates, originating from a range of disease states with heterogeneous underlying pathophysiology, is associated with significant morbidity and mortality. Although the final common pathway is a state of high right ventricular afterload leading to compromised cardiac output, multiple hemodynamic phenotypes exist in acute and chronic PH, for which cardiorespiratory treatment strategies differ. Comprehensive appraisal of pulmonary pressure, pulmonary vascular resistance, cardiac function, pulmonary and systemic blood flow, and extrapulmonary shunts facilitates delivery of individualized cardiovascular therapies in affected newborns.

Oxygen is a specific pulmonary vasodilator. Hypoxemia causes pulmonary vasoconstriction, and normoxia leads to pulmonary vasodilation. However, hyperoxia does not enhance pulmonary vasodilation but causes oxidative stress. There are no clinical trials evaluating optimal oxygen saturation or Pao_2 in pulmonary hypertension. Data from translational studies and case series suggest that oxygen saturation of 90% to 97% or Pao_2 between 50 and 80 mm Hg is associated with the lowest pulmonary vascular resistance.

Pivotal trials investigating the use of inhaled nitric oxide (iNO) in the 1990s led to approval by the Food and Drug Administration in 1999. Inhaled nitric oxide is the only approved pulmonary vasodilator for persistent pulmonary hypertension of the newborn (PPHN). Selective pulmonary vasodilation with iNO in near-term and term neonates with PPHN is safe, and targeted use of iNO in less mature neonates with pulmonary hypertension (PH) can be beneficial. This review addresses a brief history of iNO, clinical features of neonatal PH, and the clinical application of iNO.

Pulmonary hypertension in the neonatal population can be acute or chronic and carries significant risk for morbidity and mortality. It can be idiopathic but more often is associated with comorbid pulmonary and heart disease. There are several pharmacotherapeutics aimed at pulmonary vasodilation. This review highlights the most common agents as well as those on the horizon for the treatment of pulmonary hypertension in the neonate.

Neonates with a perinatal hypoxic insult and subsequent neonatal encephalopathy are at risk of acute pulmonary hypertension (aPH) in the transitional period. The phenotypic contributors to aPH following perinatal asphyxia include a combination of hypoxic vasoconstriction of the pulmonary vascular bed, right heart dysfunction, and left heart dysfunction. Therapeutic hypothermia is the standard of care for neonates with moderate-to-severe hypoxic ischemic encephalopathy. This review summarizes the underlying risk factors, causes of aPH in neonates with perinatal asphyxia, discusses the unique phenotypical contributors to disease, and explores the impact of the initial insult and subsequent therapeutic hypothermia on aPH.

This review provides a comprehensive summary of the current understanding of pulmonary hypertension (PH) in congenital diaphragmatic hernia, outlining the underlying pathophysiologic mechanisms, methods for assessing PH severity, optimal management strategies, and prognostic implications.

Pulmonary hypertension (PH) in preterm neonates has multifactorial pathogenesis with unique characteristics. Premature surfactant-deficient lungs are injured following exposure to positive pressure ventilation and high oxygen concentrations resulting in variable phenotypes of PH. The prevalence of early PH is variable and reported to be between 8% and 55% of extremely preterm infants. Disruption of the lung development and vascular signaling pathway could lead to abnormal pulmonary vascular transition. The management of early PH and the off-label use of selective pulmonary vasodilators continue to be controversial.

Preterm infants with bronchopulmonary dysplasia (BPD) are prone to develop pulmonary hypertension (PH). Strong laboratory and clinical data suggest that antenatal factors, such as preeclampsia, chorioamnionitis, oligohydramnios, and placental dysfunction leading to fetal growth restriction, increase susceptibility for BPD-PH after premature birth. Echocardiogram metrics and serial assessments of NT-proBNP provide useful tools to diagnose and monitor clinical course during the management of BPD-PH, as well as monitoring for such complicating conditions as left ventricular diastolic dysfunction, shunt lesions, and pulmonary vein stenosis. Therapeutic strategies should include careful assessment and management of underlying airways and lung disease, cardiac performance, and systemic hemodynamics, prior to initiation of PH-targeted drug therapies.

Diverse genetic developmental lung diseases can present in the neonatal period with hypoxemic respiratory failure, often associated with with pulmonary hypertension. Intractable hypoxemia and lack of sustained response to medical management should increase the suspicion of a developmental lung disorder. Genetic diagnosis and lung biopsy are helpful in establishing the diagnosis. Early diagnosis can result in optimizing management and redirecting care if needed. This article reviews normal lung development, various developmental lung disorders that can result from genetic abnormalities at each stage of lung development, their clinical presentation, management, prognosis, and differential diagnoses.

Persistent Pulmonary Hypertension of the Newborn (PPHN) is more common in Low and middle income countries (LMICs) due to high incidence of sepsis, perinatal asphyxia and meconium aspiration syndrome. Presence of hypoxic respiratory faillure and greater than 5% difference in preductal and post ductal saturation increases clinical sucipision for PPHN. The availability of Inhaled nitric oxide and extracorporaeal membrane oxygenation is limited but pulmonary vasodilators such as sildenafil are readily available in most LMICs.

Inhaled nitric oxide (iNO) is a pulmonary vasodilator considered standard of care to treat persistent pulmonary hypertension of the newborn. However, not all infants respond to iNO. The authors performed a systematic review to examine methodology, outcomes, and challenges of randomized controlled trials testing pulmonary vasodilator medications adjunctive to iNO. The 5 trials identified showed heterogeneity in eligibility criteria and outcomes assessed. No trial achieved recruitment goals, limiting conclusions regarding efficacy, safety, and pharmacology. Trial design consensus and alternative methodologic strategies such as deferred consent, real-world controls, nonrandomized database assessments, and Bayesian statistical approaches are needed.

Long-term outcomes of persistent pulmonary hypertension of newborn (PPHN) depend on disease severity, duration of ventilation, and associated anomalies. Congenital diaphragmatic hernia survivors may have respiratory morbidities and developmental delay. The presence of PPHN is associated with increased mortality in hypoxic-ischemic encephalopathy, though the effects on neurodevelopment are less clear. Preterm infants can develop pulmonary hypertension (PH) early in the postnatal course or later in the setting of bronchopulmonary dysplasia (BPD). BPD-PH is associated with higher mortality, particularly within the first year. Evidence suggests that both early and late PH in preterm infants are associated with neurodevelopmental impairment.

PROGRAM OBJECTIVE

The goal of *Clinics in Perinatology* is to keep practicing perinatologists, neonatologists, obstetricians, practicing physicians and residents up to date with current clinical practice in perinatology by providing timely articles reviewing the state of the art in patient care.

TARGET AUDIENCE

Perinatologists, neonatologists, obstetricians, practicing physicians, residents and healthcare professionals who provide patient care utilizing findings from *Clinics in Perinatology*.

LEARNING OBJECTIVES

Upon completion of this activity, participants will be able to:

1. Recognize pulmonary hypertension in the neonatal population can be acute or chronic and carries significant risk for morbidity and mortality.
2. Discuss mechanisms that contribute to the development and progression of pulmonary hypertension (PH) in infants with bronchopulmonary dysplasia (BPD).
3. Review common and emerging therapies for treating pulmonary hypertension in neonates.

ACCREDITATION

The Elsevier Office of Continuing Medical Education (EOCME) is accredited by the Accreditation Council for Continuing Medical Education (ACCME) to provide continuing medical education for physicians.

The EOCME designates this journal-based CME activity for a maximum of 14 *AMA PRA Category 1 Credit*(s)™. Physicians should claim only the credit commensurate with the extent of their participation in the activity.

All other health care professionals requesting continuing education credit for this enduring material will be issued a certificate of participation.

DISCLOSURE OF CONFLICTS OF INTEREST

The EOCME assesses conflict of interest with its instructors, faculty, planners, and other individuals who are in a position to control the content of CME activities. All relevant conflicts of interest that are identified are thoroughly vetted by EOCME for fair balance, scientific objectivity, and patient care recommendations. EOCME is committed to providing its learners with CME activities that promote improvements or quality in healthcare and not a specific proprietary business or a commercial interest.

The planning committee, staff, authors, and editors listed below have identified no financial relationships or relationships to products or devices they or their spouse/life partner have with commercial interest related to the content of this CME activity:

Steven H. Abman, MD; Gabriel Altit, MDCM, MSc, FRCPC, FAAP; Prathik Bandiya, MD, DM; Stephanie M. Boyd, MBBS (Hons), BSc (Med), MPHTM, FRACP, CCPU; Jeanne Carroll, MD; Praveen Chandrasekharan, MD; Suzan Cochius-den Otter, MD, PhD; Kristen Coletti, MD; Michael W. Cookson, MD; Olivier Danhaive, MD; Jack R.T. Darby, PhD; Ahmed Elsaie, MD; Elizabeth E. Foglia, MD, MSCE; Csaba Galambos, MD, PhD; Regan Geisinger, MD; Hannah Holmes; Ajay Raghav Joshi, MBBS, DCH, DNB (Pead); Roberta L. Keller, MD; Haresh Kirpalani, MD, MSc; Martin Kluckow, MBBS, FRACP, PhD, CCPU; Satyan Lakshminrusimha, MD, MBBS; Philip T. Levy, MD; Michelle Littlejohn; Rajeshwari Madappa, MBBS, DCH, DNB (Pead); Srinivasan Mani, MD; Patrick J. McNamara, MBBCh, MRCPCH, FASE; Hussnain Mirza, MD; Olivia J. Moir; Shiran S. Moore, MD; Janna L. Morrison, BSc, MSc, PhD; Rohit Rao, MD, MBA; Danielle R. Rios, MD, MS; Catherine Rottkamp, MD, PhD; Brahmdeep S. Saini, PhD; Deepika Sankaran, MD; Lourenco Sbragia, MD, PhD; Augusto F. Schmidt, MD, PhD, FAAP; Mike Seed, MBBS, MRCPCH, FRCR; Binoy Shivanna, MD, DM, PhD; Robin H. Steinhorn, MD; Emily Stieren, MD, PhD; Liqun Sun, MD, PhD; Jeyanthi Surendrakumar; April W. Tan, MD; K. Taylor Wild, MD; Karen C. Young, MD, MS; James Ziegler, MD

The planning committee, staff, authors, and editors listed below have identified financial relationships or relationships to products or devices they or their spouse/life partner have with commercial interest related to the content of this CME activity:

John P. Kinsella, MD: *Researcher*: Mallinckrodt

UNAPPROVED/OFF-LABEL USE DISCLOSURE

The EOCME requires CME faculty to disclose to the participants:

1. When products or procedures being discussed are off-label, unlabelled, experimental, and/or investigational (not US Food and Drug Administration [FDA] approved); and

2. Any limitations on the information presented, such as data that are preliminary or that represent ongoing research, interim analyses, and/or unsupported opinions. Faculty may discuss information about pharmaceutical agents that is outside of FDA-approved labelling. This information is intended solely for CME and is not intended to promote off-label use of these medications. If you have any questions, contact the medical affairs department of the manufacturer for the most recent prescribing information.

TO ENROLL
To enroll in the *Clinics in Perinatology* Continuing Medical Education program, call customer service at 1-800-654-2452 or sign up online at http://www.theclinics.com/home/cme. The CME program is available to subscribers for an additional annual fee of USD 254.00.

METHOD OF PARTICIPATION
In order to claim credit, participants must complete the following:
1. Complete enrolment as indicated above.
2. Read the activity.
3. Complete the CME Test and Evaluation. Participants must achieve a score of 70% on the test. All CME Tests and Evaluations must be completed online.

CME INQUIRIES/SPECIAL NEEDS
For all CME inquiries or special needs, please contact elsevierCME@elsevier.com.

CLINICS IN PERINATOLOGY

SERIES OF RELATED INTEREST

Obstetrics and Gynecology Clinics of North America
https://www.obgyn.theclinics.com

THE CLINICS ARE AVAILABLE ONLINE!
Access your subscription at:
www.theclinics.com

Foreword

Pulmonary Hypertension of the Newborn

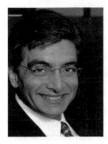

Lucky Jain, MD, MBA
Consulting Editor

The evolution of neonatology as a distinct subspeciality is deeply rooted in the physiologic underpinnings of early development, particularly the transition from fetal to neonatal life. Respiratory physiologists have led the way, with groundbreaking work on respiratory distress syndrome and its origin in surfactant deficiency dating back to the 1950s.[1] Since then, much effort has been focused on understanding extrauterine lung development in the premature newborn. Meanwhile, persistent pulmonary hypertension of the newborn (PPHN) continues to torment clinicians and physiologists alike with its complexity and propensity to do harm if not managed properly. While the introduction of inhaled nitric oxide ushered in an era of better outcomes in many sick neonates with this malady, options for a subset of neonates who do not respond to the treatment remain limited. Unlike surfactant and respiratory distress syndrome, our understanding of the molecular mechanisms behind PPHN also remains limited. Indeed, the success of inhaled nitric oxide may have led to slowing down of research into pathways contributing to various types of pulmonary hypertension and the quest for other treatment options.

The transition of pulmonary circulation at birth from a high-resistance–low-flow circuit to a significantly higher blood flow system once the resistance goes down, is a physiologic miracle. While my own laboratory spent years looking at the clearance of lung fluid as a prerequisite for successful neonatal respiratory transition, distension of the lung with inhaled gases, introduction of oxygen, and many other downstream effects are all linked to release of endogenous vasodilators that lead to a precipitous drop in vascular resistance.[2] There is a significant body of information about the vasodilators involved in the pulmonary vascular transition; however, much less is known about how the signals are being processed at the cellular level, and how a precise ventilation-perfusion balance is maintained. Even though hypoxic pulmonary

Clin Perinatol 51 (2024) xv–xvii
https://doi.org/10.1016/j.clp.2023.12.004
0095-5108/24/© 2023 Published by Elsevier Inc.

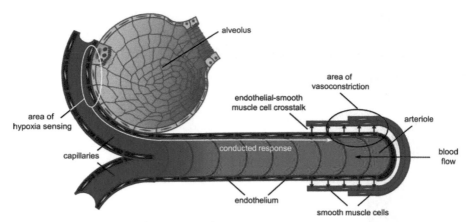

Fig. 1. Schematic concept for the role of the endothelium in hypoxic pulmonary vasoconstriction. Alveolar hypoxia is primarily sensed at the level of the alveolocapillary barrier from where the hypoxic signal is propagated retrogradely along the vascular endothelium as a conducted response via gap junctions composed of connexin 40 to the area of vasoconstriction in the upstream arterioles and subsequently triggers contraction of adjacent pulmonary artery smooth muscle cells via endothelial–smooth muscle cell crosstalk. (With permission from Grimmer B, Kuebler W. The endothelium in hypoxic pulmonary vasoconstriction. J Appl Physiol 2017;123:1635-1646. (Page 1637).)

vasoconstriction was first identified more than a century ago, much remains to be determined about the site and mechanism of initial oxygen sensing.[3] Attention has been drawn to how reactive oxygen species in pulmonary arterial smooth muscle cells trigger the downstream redox changes, and subsequent changes in ion transporters, including oxygen-sensitive potassium channels and voltage-gated calcium channels. New evidence also points to a role for endothelial cells in oxygen sensing and triggering of pulmonary artery smooth muscle cell contraction (**Fig. 1**).[3]

I am delighted to see an entire issue of the *Clinics in Perinatology* devoted to pulmonary hypertension. This malady requires us to be at the top of our game; it also brings out the "physiologist" in clinicians everywhere. In this issue of the *Clinics in Perinatology*, Drs Lakshminrusimha and Abman have brought many aspects of this important clinical entity to life by assembling an extraordinary list of experts in the field. They are all to be congratulated for a truly state-of-the-art offering deeply steeped in physiologic underpinnings of this subject. As always, I am grateful to the authors for their valuable contributions, and to my publishing partners at Elsevier (Kerry Holland and Nitesh Barthwal) for their help in bringing this amazing issue of the *Clinics in Perinatology* to you.

Lucky Jain, MD, MBA
Emory University School of Medicine, and
Children's Healthcare of Atlanta
1760 Haygood Drive, W409
Atlanta, GA 30322, USA

E-mail address:
ljain@emory.edu

REFERENCES

1. Avery ME, Mead J. Surface properties in relation to atelectasis and hyaline membrane disease. Am J Dis Child 1959;97:517–23.
2. Jain L, Eaton DC. Alveolar fluid transport: a changing paradigm. Am J Physiol Lung Cell Mol Physiol 2006;290(4):L646–8.
3. Grimmer B, Kuebler W. The endothelium in hypoxic pulmonary vasoconstriction. J Appl Physiol 2017;123:1635–46.

Preface

Neonatal Pulmonary Hypertension: Phenotypes, Physiology, and Management

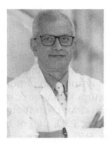
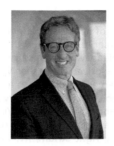

Satyan Lakshminrusimha, MD, FAAP   Steven H. Abman, MD
Editors

In the early 1970s, several case reports and series outlined neonates with cyanosis, respiratory distress associated with right-to-left shunt across the ductus arteriosus, right ventricular hypertrophy, and pulmonary hypertension (PH) diagnosed by cine-radiography, ECG, or cardiac catheterization.[1,2] These infants had either paren-chymal lung disease or pulmonary oligemia on chest radiograph and were called persistent pulmonary vascular obstruction in newborn[3] or persistent transitional cir-culation,[1] persistent fetal circulation, and subsequently, persistent pulmonary hy-pertension of the newborn.[4] During the subsequent years, the presence of acute PH was observed in preterm infants. Over the last 15 years, our understanding of the incidence, echocardiographic features, and management of early PH in extremely preterm infants continues to advance. Chronic PH is associated with con-ditions such as congenital diaphragmatic hernia (CDH) or bronchopulmonary dysplasia (BPD).

Instead of classifying neonatal PH based on infants' gestation, timing, or underlying disease, we prefer an approach using physiology to classify various phenotypes: resis-tance-driven, flow-driven, and postcapillary (**Fig. 1**). Such a physiologic approach guides therapeutic management. For example, inhaled nitric oxide (iNO) is indicated in resistance-driven PH but may worsen pulmonary edema in flow-driven and postca-pillary PH. The increased availability of bedside echocardiography enables us to target therapy to individual patients ("precision-medicine" approach).

Previous clinical trials in neonatal PH have focused on hypoxemic respiratory failure with oxygenation indices as inclusion criteria and also as primary endpoints. This approach led to the inclusion of hypoxic preterm and term neonates secondary to

Clin Perinatol 51 (2024) xix–xxii
https://doi.org/10.1016/j.clp.2023.11.010
0095-5108/24/© 2023 Published by Elsevier Inc.

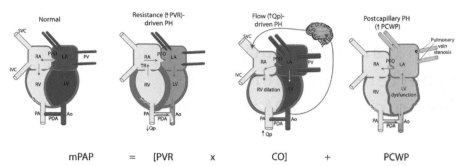

$$mPAP \quad = \quad [PVR \quad x \quad CO] \quad + \quad PCWP$$

Fig. 1. Physiologic phenotypes of neonatal PH. Mean pulmonary arterial pressure (mPAP) is influenced by pulmonary vascular resistance (PVR), cardiac output (CO) or pulmonary blood flow (Qp), and pulmonary capillary wedge pressure (PCWP). Each of these components, PVR (resistance-driven PH), CO (flow-driven PH, as seen with vein of Galen and other left-to-right shunts), and PCWP (postcapillary PH secondary to left ventricular dysfunction or pulmonary vein stenosis) can contribute to elevated pulmonary arterial pressure. Therapeutic management is dependent on the phenotype. Ao, aorta; IVC, inferior vena cava; LA, left atrium; LV, left ventricle; PA, pulmonary artery; PDA, patent ductus arteriosus; PFO, patent foramen ovale; PV, pulmonary vein; RA, right atrium; RV, right ventricle; SVC, superior vena cava; TR, tricuspid regurgitation. (Image courtesy of Dr Satyan Lakshminrusimha.)

parenchymal lung disease, PH, cardiac dysfunction resulting in mixed results limiting clinical applicability. Future trials need to precisely identify the physiologic phenotype of neonatal PH to evaluate newer therapeutic options.

New insights into pathophysiology of neonatal PH, understanding the role of vascular mediators such as nitric oxide, prostacyclin, endothelin and oxygen free radicals, genetic and developmental pathways, and cardiopulmonary interactions have enabled us to advance diagnostic and therapeutic approaches.

Therapeutic management of neonatal PH has evolved from hyperoxia and alkalosis[5] and nonspecific intravenous pulmonary vasodilators, such as tolazoline.[6,7] The discovery of the key role played by endothelium-derived nitric oxide in normal pulmonary vascular transition at birth[8] led to the advent of iNO, a selective pulmonary vasodilator as a therapeutic agent, and revolutionized the management of neonatal PH.[9,10] However, high cost, lack of availability in some settings, and 10% to 15% incidence of poor or lack of sustained improvement to iNO have led to further investigation of pulmonary vasodilator therapy in neonatal PH. Enteral sildenafil has emerged as an effective alternate therapy of PH in resource-limited settings without access to iNO.[11] Newer therapeutic advances, such as newer prostacyclin analogs, endothelin antagonists, and soluble guanylate cyclase activators, may provide us with more tools to tackle iNO-resistant PH.

In this illustrated issue of the *Clinics in Perinatology*, internationally acclaimed authorities in the field of neonatal PH discuss pathophysiology, diagnosis, and management of neonatal PH secondary to parenchymal lung disease in both term and preterm infants, asphyxia, therapeutic hypothermia, CDH, BPD, and genetic and developmental lung disease in both high-income and low- and middle-income countries.

In addition to our appreciation of these authors, we would like to thank the editorial team at Elsevier, Mr Nitesh Barthwal, and Kerry K. Holland for their patience and support. We sincerely appreciate Dr Lucky Jain for assigning us with the important task of bringing out this issue dedicated to the management of neonatal PH.

With fond remembrance, we dedicate this issue in memory of Dr Regan Giesinger, our angel of Neonatal Hemodynamics. During her short life, she revolutionized the hemodynamic monitoring and finetuning of the management of neonatal PH. We both have shared panel discussions and state-of-the-art sessions with Regan and miss her astute observations and contributions to the field of neonatal PH. We feel honored to have an article authored by her as part of this issue of *Clinics in Perinatology*.

Satyan Lakshminrusimha, MD, FAAP
Department of Pediatrics
University of California, Davis
UC Davis Children's Hospital, Sacramento
2516, Stockton Boulevard
Sacramento, CA 95817, USA

Steven H. Abman, MD
Department of Pediatrics
Pediatric Heart Lung Center
University of Colorado Denver
Anschutz School of Medicine
Children's Hospital Colorado
Mail Stop B395, 13123 East 16th Avenue
Aurora, CO 80045, USA

E-mail addresses:
slakshmi@ucdavis.edu (S. Lakshminrusimha)
Steven.Abman@cuanschutz.edu (S.H. Abman)

REFERENCES

1. Brown R, Pickering D. Persistent transitional circulation. Arch Dis Child 1974; 49(11):883–5.

2. Siassi B, Goldberg SJ, Emmanouilides GC, et al. Persistent pulmonary vascular obstruction in newborn infants. J Pediatr 1971;78(4):610–5.

3. Shannon DC, Lusser M, Goldblatt A, et al. The cyanotic infant–heart disease or lung disease. New Engl J Med 1972;287(19):951–3.

4. Haworth SG, Reid L. Persistent fetal circulation: newly recognized structural features. J Pediatr 1976;88(4 Pt 1):614–20.

5. Peckham GJ, Fox WW. Physiologic factors affecting pulmonary artery pressure in infants with persistent pulmonary hypertension. J Pediatr 1978;93(6):1005–10.

6. Goetzman BW, Sunshine P, Johnson JD, et al. Neonatal hypoxia and pulmonary vasospasm: response to tolazoline. J Pediatr 1976;89(4):617–21.

7. Drummond WH, Gregory GA, Heymann MA, et al. The independent effects of hyperventilation, tolazoline, and dopamine on infants with persistent pulmonary hypertension. J Pediatr 1981;98(4):603–11.

8. Abman SH, Chatfield BA, Hall SL, et al. Role of endothelium-derived relaxing factor during transition of pulmonary circulation at birth. Am J Physiol 1990;259(6 Pt 2):H1921–7.

9. Roberts JD Jr, Fineman JR, Morin FC 3rd, et al. Inhaled nitric oxide and persistent pulmonary hypertension of the newborn. The Inhaled Nitric Oxide Study Group. New Engl J Med 1997;336(9):605–10.

10. NINOS. Inhaled nitric oxide in full-term and nearly full-term infants with hypoxic respiratory failure. The Neonatal Inhaled Nitric Oxide Study Group. New Engl J Med 1997;336(9):597–604.
11. Baquero H, Soliz A, Neira F, et al. Oral sildenafil in infants with persistent pulmonary hypertension of the newborn: a pilot randomized blinded study. Pediatrics 2006;117(4):1077–83.

Pulmonary Vascular Regulation in the Fetal and Transitional Lung

Hannah Holmes[a], Brahmdeep S. Saini[a], Olivia J. Moir[a],
Jack R.T. Darby[b], Janna L. Morrison[b,c,d,1], Liqun Sun[a,1],
Mike Seed[a,c,d,e,f,*,1]

KEYWORDS

- Pulmonary circulation • Pulmonary vasculature • Regulatory factors • Fetal lung
- Transitional lung • Vascular development • Pulmonary blood flow
- Pulmonary vascular tone

KEY POINTS

- The fetal pulmonary circulation transitions from a high-resistance low-flow system to a low-resistance high-flow system in the newborn.
- Pulmonary blood flow is regulated by vasoconstrictive and vasodilatory factors that mediate pulmonary vascular tone.
- The pulmonary vasculature develops in parallel with the lungs, undergoing maturational changes in endothelial and smooth muscle cell function that also regulate *in utero* pulmonary vascular resistance and prepare for the transition.

INTRODUCTION

Successful transition of a fetus to a newborn is influenced by several factors, including maternal and fetal health, gestational age, and delivery management.[1] Approximately 10% of newborns require intervention at birth and with insight into how and why such challenges develop, clinicians may better navigate the management of these patients.[1,2]

[a] Division of Cardiology, Department of Pediatrics, The Hospital for Sick Children, University of Toronto, Toronto, Ontario, M5G 1X8, Canada; [b] Early Origins of Adult Health Research Group, University of South Australia, Adelaide, South Australia, 5001, Australia; [c] Department of Physiology, Faculty of Medicine, University of Toronto, 555 University Avenue, Toronto, Ontario, M5G 1X8 Canada; [d] Translational Medicine Program, The Hospital for Sick Children, University of Toronto, 555 University Avenue, Toronto, Ontario, M5G 1X8 Canada; [e] Research Institute, The Hospital for Sick Children, University of Toronto, 555 University Avenue, Toronto, Ontario, M5G 1X8 Canada; [f] Department of Diagnostic Imaging, The Hospital for Sick Children, University of Toronto, 555 University Avenue, Toronto, Ontario, M5G 1X8 Canada
[1] These authors have contributed equally to this work and share senior authorship.
* Corresponding author. Division of Cardiology, Department of Pediatrics, The Hospital for Sick Children, University of Toronto, Toronto, Ontario, Canada.
E-mail address: mike.seed@sickkids.ca

Clin Perinatol 51 (2024) 1–19
https://doi.org/10.1016/j.clp.2023.11.003
perinatology.theclinics.com

The placenta is responsible for supplying the fetus with oxygen prenatally and therefore the pulmonary circulation need not receive the entire right ventricular output. After birth, pulmonary vascular resistance (PVR) decreases with ventilation of the lungs. Oxygen plays a major role in the reduction in PVR, which results in increased pulmonary blood flow (PBF) and establishes the lungs as the organ of gas exchange.[3] As tissues and organs develop, they exhibit plasticity that allows a range of physiologic and morphologic states in response to the various environmental conditions they encounter.[4,5] However, stimuli or insults experienced during this period may generate permanent structural or physiologic alterations that can predispose the fetus to certain postnatal diseases.[4–8]

Evidence from animal models and human pregnancies supports a strong association between developmental programming and pulmonary arterial remodeling and dysfunction.[7,9–11] Fetal stressors, such as the hypoxia experienced in the setting of certain congenital heart diseases (CHDs), can directly or indirectly act at cellular and molecular levels, altering cardiopulmonary development and manifesting in diverse cardiopulmonary pathologies.[4,5,12–15] This review focuses on the key events and determinants of fetal pulmonary vascular development and transitional physiology providing examples from preclinical and clinical studies, including research conducted by our group.

PULMONARY CIRCULATION: STRUCTURE AND FUNCTION

The pulmonary arterial circulation is the assembly of vessels that carry deoxygenated blood to the alveoli, enabling gas exchange.[16] Pulmonary veins subsequently return oxygenated blood to the heart to be distributed by the systemic circulation.[16] These vessels have 3general layers, from inner-to outer-most the intima, media, and adventitia; although morphology varies depending on vessel size and function.[17,18] The main pulmonary artery (MPA) has a thick layer of smooth muscle cells (SMCs) forming its media, while in small arterioles, this becomes a thinner, non-uniform layer of SMCs.[16] Moreover, distal to these are non-muscular arterioles, which lack this layer entirely.[16] The arterioles ultimately divide into a network of capillaries that connect with the alveoli.[16] Capillary walls comprise only a single layer of endothelial cells (ECs), which enables their capability for gas exchange.[16] The structure of pulmonary capillaries is an example of how the cellular composition of the vasculature contributes to its function, and this similarly depends on location.[17,18]

In addition to gas exchange, pulmonary circulation has other functions, including regulating the rate at which blood flows through its vessels.[16] PBF is determined by vascular tone, which is controlled through communication between ECs and SMCs of the pulmonary vasculature (**Fig. 1**). This is realized through the production and modulation of vasoactive substances, some of which are synthesized by ECs and others that bind cell surface receptors (see **Fig. 1**).[16] These initiate cell signaling cascades that modify the intracellular calcium concentration ($[Ca^{2+}]_i$) of SMCs.[19] As is a common feature across muscle physiology, increases in SMC $[Ca^{2+}]_i$ result in contraction while decreases cause relaxation.[19] The multiple pathways involved in governing SMC $[Ca^{2+}]_i$ and thus pulmonary vascular tone (see **Fig. 1**) are explored in the following paragraphs.[19]

Pathways Regulating Pulmonary Vascular Tone

Pulmonary vascular tone is typically controlled by pathways that act through the production of the vasoactive substances: nitric oxide (NO), endothelin-1 (ET-1), and arachidonic acid (AA) derivatives, as shown in **Fig. 1**. NO is synthesized within ECs

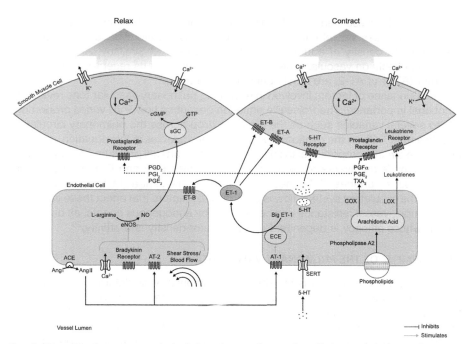

Fig. 1. Signaling between endothelial and smooth muscle cells in modulating pulmonary vascular tone. Stimulatory interactions are shown in green and inhibitory interactions are shown in red. The vasoactive substances are shown within the diagram. 5-HT, serotonin; ACE, angiotensin converting enzyme; AngI, angiotensin I; AngII, angiotensin II; AT-1/2, angiotensin receptor 1/2; cGMP, cyclic guanosine monophosphate; COX, cyclooxygenase; ECE, endothelin converting enzyme; eNOS, endothelial nitric oxide synthase; ET-1, endothelin; ET-A/B, endothelin receptor A/B; GTP, guanosine triphosphate; LOX, lipoxygenase; NO, nitric oxide; SERT, serotonin transporter; sGC, soluble guanylate cyclase.

through activation of the enzyme NO synthetase, which facilitates oxygenation of L-arginine to generate NO.[20,21] Following its synthesis, NO diffuses into SMCs where it activates its target, soluble guanylyl cyclase (sGC).[20,22] This reaction initiates a cascade that induces SMC relaxation and pulmonary vasodilation.[20,22] NO production and release by ECs are modulated by various factors (see **Fig. 1**). These include, but are not limited to, shear stress associated with increased blood flow within the vessel or receptor binding of vasodilatory molecules such as bradykinin.[20,21,23]

The production of AA mediates another pathway involved in modulating vascular tone. This fatty acid is a stepping stone in the creation of eicosanoids and is derived from phospholipids situated within the cell membrane.[20] Lipoxygenase (LOX) and cyclooxygenase (COX) enzymes then convert AA into leukotrienes and prostaglandins, respectively, which signal changes in vascular tone (see **Fig. 1**).[20] Prostaglandin E_2 (PGE_2) can either cause the SMC to relax or constrict, depending upon the receptor type present.[20] As with the NO pathway, eicosanoid production is under the influence of other circulating factors.[20] For example, prostaglandin I_2 aka prostacyclin (PGI_2) production is increased by higher oxygen tension or the action of angiotensin II (AngII).[20]

Another critical pathway in the regulation of pulmonary vascular tone involves ET-1, which is also produced by ECs.[20] It primarily acts on its receptors, ET-A and ET-B, which are present on the SMC and induce contraction.[20,22,24] ET-B, however, is also present on ECs, where its activation stimulates NO production and therefore vasodilation. ECs also clear ET-1 from the circulation.[20,22,24] The effect of ET-1, that is whether it induces vessel dilation or constriction, is therefore dependent upon the presence and density of endothelial ET-B receptors.[24–26] Similarly, AngII can have opposing effects on vascular tone, depending on which of its receptors, angiotensin receptor (AT)-1 or AT-2, are most abundant (see **Fig. 1**).[27]

The abundance of factors involved in regulating pulmonary vascular tone reveals its functional importance. The Poiseuille equation describes how PVR varies proportionally to several variables such as the pressure drop across the pulmonary circulation and flow rate.[28] Given the relationship between the variables in this equation, changes in PVR are directly proportional to shifts in pulmonary arterial pressure (P_{PA}) and blood viscosity, while an inverse relationship exists between PVR and PBF, vessel radius, and number of arteries.[20] As these relationships are central to the flow of blood through the circulatory system, flow is controlled by factors that affect these variables. For example, vessel resistance can be affected by endogenous agents, as discussed earlier, whose efficacy is dependent upon receptor density and affinity.[29]

DEVELOPMENT OF THE PULMONARY VASCULATURE

There are 2 main mechanisms by which the pulmonary vasculature forms: vasculogenesis and angiogenesis.[30–32] Vasculogenesis describes the development of new blood vessels. This begins with endothelial progenitors, known as angioblasts, forming blood islands before differentiating into ECs (**Fig. 2**).[30] Angiogenesis rather describes blood vessels forming through the remodeling and expansion of pre-existing vessels.[30,33] Thus, once a vascular plexus has been assembled, it can be refined into a functional network by angiogenesis.[34] These endothelial-lined vessels must then mature, acquiring a basement membrane and outer layer.[35,36] This process, termed "arteriogenesis," stabilizes new vessels through the recruitment of pericytes, SMCs, and extracellular matrix.[35] This provides vessels with strength and facilitates their function, enabling the regulation of vessel perfusion.[35] Enticed by EC-secreted growth factors, pericytes are the first recruited to envelop newly formed vessels.[34,37,38] ECs and pericytes are then able to modulate vessel formation by coordinating tightly regulated molecules.[34,37]

A principal guiding factor for pulmonary vascular growth is alveolarization, as lung tissue and its vessels are functionally and structurally intertwined.[30] While the

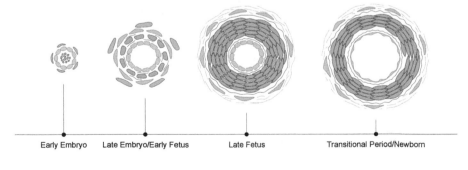

Early Embryo   Late Embryo/Early Fetus   Late Fetus   Transitional Period/Newborn

⊙ Endothelial Cells   ⊙ Smooth Muscle Cells   ⊙ Pericytes   ⊙ Fibroblasts/Fibrocytes   ⊙ Hematopoietic Stem Cells   ∼ Elastic Fibres   ∼ Collagen Fibres

Fig. 2. Structure and cellular makeup of pulmonary blood vessels throughout development. These are generalized to depict the changes the vessels undergo over various stages of development. The early embryo represents a blood island and the transitional period/newborn a mature pulmonary vessel.

mechanisms are not fully understood, an interaction between vascular growth and alveolarization exists wherein the airway acts as a template for vessel development.[18] This entwinement is best illustrated through alignment of vessel growth and the stages of lung development (**Table 1**). Initially, during the embryonic stage, the lung bud grows and repeatedly branches, forming the respiratory tree.[17,30,39] By 28 days gestation, there are already ECs within the mesenchyme that surround the lung bud and are the cornerstone from which the first pulmonary blood vessels arise.[30,32,39] By 34 days gestation, a plexus of capillaries surround the lung buds and connect to the pulmonary artery and vein.[18,40] The completion of conducting airway branching during the pseudoglandular stage aligns with all pre-acinar arteries being present by week 16.[17,18,41] Conversely, intra-acinar vessels only develop as the alveoli form; this occurs during fetal life and continues after birth, with arteries multiplying rapidly to keep pace with alveolar multiplication.[41] During the canalicular stage, the respiratory airways form and the vascular plexus similarly enlarges.[17,30,32] Concurrently, airway epithelium thins and by the end of this stage, a blood-gas barrier sufficient to sustain life is established.[18] As gestation continues, vessels grow in length and diameter but not in number.[41] Further changes are characterized as remodeling, which comprises changes in wall thickness and in the distribution of cells within these vessels.[41] Therefore, capillary remodeling transpires during the saccular stage.[17,30,32,39] This occurs simultaneously with alveolar cell differentiation.[17,30,32,39] The alveolar stage is last, when alveolar septation as well as capillary proliferation and remodeling take place.[30,39] This parallel and reciprocal development ensures close proximity of the vascular and alveolar beds.[30]

As the pulmonary vascular system evolves, its cellular structure must follow suit, as illustrated in **Fig. 2.**[42] Following initial vessel formation, ECs must mature and remodel. These are highly plastic cells that constantly undergo changes to meet the requirements of the developing vessel.[42] This extends to structural changes as the ECs of the pulmonary arteries enter the fetal period cuboidal in shape and become flat and overlapping by the end of gestation.[42,43] ECs also promote vascular growth and maturation by secreting chemotactic factors to attract SMCs, fostering their migration and division.[42] The extent of muscularized arteries increases throughout gestation as the total number of SMCs increases.[41] The pulmonary arteries are completely muscularized to the level of the terminal bronchioles during the fetal period and only after birth does the muscle extend to the alveolar ducts.[41,44] The cytoskeletal structure of these pulmonary vascular SMCs also matures as gestation advances.[18] As stretch upregulates myogenic differentiation, stretch from the fluid present in the airways from 8 weeks gestation supports this differentiation.[18,45] As the lungs increase in size with age, the volume of blood flowing through the pulmonary circulation concurrently increases, thus causing more stretch.[18] As such, blood flow and shear stress are important factors in SMC differentiation during arteriogenesis.[35,37,46] As the muscle tissue develops, it works to stabilize the vessel wall, in part by stimulating the production of extracellular matrix, while protecting these new vessels from rupture.[36]

Table 1 Stages of lung development	
Lung Development Stage	**Gestational Age**
Embryonic	4–7 wk
Pseudoglandular	5–17 wk
Canalicular	16–26 wk
Saccular	26–36 wk
Alveolar	36 wk–2 y

Fetal lungs have fewer and smaller arteries, and thus a smaller cross-sectional vascular area compared to those of a newborn or adult (**Fig. 3**).[20] PVR is therefore higher earlier in gestation, balancing out the variables of the Poiseuille equation.[20] Low PBF is maintained throughout gestation and PVR remains high as the lungs are not responsible for gas exchange. The cuboidal shape of endothelial cells and the thick muscular layer present in fetal pulmonary arteries (see **Fig. 3**) are in part responsible for the high PVR during this period.[43] However, as new pulmonary arteries grow and the cross-sectional area of the vascular bed increases during fetal life, PVR correspondingly decreases.[20] With PVR decreasing with advancing gestation, the rate of PBF correspondingly increases.[41] During the last few weeks of gestation, the fetal pulmonary vasculature is more sensitive to oxygen and relative fetal "hypoxemia" results in high PVR (see **Fig. 3**). After birth, SMCs within these arteries involute, rapidly decreasing wall thickness, thus helping lower PVR to allow more blood to flow to the lungs.[20,43]

Factors Regulating Pulmonary Blood Flow Throughout Gestation

In human fetuses, PBF increases exponentially throughout gestation, as demonstrated by Sutton and colleagues with a reported 4-fold increase between 20 and 35 weeks.[47] Such changes in blood flow and the factors responsible are depicted in **Fig. 3**. As early as 6 weeks gestation, the lung epithelium begins producing fluid.[19] This expands the lungs while simultaneously compressing the small pulmonary arteries, helping maintain high PVR.[41] Elevated PVR is otherwise achieved with high pulmonary vascular tone, which is largely mediated by vasoconstrictive pathways. During

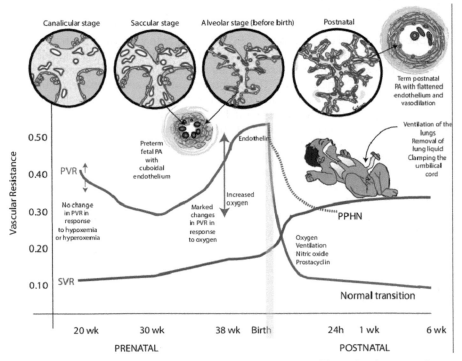

Fig. 3. Changes in vascular resistance throughout the stages of lung development. (Image Courtesy of Dr. Satyan Lakshminrusimha.)

the pseudoglandular phase, angiotensin converting enzyme (ACE) first presents on the endothelium.[20] This enables its product, AngII, to contribute to pulmonary vessel constriction.[20] Moreover, beginning in the canalicular stage, ET-1 and ET-A expression increases, remaining so throughout gestation.[25,26] These ET-1 levels are understood to mediate vasoconstriction throughout the fetal period as weak ET-B expression was found during early stages.[20,26] Thus, the ET-A pathway assists in preserving high PVR in prenatal life. Metabolites of AA also help maintain pulmonary vasoconstriction during the fetal period as COX activity increases.[20,48]

While pulmonary vasoconstriction is mainly responsible for the high PVR typical of prenatal life, this is dependent on the action of calcium on SMC contraction.[19] The response of SMCs to calcium differs between fetus and newborn, which is partly due to changes in ion flow.[19] During early stages of fetal development, hypoxia induces production of potassium ion channels, which play a role in establishing the cell's membrane potential.[19,49] Oxygen increases transmembrane potassium flow, which has downstream effects leading to decreased $[Ca^{2+}]_i$ and thus vasodilation.[19,49,50] With oxygen as a stimulus, this response is minimized in the hypoxic state of the fetal pulmonary circulation. With advancing gestation, the pulmonary vasculature becomes more responsive to changes in oxygen tension, whereby vasodilation is induced by higher oxygen tension.[19,49]

SMC responsiveness to NO depends on the activity of its target enzyme, sGC, the expression of which increases in late gestation.[20] This makes the pulmonary vasculature more responsive to vasodilatory stimuli as birth approaches, and levels of these mediators congruently increase as the fetus approaches term.[20] Furthermore, ET-B plays an important vasodilatory role in the perinatal period as its expression increases in midgestation and remains high after birth.[25,26] Production of PGI_2, another dilatory mediator, increases throughout the fetal period.[41] Reduction of alveolar surface tension is achieved with increased surfactant production in later stages of gestation.[51] This enables capillary shape to be maintained and in turn influences PBF.[51] Overall, a series of changes transpiring in late gestation work in concert to prepare for ex-utero life.

TRANSITION AT BIRTH

Fetal and neonatal physiology are fundamentally different, especially with respect to the cardiopulmonary system, requiring rapid, complex, and well-timed steps to successfully adapt from intra-to extrauterine life, in a process known as "transition."[40] The lungs must be prepared to promptly takeover gas exchange at birth, and thus this transition begins before the onset of labor, requiring changes to the pulmonary vasculature.[1]

Near the end of term, the adrenal glands mature, at which point cortisol production dramatically increases and the process of preparing the fetus for transition begins.[1] This prepartum cortisol surge is followed by clearance of fetal lung fluid, inducing pulmonary maturation.[1,52–54] Lung epithelium increases its production of sodium channels, transitioning the lung into a state of sodium reabsorption, pulling fluid out of the alveoli.[1] Increased oxygen tension after birth further increases the number of sodium channels in the epithelium and allows the remaining fluid to be cleared from the lungs.[1] Together, fluid clearance and air entering the lungs establishes an air-liquid interface.[55,56] Consequently, surface tension develops within the alveoli, increasing lung recoil.[56] As alveoli and capillary units are connected, the increase in alveolar recoil causes capillary distention, and as such, contributes to the fall in PVR at birth.[1,56] Lung inflation through the first few breaths initiates a cascade wherein the pulmonary vasculature dilates, rapidly decreasing PVR, allowing receipt of more blood flow.[16,57] Therefore, transitioning the newborn pulmonary vasculature out of the high-resistance low-flow state of the fetus.[16] This forms a mature pulmonary circulation in which deoxygenated blood entering the right heart is sent to the lungs for gas exchange and then returned to the left heart to be circulated to the entire body.[57,58]

At birth, simultaneous increase in PBF, reduction in PVR, clearance of lung fluid, and lung oxygenation induce adaptations on a cellular level, facilitating vessel wall changes that are critical to transition.[42] For example, after birth, ECs thin within the first minutes while SMCs also progressively thin (see **Figs. 2** and **3**).[42,55] These changes allow the lumen to increase in size and flow capacity.[42] With increased flow, ECs endure shearing forces, stimulating production of vasodilatory substances and inhibiting those mediating vasoconstriction.[55,59] Increased circulating bradykinin levels and release of PGI_2 and NO have therefore been found.[42] This creates a positive feedback loop, enhancing PBF until the point by which the increase in shear stress from increased flow is offset by the decrease in shear stress from increased vessel diameter.[59]

While the dramatic fall in pulmonary vascular resistance initiates and maintains the transition from the parallel fetal to in-series postnatal circulation, completion of the transition also requires the closure of the 3 fetal shunts at the foramen ovale, ductus arteriosus (DA), and ductus venosus.[60] The increase in left atrial pressure resulting from increased pulmonary blood flow (and therefore pulmonary venous return) helps to close the foramen flap.[60] Meanwhile, exposure of the umbilical cord leads to umbilical artery vasoconstriction and a drop in flow in the ductus venosus.[60] Separation from the placenta also results in a drop in circulating prostaglandin E1, allowing vasoconstriction in the DA, which is also triggered by exposure to the higher oxygen tensions in circulating blood.[60] To some extent, these events occur simultaneously, although clamping of the umbilical cord results in an acute drop in right ventricular preload.[60] If cord clamping precedes the establishment of pulmonary ventilation, this may induce a transient drop in cardiac output and cerebral blood flow.[60] Thus, delayed cord clamping is now generally recommended for routine term and preterm deliveries.[61]

Pulmonary Blood Flow Regulators at Transition

Increased capacity for NO-mediated processes in late fetal and early postnatal life optimizes pulmonary vasodilation at transition.[48,62] Shaul and colleagues reported a 2-fold rise in basal NO production between late gestation and 1 week of age, and another 1.6-fold over the following 4 weeks.[48] Oxygen tension increases from 20 to 30 mm Hg in the fetus to 80 to 100 mm Hg in the adult, and increases in vessel wall shear stress are likely responsible for inducing this rise in NO production.[20,56,63] Moreover, Hanson and colleagues found less deactivation of the pathway through which NO acts within the first hour after birth.[64] As such, the vasodilatory effect of NO is thought to be potentiated, correlating with the rapid decrease in PVR in early transition.[62,64] Secondary to this vasodilation, ventilation-perfusion matching improves.[1]

PRECLINICAL AND CLINICAL APPLICATIONS OF PULMONARY VASCULAR REGULATION

Hyperoxia, Normoxia, and Hypoxia

Maternal hyperoxygenation increases placental oxygen transfer and fetal oxygen content.[65,66] Investigations of acute maternal hyperoxygenation in sheep fetuses demonstrate the vasodilatory response of the fetal pulmonary circulation to acute oxygen challenges. Changes in blood flow and oxygen saturations in major fetal vessels can be detected using MRI methods in humans and sheep.[67–70] Sheep are an appropriate preclinical model because they are of similar size to humans and thus the same MRI procedures and scanners can be used in sheep and humans. There is also a similar timing of cardiorespiratory maturation before birth in both species.[71] At 126 days gestation (term, 150 days), maternal hyperoxygenation changes blood flow and oxygen saturations in the major fetal vessels (**Fig. 4**). In keeping with prior reports,[72–74] PBF doubled under these conditions resulting in increased pulmonary venous return to the left atrium, and reduced foramen ovale shunting due to increased left atrial pressure. Consequently, shunting in the DA and ductus venosus was also reduced. Conversely, a relative reduction in PBF was observed with acute hypoxemia at 118 days gestation, while in contrast to hyperoxemia the flows in the fetal shunts trended higher (**Fig. 5**). These findings are consistent with other fetal sheep studies.[75–77] **Fig. 6** further illustrates how such variations in fetal blood oxygen levels impact the distribution of PBF and across fetal shunts.

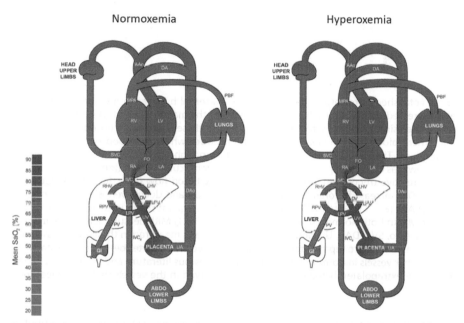

Fig. 4. Fetal sheep circulatory changes to acute maternal hyperoxygenation measured by MRI. The oxygen saturations (SaO$_2$) increased significantly in hyperoxemia in each of the major vessels in which measurements were made using T2 relaxometry MRI technique, and these changes are encoded via the color scale where blood with higher SaO$_2$ is brighter/redder while the blood with lower SaO$_2$ is darker/bluer. The blood flows were measured using phase contrast MRI technique and when flow was derived as percentage of combined ventricular output (left + right ventricular output), significant changes were observed in pulmonary blood flow (PBF; increased), ductus arteriosus (DA, decreased), foramen ovale (FO, decreased) and ductus venosus (DV, decreased). Note: (1) At 126 ± 1 day (term 150 day) gestation, 6 pregnant sheep underwent fetal cardiovascular MRI in both normoxemia and hyperoxemia. (2) SaO$_2$ MRI measurements were made in main pulmonary artery (MPA), DA, ascending aorta (AAo), superior vena cava (SVC), descending aorta (DAo), umbilical vein (UV), and DV. (3) Blood flow was measured in these same vessels and the changes in flow are represented with a change in vessel diameter between the 2 states. (4) SaO$_2$ in other vessels in normoxemia is based on previous literature and their values in hyperoxemia are extrapolated based on the changes observed in the vessels that were measured.

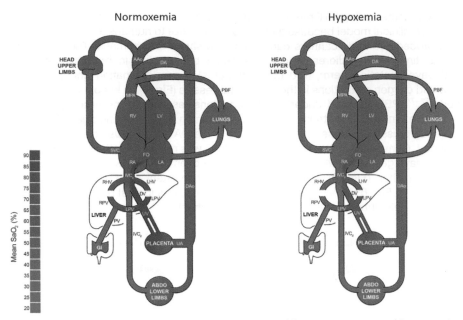

Fig. 5. Fetal sheep circulatory changes to acute maternal hypoxemia measured by MRI. The SaO$_2$ decreased significantly in hypoxemia in each of the major vessels in which measurements were made using T2 relaxometry MRI technique, and these changes are encoded via the color scale where blood with higher SaO$_2$ is brighter/redder while the blood with lower SaO$_2$ is darker/bluer. The blood flows were measured using phase contrast MRI technique and when flow was derived as percentage of combined ventricular output (left + right ventricular output), relative trends were observed in pulmonary blood flow (PBF; decreased), ductus arteriosus (DA, increased), foramen ovale (FO, increased), and ductus venosus (DV, increased). Note: (1) At 118 ± 1 day (term 150 day) gestation, 12 pregnant sheep underwent fetal cardiovascular MRI in both normoxemia and hypoxemia. (2) SaO$_2$ MRI measurements were made in MPA, DA, AAo, SVC, DAo, UV, and DV. (3) Blood flow was measured in these same vessels and the changes in flow are represented with a change in vessel diameter between the 2 states. (4) SaO$_2$ in other vessels in normoxemia are based on previous literature and their values in hypoxemia are extrapolated based on the changes observed in the vessels that were measured.

The response of the fetal pulmonary circulation to hyperoxia includes a rapid reduction in PVR and increase in PBF, which reflects an optimal adaptation to postnatal life with PaO$_2$ rising dramatically at birth.[78] The reactivity of the fetal pulmonary circulation to maternal hyperoxygenation increases with advancing gestational age.[77,78] Rasanen and colleagues studied human fetuses using Doppler ultrasound and demonstrated that while maternal hyperoxygenation did not impact the distribution of blood flow between 20 and 26 weeks, changes were observed between 31 and 36 weeks (see **Fig. 3**).[77] Other ultrasound evidence suggests that human fetal pulmonary reactivity to oxygen may start earlier, during the second trimester, whereas in sheep fetuses the hypoxic vasoconstrictive response develops after 121 days.[79–81] A diagnostic challenge of acute maternal hyperoxygenation to help evaluate any disturbance of pulmonary vascular development has been proposed in the setting of various conditions including congenital diaphragmatic hernia and hypoplastic left heart with restrictive atrial septum.[82,83]

The pulmonary vasodilatory impact of maternal hyperoxygenation has also been explored as a therapeutic agent in the setting of congenital heart disease, whereby

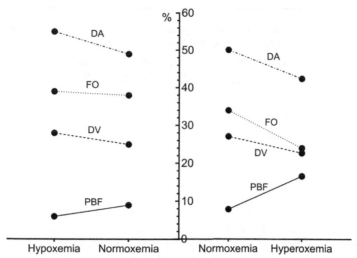

Fig. 6. Changes in pulmonary blood flow and in the shunts in sheep fetuses measured by MRI. The flow measurements are represented as a percentage of combined ventricular output. Blood flow was measured using cine phase contrast technique in DA, DV, right and left branch pulmonary arteries (PBF), AAo, and MPA. FO flow was derived by subtracting PBF from ascending aortic flow. Combined ventricular output was derived as a sum of AAo and MPA flows. Note: hypoxemia MRI experiment was performed in 12 sheep fetuses at 118 ± 1 day gestation (term 150 day) while hyperoxemia MRI experiment was performed in 6 sheep fetuses at 126 ± 1 day gestation.

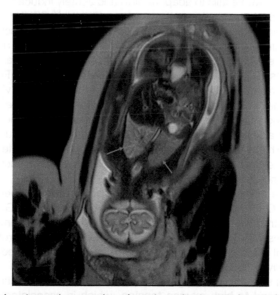

Fig. 7. Fetal MRI showing pulmonary lymphangiectasia. An MRI image depicting fetal pulmonary lymphangiectasia in the setting of hypoplastic left heart syndrome in late gestation. The arrows point to the hyperintense signal extending from the hila and pleural effusion.

Table 2
Pulmonary blood flow in the setting of late gestational hypoplastic left heart syndrome and transposition of the great arteries compared to normal control fetuses

	Normal Controls (n = 40)	HLHS RAS (n = 7)	HLHS UAS (n = 34)	TGA RAS (n = 2)	TGA UAS (n = 61)
Pulmonary blood flow (mL/min/kg)	79 (53,97)	26 (22,43)	71 (47, 93)	175 (112, 238)	75 (49, 114)

Data reported as mean and interquartile range.
 The difference between HLHS RAS vs. normal controls (P < .0001) and HLHS RAS vs. UAS (P < .01) was statistically significant; P < .05.
 Abbreviations: HLHS, hypoplastic left heart syndrome; RAS, restrictive atrial septum; TGA, transposition of the great arteries; UAS, unrestricted atrial septum.

increased pulmonary venous return has been proposed to improve left heart filling and growth in the setting of underdevelopment of left heart structures.[84,85] However, following an initial pulmonary vasodilatory response to an increase in pulmonary artery oxygen tension, fetal pulmonary vascular resistance increases to normal levels over a matter of hours, indicating that other mechanisms promote high PVR beyond simply oxygen tension.[73]

Persistent Pulmonary Hypertension of the Newborn and Congenital Heart Disease

As abnormal cardiovascular physiology impacts the respiratory system, infants with CHDs may exhibit variations to normal pulmonary vascular physiology during prenatal development, transition, and postnatally.[86] In postnatal pulmonary vascular obstructive disease, vascular remodeling is characterized largely by fibroblast, SMC, and EC proliferation, which results in lumen obliteration.[87] This contributes to the development of pulmonary hypertension (PH), a common comorbidity associated with many CHDs.[86,87] If the pulmonary vasculature fails to adapt at birth and acutely induces PH, it is known as persistent pulmonary hypertension of the newborn (PPHN).[86] PPHN manifests secondary to delayed or impaired relaxation of the neonatal pulmonary vasculature.[88,89] Factors such as impaired vasoreactivity or altered vascular structure in development may contribute to the elevated PVR at birth seen in this condition.[90] Failure to decrease PVR at birth results in right-to-left shunting across the foramen ovale (FO) and/or ductus arteriosus and consequentially hypoxemia.[88,90,91] In this setting, a vicious cycle may ensue, whereby the resulting acidosis and hypoxia both further induce pulmonary vasoconstriction and increase PVR.[86] As low PBF results, oxygen saturation and pulmonary venous return are also reduced, and the resulting systemic hypoperfusion fosters a cycle of persistently high PVR.[86] Furthermore, hypoxia induces transdifferentiation of ECs into smooth muscle-like cells.[92] This results in the thickening and muscularization of pulmonary vessels and development of PH.[92,93]

The importance of the concepts discussed throughout this paper is well demonstrated through 2 CHD models: transposition of the great arteries (TGA) and hypoplastic left heart syndrome (HLHS). **Table 2** provides MRI measurements of PBF in late gestational fetuses with TGA and HLHS compared to normal controls. In the setting of restrictive atrial septum (RAS), both of these CHDs are associated with pulmonary vascular pathology at birth.[94]

In TGA, normal streaming of oxygenated blood across the FO initially results in the lungs being exposed to high oxygen tension, which is associated with pulmonary vasodilation.[95–97] However, in a small proportion of fetuses with TGA, the combination of pulmonary vasodilation and discordant ventriculo-arterial connections appears to cause restriction at the DA and FO.[95–97] Under these circumstances, reversal of the normal gradient of oxygen saturations between the right and left sides of the heart has been observed, with the left heart exhibiting lower oxygen saturations due to isolation from the placental supply of oxygenated blood.[97,98] It is likely that under these conditions, the bronchial arteries become enlarged to restore a supply of oxygen to the lungs, resulting in high PBF.[96,99] It is possible that the combination of in utero pulmonary artery hypoxemia and high PBF is responsible for the severe pulmonary vascular disease that occasionally complicates neonatal transition physiology.[95,99–101] While this situation occurs in less than 5% of babies with TGA, it is associated with high morbidity and mortality.[100]

In HLHS, the left side of the heart is obstructed, resulting in mixing of the venous return in the right heart and the whole circulation being supplied with blood of the same oxygen content via the MPA and DA.[102–104] PBF was found to be higher in this population, which may result from the disruption of the normal streaming of oxygen away from the pulmonary arteries (see **Table 2**).[102] However, PBF is reduced in the setting of HLHS RAS.[105,106] In complete left heart obstruction, pulmonary venous blood must return to the circulation via a left-to-right shunt at atrial level.[105,106] Thus, restriction at the FO results in increased LA pressure and pulmonary venous obstruction.[105–107] This significantly increases the pressure within the pulmonary vasculature.[105–107] In consequence, the lymphatic vessels endure increased hydrostatic forces and have been found to dilate as a result, a condition known as "pulmonary lymphangiectasia," which can be seen on fetal MRI (**Fig. 7**).[79,107,108] Maladaptive pulmonary vascular development has also been described in this setting, with muscularization of the pulmonary veins and hypoplasia and wall thickening of the small pulmonary arteries.[105,106] By contrast with an unrestrictive atrial septum, newborns with HLHS RAS typically present with low PBF at birth requiring emergency catheter or surgical intervention.[105,106] Subsequent problems with inadequate pulmonary artery growth and the development of pulmonary vein stenosis are associated with very high mortality in this population.[105,106]

SUMMARY

Pulmonary vascular structure evolves over gestation; endothelial-lined vessels mature to facilitate vessel function and regulate perfusion. With complex mechanisms at play, an appreciation for the regulation of this system may reveal opportunities for better clinical management when complications arise, such as occur in the setting of PPHN and CHDs such as TGA and HLHS. A better understanding of such with the utilization of imaging tools like MRI, and fetal interventions such as balloon atrial septostomy may prove beneficial for these clinical populations.

Best Practice Box

- In the presence of conditions interfering with normal pulmonary vascular transition at birth (such as birth asphyxia), close monitoring of gas exchange and pulmonary hemodynamics by echocardiography may be needed for early detection and management of pulmonary hypertension.

- The ontogeny and maturational differences in enzyme pathways of pulmonary vasoactive mediators may influence choice of pulmonary vasodilator therapy. Endothelium-dependent pulmonary vasodilators such as oxygen may be less effective at lower gestation compared to endothelium-independent pulmonary vasodilators.

- In the presence of congenital heart disease such as TGA or HLHS, recognizing anatomic features such as a restrictive FO may enable assessment of risk for pulmonary hypertension.

DISCLOSURE

The authors have nothing to disclose.

REFERENCES

1. Swanson JR, Sinkin RA. Transition from fetus to newborn. Pediatr Clin North Am 2015;62(2):329–43.
2. Kattwinkel J, Perlman JM, Aziz K, et al. Part 15: neonatal resuscitation: 2010 american heart association guidelines for cardiopulmonary resuscitation and emergency cardiovascular care. Circulation 2010;122(18 Suppl 3):S909–19.
3. Clark AR, Burrowes KS, Tawhai MH. Translational research: multi-scale models of the pulmonary circulation in health and disease. In: Gefen A, editor. Multiscale computer modeling in biomechanics and biomedical engineering. studies in mechanobiology, tissue engineering and biomaterials. Springer; 2013. p. 259–86. https://doi.org/10.1007/8415_2012_152.
4. Kwon EJ, Kim YJ. What is fetal programming?: a lifetime health is under the control of in utero health. Obstet Gynecol Sci 2017;60(6):506–19.
5. Barker DJP. The developmental origins of well-being. Philos Trans R Soc Lond B Biol Sci 2004;359(1449):1359–66.
6. Darby JRT, Varcoe TJ, Orgeig S, et al. Cardiorespiratory consequences of intrauterine growth restriction: influence of timing, severity and duration of hypoxaemia. Theriogenology 2020;150:84–95.
7. Sartori C, Allemann Y, Trueb L, et al. Augmented vasoreactivity in adult life associated with perinatal vascular insult. Lancet 1999;353(9171):2205–7.
8. Lock M, McGillick EV, Orgeig S, et al. Regulation of fetal lung development in response to maternal overnutrition. Clin Exp Pharmacol Physiol 2013;40(11): 803–16.
9. Lamireau D, Nuyt AM, Hou X, et al. Altered vascular function in fetal programming of hypertension. Stroke 2002;33(12):2992–8.
10. Papamatheakis DG, Blood AB, Kim JH, et al. Antenatal hypoxia and pulmonary vascular function and remodeling. Curr Vasc Pharmacol 2013;11(5):616–40.
11. Rexhaj E, Bloch J, Jayet PY, et al. Fetal programming of pulmonary vascular dysfunction in mice: role of epigenetic mechanisms. Am J Physiol Heart Circ Physiol 2011;301(1):H247–52.
12. McGillick EV, Orgeig S, Allison BJ, et al. Maternal chronic hypoxia increases expression of genes regulating lung liquid movement and surfactant maturation in male fetuses in late gestation. J Physiol 2017;595(13):4329–50.
13. Orgeig S, Crittenden TA, Marchant C, et al. Intrauterine growth restriction delays surfactant protein maturation in the sheep fetus. Am J Physiol Lung Cell Mol Physiol 2010;298(4):L575–83.
14. McGillick EV, Orgeig S, Morrison JL. Structural and molecular regulation of lung maturation by intratracheal vascular endothelial growth factor administration in the normally grown and placentally restricted fetus. J Physiol 2016;594(5): 1399–420.
15. McGillick EV, Orgeig S, Morrison JL. Regulation of lung maturation by prolyl hydroxylase domain inhibition in the lung of the normally grown and placentally restricted fetus in late gestation. Am J Physiol Regul Integr Comp Physiol 2016;310(11):R1226–43.
16. Suresh K, Shimoda LA. Lung circulation. Compr Physiol 2016;6(2):897–943.
17. Nikolić MZ, Sun D, Rawlins EL. Human lung development: recent progress and new challenges. Development 2018;145(16):dev163485.

18. Hislop AA. Airway and blood vessel interaction during lung development. J Anat 2002;201(4):325–34.
19. Gao Y, Raj JU. Regulation of the pulmonary circulation in the fetus and newborn. Physiol Rev 2010;90(4):1291–335.
20. Fineman JR, Soifer SJ, Heymann MA. Regulation of pulmonary vascular tone in the perinatal period. Annu Rev Physiol 1995;57:115–34.
21. Heymann MA. Control of the pulmonary circulation in the fetus and during the transitional period to air breathing. Eur J Obstet Gynecol Reprod Biol 1999; 84(2):127–32.
22. Lo CCW, Moosavi SM, Bubb KJ. The regulation of pulmonary vascular tone by neuropeptides and the implications for pulmonary hypertension. Front Physiol 2018;9:1167.
23. Shen JK, Zhang HT. Function and structure of bradykinin receptor 2 for drug discovery. Acta Pharmacol Sin 2023;44(3):489–98.
24. Mazzuca MQ, Khalil RA. Vascular endothelin receptor type b: structure, function and dysregulation in vascular disease. Biochem Pharmacol 2012;84(2):147–62.
25. Lévy M, Maurey C, Dinh-Xuan AT, et al. Developmental expression of vasoactive and growth factors in human lung. role in pulmonary vascular resistance adaptation at birth. Pediatr Res 2005;57(5 Pt 2):21R–5R.
26. Levy M, Maurey C, Chailley-Heu B, et al. Developmental changes in endothelial vasoactive and angiogenic growth factors in the human perinatal lung. Pediatr Res 2005;57(2):248–53.
27. Chai W, Wang W, Liu J, et al. Angiotensin AT1 and AT2 receptors regulate basal skeletal muscle microvascular volume and glucose utilization. Hypertension 2010;55(2):523.
28. Roos A. Poiseuille's law and its limitations in vascular systems. Med Thorac 1962;19:224–38.
29. Keith IM. The role of endogenous lung neuropeptides in regulation of the pulmonary circulation. Physiol Res 2000;49(5):519–37.
30. Woik N, Kroll J. Regulation of lung development and regeneration by the vascular system. Cell Mol Life Sci 2015;72(14):2709–18.
31. Semenza GL. Vasculogenesis, angiogenesis, and arteriogenesis: mechanisms of blood vessel formation and remodeling. J Cell Biochem 2007;102(4):840–7.
32. Cardoso WV. Molecular regulation of lung development. Annu Rev Physiol 2001; 63:471–94.
33. Carmeliet P. Angiogenesis in life, disease and medicine. Nature 2005; 438(7070):932–6.
34. Garrison AT, Bignold RE, Wu X, et al. Pericytes: the lung-forgotten cell type. Front Physiol 2023;14. https://doi.org/10.3389/fphys.2023.1150028.
35. Carmeliet P. Manipulating angiogenesis in medicine. J Intern Med 2004;255(5): 538–61.
36. Carmeliet P. Mechanisms of angiogenesis and arteriogenesis. Nat Med 2000; 6(4):389–95.
37. Bergers G, Song S. The role of pericytes in blood-vessel formation and maintenance. Neuro Oncol 2005;7(4):452–64.
38. Betsholtz C. Insight into the physiological functions of PDGF through genetic studies in mice. Cytokine Growth Factor Rev 2004;15(4):215–28.
39. Joshi S, Kotecha S. Lung growth and development. Early Hum Dev 2007;83(12): 789–94.
40. Morton SU, Brodsky D. Fetal physiology and the transition to extrauterine life. Clin Perinatol 2016;43(3):395–407.

41. Laudy JA, Wladimiroff JW. The fetal lung. 1: developmental aspects. Ultrasound Obstet Gynecol 2000;16(3):284–90.
42. Wojciak-Stothard B, Haworth SG. Perinatal changes in pulmonary vascular endothelial function. Pharmacol Ther 2006;109(1–2):78–91.
43. Vali P, Lakshminrusimha S. The fetus can teach us: oxygen and the pulmonary vasculature. Children 2017;4(8):67.
44. Hislop A, Reid L. Intra-pulmonary arterial development during fetal life-branching pattern and structure. J Anat 1972;113(Pt 1):35–48.
45. Yang Y, Beqaj S, Kemp P, et al. Stretch-induced alternative splicing of serum response factor promotes bronchial myogenesis and is defective in lung hypoplasia. J Clin Invest 2000;106(11):1321–30.
46. Vrancken Peeters MP, Gittenberger-de Groot AC, Mentink MM, et al. Differences in development of coronary arteries and veins. Cardiovasc Res 1997;36(1):101–10.
47. Sutton MS, Groves A, MacNeill A, et al. Assessment of changes in blood flow through the lungs and foramen ovale in the normal human fetus with gestational age: a prospective Doppler echocardiographic study. Br Heart J 1994;71(3):232–7.
48. Shaul PW. Regulation of vasodilator synthesis during lung development. Early Hum Dev 1999;54(3):271–94.
49. Cornfield DN. Developmental regulation of oxygen sensing and ion channels in the pulmonary vasculature. Adv Exp Med Biol 2010;661:201–20.
50. Jackson WF. Potassium channels in regulation of vascular smooth muscle contraction and growth. Adv Pharmacol 2017;78:89–144.
51. Ikegami M, Weaver TE, Grant SN, et al. Pulmonary surfactant surface tension influences alveolar capillary shape and oxygenation. Am J Respir Cell Mol Biol 2009;41(4):433–9.
52. Bland RD, Nielson DW. Developmental changes in lung epithelial ion transport and liquid movement. Annu Rev Physiol 1992;54:373–94.
53. Bland RD, Hansen TN, Haberkern CM, et al. Lung fluid balance in lambs before and after birth. J Appl Physiol Respir Environ Exerc Physiol 1982;53(4):992–1004.
54. Hillman NH, Kallapur SG, Jobe AH. Physiology of transition from intrauterine to extrauterine life. Clin Perinatol 2012;39(4):769–83.
55. Deshpande P, Baczynski M, McNamara PJ, et al. Patent ductus arteriosus: the physiology of transition. Semin Fetal Neonatal Med 2018;23(4):225–31.
56. Hooper SB, Polglase GR, Roehr CC. Cardiopulmonary changes with aeration of the newborn lung. Paediatr Respir Rev 2015;16(3):147–50.
57. Finnemore A, Groves A. Physiology of the fetal and transitional circulation. Semin Fetal Neonatal Med 2015;20(4):210–6.
58. Hines MH. Neonatal cardiovascular physiology. Semin Pediatr Surg 2013;22(4):174–8.
59. Ghanayem NS, Gordon JB. Modulation of pulmonary vasomotor tone in the fetus and neonate. Respir Res 2001;2(3):139–44.
60. Bhatt S, Alison BJ, Wallace EM, et al. Delaying cord clamping until ventilation onset improves cardiovascular function at birth in preterm lambs. J Physiol 2013;591(8):2113–26.
61. American College of Obstetricians and Gynecologists' Committee on Obstetric Practice. Delayed umbilical cord clamping after birth: ACOG committee opinion, number 814. Obstet Gynecol 2020;136(6):e100–6.

62. Abman SH, Chatfield BA, Hall SL, et al. Role of endothelium-derived relaxing factor during transition of pulmonary circulation at birth. Am J Physiol 1990; 259(6 Pt 2):H1921–7.

63. Chandrasekharan P, Rawat M, Lakshminrusimha S. How do we monitor oxygenation during the management of pphn? alveolar, arterial, mixed venous oxygen tension or peripheral saturation? Children 2020;7(10):180.

64. Hanson KA, Burns F, Rybalkin SD, et al. Developmental changes in lung cGMP phosphodiesterase-5 activity, protein, and message. Am J Respir Crit Care Med 1998;158(1):279–88.

65. Sørensen A, Peters D, Simonsen C, et al. Changes in human fetal oxygenation during maternal hyperoxia as estimated by BOLD MRI. Prenat Diagn 2013; 33(2):141–5.

66. Porayette P, Madathil S, Sun L, et al. MRI reveals hemodynamic changes with acute maternal hyperoxygenation in human fetuses with and without congenital heart disease. Prenat Diagn 2016;36(3):274–81.

67. Darby JRT, Schrauben EM, Saini BS, et al. Umbilical vein infusion of prostaglandin I2 increases ductus venosus shunting of oxygen-rich blood but does not increase cerebral oxygen delivery in the fetal sheep. J Physiol 2020; 598(21):4957–67.

68. Zhu MY, Milligan N, Keating S, et al. The hemodynamics of late-onset intrauterine growth restriction by MRI. Am J Obstet Gynecol 2016;214(3):367.e1–17.

69. Duan AQ, Darby JRT, Soo JY, et al. Feasibility of phase-contrast cine magnetic resonance imaging for measuring blood flow in the sheep fetus. Am J Physiol Regul Integr Comp Physiol 2019;317(6):R780–92.

70. Saini BS, Darby JRT, Portnoy S, et al. Normal human and sheep fetal vessel oxygen saturations by T2 magnetic resonance imaging. J Physiol 2020;598(15): 3259–81.

71. Morrison JL, Berry MJ, Botting KJ, et al. Improving pregnancy outcomes in humans through studies in sheep. Am J Physiol Regul Integr Comp Physiol 2018; 315(6):R1123–53.

72. Rudolph A. Congenital diseases of the heart: clinical-physiological considerations. 3rd edition. NJ, USA: Wiley-Blackwell; 2009.

73. Accurso FJ, Alpert B, Wilkening RB, et al. Time-dependent response of fetal pulmonary blood flow to an increase in fetal oxygen tension. Respir Physiol 1986; 63(1):43–52.

74. Storme L, Rairigh RL, Parker TA, et al. In vivo evidence for a myogenic response in the fetal pulmonary circulation. Pediatr Res 1999;45(3):425–31.

75. Cohn HE, Sacks EJ, Heymann MA, et al. Cardiovascular responses to hypoxemia and acidemia in fetal lambs. Am J Obstet Gynecol 1974;120(6):817–24.

76. Moore PJ, Hanson MA. The role of peripheral chemoreceptors in the rapid response of the pulmonary vasculature of the late gestation sheep fetus to changes in PaO2. J Dev Physiol 1991;16(3):133–8.

77. Rasanen J, Wood DC, Debbs RH, et al. Reactivity of the human fetal pulmonary circulation to maternal hyperoxygenation increases during the second half of pregnancy: a randomized study. Circulation 1998;97(3):257–62.

78. McHugh A, Breatnach C, Bussmann N, et al. Prenatal prediction of neonatal haemodynamic adaptation after maternal hyperoxygenation. BMC Pregnancy Childbirth 2020;20(1):706.

79. Lee FT, Marini D, Seed M, et al. Maternal hyperoxygenation in congenital heart disease. Transl Pediatr 2021;10(8):2197–209.

80. Tulzer A, Huhta JC, Hochpoechler J, et al. Hypoplastic left heart syndrome: is there a role for fetal therapy? Front Pediatr 2022;10:944813.
81. Lewis AB, Heymann MA, Rudolph AM. Gestational changes in pulmonary vascular responses in fetal lambs in utero. Circ Res 1976;39(4):536–41.
82. Done E, Allegaert K, Lewi P, et al. Maternal hyperoxygenation test in fetuses undergoing FETO for severe isolated congenital diaphragmatic hernia. Ultrasound Obstet Gynecol 2011;37(3):264–71.
83. Szwast A, Tian Z, McCann M, et al. Vasoreactive response to maternal hyperoxygenation in the fetus with hypoplastic left heart syndrome. Circ Cardiovasc Imaging 2010;3(2):172–8.
84. Kohl T. Chronic intermittent materno-fetal hyperoxygenation in late gestation may improve on hypoplastic cardiovascular structures associated with cardiac malformations in human fetuses. Pediatr Cardiol 2010;31(2):250–63.
85. Lara DA, Morris SA, Maskatia SA, et al. Pilot study of chronic maternal hyperoxygenation and effect on aortic and mitral valve annular dimensions in fetuses with left heart hypoplasia. Ultrasound Obstet Gynecol 2016;48(3):365–72.
86. Singh Y, Tissot C. Echocardiographic evaluation of transitional circulation for the neonatologists. Front Pediatr 2018;6:140.
87. Pak O, Aldashev A, Welsh D, et al. The effects of hypoxia on the cells of the pulmonary vasculature. Eur Respir J 2007;30(2):364–72.
88. Cookson MW, Abman SH, Kinsella JP, et al. Pulmonary vasodilator strategies in neonates with acute hypoxemic respiratory failure and pulmonary hypertension. Semin Fetal Neonatal Med 2022;27(4):101367.
89. Nair J, Lakshminrusimha S. Update on PPHN: mechanisms and treatment. Semin Perinatol 2014;38(2):78–91.
90. Mandell E, Kinsella JP, Abman SH. Persistent pulmonary hypertension of the newborn. Pediatr Pulmonol 2021;56(3):661–9.
91. Lakshminrusimha S, Konduri GG, Steinhorn RH. Considerations in the management of hypoxemic respiratory failure and persistent pulmonary hypertension in term and late preterm neonates. J Perinatol 2016;36(Suppl 2):S12–9.
92. Zhu P, Huang L, Ge X, et al. Transdifferentiation of pulmonary arteriolar endothelial cells into smooth muscle-like cells regulated by myocardin involved in hypoxia-induced pulmonary vascular remodelling. Int J Exp Pathol 2006;87(6):463–74.
93. Zhang B, Niu W, Dong HY, et al. Hypoxia induces endothelial-mesenchymal transition in pulmonary vascular remodeling. Int J Mol Med 2018;42(1):270–8.
94. Patel SR, Madan N, Jone PN, et al. Utility of fetal echocardiography with acute maternal hyperoxygenation testing in assessment of complex congenital heart defects. Children 2023;10(2):281.
95. Porayette P, van Amerom JFP, Yoo SJ, et al. MRI shows limited mixing between systemic and pulmonary circulations in foetal transposition of the great arteries: a potential cause of in utero pulmonary vascular disease. Cardiol Young 2015;25(4):737–44.
96. Maeno YV, Kamenir SA, Sinclair B, et al. Prenatal features of ductus arteriosus constriction and restrictive foramen ovale in d-transposition of the great arteries. Circulation 1999;99(9):1209–14.
97. Sun L, van Amerom JFP, Marini D, et al. MRI characterization of hemodynamic patterns of human fetuses with cyanotic congenital heart disease. Ultrasound Obstet Gynecol 2021;58(6):824–36.

98. Sun L, Lee FT, van Amerom JFP, et al. Update on fetal cardiovascular magnetic resonance and utility in congenital heart disease. Journal of Congenital Cardiology 2021;5(1):4.
99. Rudolph AM. Aortopulmonary transposition in the fetus: speculation on pathophysiology and therapy. Pediatr Res 2007;61(3):375–80.
100. Kumar A, Taylor GP, Sandor GG, et al. Pulmonary vascular disease in neonates with transposition of the great arteries and intact ventricular septum. Br Heart J 1993;69(5):442–5.
101. Hoshino S, Somura J, Furukawa O, et al. The histological findings in transposition of the great artery with severe persistent pulmonary hypertension of the newborn. Journal of Cardiology Cases 2018;17(5):159–62.
102. Sun L, Marini D, Saini B, et al. Understanding fetal hemodynamics using cardiovascular magnetic resonance imaging. Fetal Diagn Ther 2020;47(5):354–62.
103. Feinstein JA, Benson DW, Dubin AM, et al. Hypoplastic left heart syndrome. J Am Coll Cardiol 2012;59(1 Suppl):S1–42.
104. Kritzmire SM, Cossu AE. Hypoplastic left heart syndrome. In: StatPearls. StatPearls Publishing; 2023. Available at: http://www.ncbi.nlm.nih.gov/books/NBK554576/. Accessed June 20, 2023.
105. Rychik J, Rome JJ, Collins MH, et al. The hypoplastic left heart syndrome with intact atrial septum: atrial morphology, pulmonary vascular histopathology and outcome. J Am Coll Cardiol 1999;34(2):554–60.
106. Maeda K, Yamaki S, Kado H, et al. Hypoplasia of the small pulmonary arteries in hypoplastic left heart syndrome with restrictive atrial septal defect. Circulation 2004;110(11_suppl_1):II–139.
107. Al Nafisi B, van Amerom JFP, Forsey J, et al. Fetal circulation in left-sided congenital heart disease measured by cardiovascular magnetic resonance: a case-control study. J Cardiovasc Magn Reson 2013;15(1):65.
108. Serrano RM, Hussain S, Brown B, et al. Risk stratification of patients with hypoplastic left heart syndrome and intact atrial septum using fetal MRI and echocardiography. Cardiol Young 2020;30(6):790–8.

Pathogenesis and Physiologic Mechanisms of Neonatal Pulmonary Hypertension: Preclinical Studies

Karen C. Young, MD, MS[a],*, Augusto F. Schmidt, MD, PhD[a],
April W. Tan, MD[a], Lourenco Sbragia, MD, PhD[b],
Ahmed Elsaie, MD[c,d], Binoy Shivanna, MD, DM, PhD[e]

KEYWORDS

- Neonatal pulmonary hypertension • PH • Pulmonary vascular resistance • PVR
- Bronchopulmonary dysplasia • BPD

KEY POINTS

- Creation of animal models of neonatal PH require a thorough understanding of embryology and growth factors that play an important role in lung development.
- Small animall models have the advantage of providing a targeted approach for studying specific genes and identifying novel therapeutic targets.
- Caution must be excercised while interpreting data from animal models while developing clinical guidelines. Limitations such as species differences, lack of multifactorial etiology in the development of the disease model must be taken into consideration.

PULMONARY VASCULAR DEVELOPMENT

The pulmonary vascular network comprising highly specialized cells develops through a tightly coordinated process of vasculogenesis and angiogenesis through all stages of lung development.[1] The development of the pulmonary arterial system and airways mirror each other, involving branching morphogenesis, whereas pulmonary venous

[a] Division of Neonatology, Department of Pediatrics, University of Miami Miller School of Medicine, Batchelor Children's Research Institute, 1580 North West 10th Avenue, RM-345, Miami, Fl 33136, USA; [b] Ribeirao Preto Medical School, University of Sao Paulo, Av. Bandeirantes 3900, 10th Floor, Monte Alegre14049-900, Ribeirao Preto SP, Brazil; [c] Ascension Via Christi St.Joseph Hospital, 3rd Floor, section of Neonatology, 3600 East Harry StreetWichita, KS 67218, USA; [d] Department of Pediatrics, Cairo University, Cairo 11956, Egypt; [e] Division of Neonatology, Department of Pediatrics, 6621 Fannin Street, MC: WT 6-104, Houston, TX 77030, USA
* Corresponding author. 1580 NorthWest 10th Avenue, RM-345, Miami, FL 33136.
E-mail address: Kyoung3@med.miami.edu

Clin Perinatol 51 (2024) 21–43
https://doi.org/10.1016/j.clp.2023.11.004
0095-5108/24/© 2023 Elsevier Inc. All rights reserved.
perinatology.theclinics.com

and lymphatic systems have different patterning and locations within the lung. Further, the lung capillary endothelial cells form a microenvironment called vascular niche where they interact with other resident cells, including epithelial, mesenchymal, and immune cells, to regulate the development and regeneration of the lungs.[2] The cross-sectional area of the pulmonary vasculature and its sensitivity to oxygen increase with advancing stages of lung development.

Embryonic Phase

The pulmonary vasculature starts developing during the embryonic phase as the lung buds grow from the foregut endoderm. The initial process through which pulmonary arteries are formed is vasculogenesis entailing the formation of new vessels de novo by differentiation of mesoderm progenitor cells into endothelial cells. During this phase, hemangioblasts form blood lakes in the mesenchyme, predominantly around the distal epithelial buds.[3] Angiogenesis, the other process that contributes to pulmonary vascular development in the embryonic phase, involves the formation of new vessels from a preexisting vessel. During proximal angiogenesis, blood vessels sprout from larger vessels surrounding the trachea.[3] In contrast, distal angiogenesis involves proliferation, migration, and coalescence of the endothelial cells in the mesenchymal blood lakes surrounding the epithelial buds.[3,4] A third process that may contribute to pulmonary vascular development is intussusceptive angiogenesis, which involves new vessel generation by the formation of tissue pillars dividing preexisting vessels. The endothelial cells form the vascular niche with epithelial and mesenchymal cells, contributing to embryonic lung development through vascular endothelial growth factor (VEGF) signaling. The epithelial cell secreted growth factors such as fibroblast growth factor (FGF) 9 and sonic hedgehog instruct the surrounding mesenchymal cells to increase the expression of VEGF[5] that acts on the VEGF receptor 2 (VEGFR2) present on the endothelial cells to promote vasculogenesis and angiogenesis.[6,7]

Pseudoglandular Phase

The proximal vasculature arising from the sixth aortic arch develops in parallel to the bronchial tree giving rise to preacinar arteries and veins by vasculogenesis during this phase.[8] The pulmonary vascular network present predominantly in the mesenchyme[8,9] becomes increasingly organized.[8] The epithelium, rather than the mesenchyme, becomes the primary source of VEGF resulting in a close approximation of endothelial cells with the epithelium.[4] Cross-talk between the epithelial, mesenchymal, and endothelial cells in the niche through growth factors such as FGF9 (secreted by epithelium),[5] FGF10 (secreted by mesenchyme),[5] and hepatocyte growth factor (secreted by the alveolar capillaries)[10] regulate epithelial and capillary development during this phase.

Canalicular Phase

The initial air-blood barriers are formed during this stage as the type I alveolar epithelial cells closely approximate with the mesenchymal capillary network from complex interactions between the endodermal-derived epithelium and the mesodermally-derived endothelium.[8,11] The capillary endothelial cells further approximate the epithelial cells as the latter cells, mostly alveolar type 2 epithelial cells, and not the mesenchymal cells are the source of VEGF during this stage.[12] Cross-talk between the epithelial and endothelial cells promotes the formation of acinar units. In patients with alveolar capillary dysplasia with misalignment of the pulmonary veins, the formation of air-blood barriers during this phase is disrupted as the mesenchyme surrounding the airways mainly contains small blood vessels instead of capillaries and the alveolar septa are thickened.[13]

Saccular Phase

During the early saccular phase of lung development, the pulmonary vessels rapidly proliferate, resulting in an increased cross-sectional area of the pulmonary vascular bed and expansion of the gas exchange site. The primary septa formed between 2 airspaces contain a double-layered capillary network. The endothelial cells display significant heterogeneity.[14] Additionally, the pulmonary vessels, including the pulmonary veins become more reactive to vasoconstrictors and vasodilators.

Alveolar Phase

The surface area of the pulmonary capillary network increases by 20-fold, and the volume of the pulmonary capillaries increase by 35-fold through adulthood.[15] Microvascular maturation and alveolarization occur in parallel and continue through young adulthood. Microvascular maturation is characterized by extensive development of the pulmonary capillary bed in the distal lung. The double-capillary network becomes a single capillary layer, and the lung mesenchyme and epithelial layers become thinner, decreasing the distance between distal airways and the capillaries and improving gas exchange efficiency.[8] Cross-talk between the myofibroblasts, pericytes, and endothelial cells in the niche drives secondary septation, alveolarization, continued angiogenesis, and microvascular maturation by secretion of elastin by myofibroblasts,[16] retinoic acid by endothelial cells,[17] and via Tie2[18] and VEGF-VEGFR signaling.[2]

Regulation of Fetal Pulmonary Vascular Tone

Despite an increase in lung vascular density throughout the saccular and alveolar stages of lung development, intrauterine pulmonary vascular resistance (PVR) is high. Low oxygen tension, fluid-filled lungs, along with an imbalance of vasoconstrictors such as endothelin-1 and leukotrienes and low levels of vasodilators, such as nitric oxide (NO) and prostacyclins are key contributors to this high fetal PVR.[19,20] With birth, oxygen tension increases, lung fluid clears, PVR decreases and pulmonary blood flow increases.[21] Increased oxygen tension and endothelial sheer stress along with increased ATP promote NO production which increases cyclic guanosine monophosphate (cGMP) production leading to smooth muscle relaxation.[22,23] Prostacyclin levels also increase with lung inflation and following binding to its receptor, adenyl cyclase is activated, leading to increased cyclic adenosine monophosphate (cAMP) and smooth muscle cell relaxation.[24,25]

PERSISTENT PULMONARY HYPERTENSION OF THE NEWBORN

Failure of pulmonary vascular adaptation at birth results in persistent pulmonary hypertension of the newborn (PPHN).[26] PPHN is characterized by elevated PVR, right to left shunting of deoxygenated blood across the foramen ovale or ductus arteriosus, hypoxemia, and decreased perfusion of systemic organs.[27]

PPHN may be classified as idiopathic or secondary.[28] Newborns with idiopathic PPHN have no apparent parenchymal lung disease. However, autopsy findings of infants who die shortly after birth secondary to idiopathic PPHN reveal pulmonary vascular smooth muscle cell proliferation and extension of muscle into normally nonmuscular peripheral pulmonary vessels.[29,30] In utero constriction of the ductus leading to increased pulmonary vascular endothelial stress and remodeling is a contributor to idiopathic PPHN. Non-steroidal anti-inflammatory drugs and serotonin reuptake inhibitor (SSRI) use in pregnancy has been associated with idiopathic PPHN risk but data have been mixed.[31,32] Both drugs constrict the ductus prematurely and SSRIs directly induce pulmonary vascular smooth muscle cell proliferation.[33,34] Secondary PPHN accounts for 80% to 90% of all PPHN cases. Lung parenchymal diseases such as pneumonia, sepsis, meconium aspiration syndrome, respiratory distress syndrome, abnormal transition as occurs in perinatal asphyxia, and lung hypoplasia (discussed in section 4.0) are often complicated by PPHN.

Lessons Learnt from Animal Models

Large and small animal models have provided invaluable insight into PPHN pathogenesis. Large animal models such as fetal lambs and newborn piglets are attractive as they have similar size and maturation as human newborns and technically, they allow for easier instrumentation, hemodynamic studies and testing of therapeutic interventions. Pregnant sheep are also relatively less likely to have preterm labor and newborn piglets have a very reactive pulmonary vasculature, prone to remodeling. **Table 1** summarizes these animal models and their associated biochemical alterations. Disrupted NO-cGMP, prostacyclin-cAMP, endothelin-1, Rho-kinase signaling pathways, as well as oxidative and nitrosative stress are now recognized as key contributors to the pathophysiological features seen in PPHN (**Fig. 1**).[35–39]

Antenatal ductal constriction in large animals is 1 of the most reproducible models of idiopathic PPHN. In utero, the ductus arteriosus diverts blood flow away from the lungs and antenatal ductal constriction forces blood into a constricted pulmonary vasculature, leading to endothelial sheer stress and vascular remodeling. In fetal lambs, ductal constriction is performed at 125 to 127 days gestation, and within 8 to 14 days of ductal constriction, pulmonary vascular maldevelopment is evident.[40] Large animals are, however, expensive to maintain.

Small animal PPHN models, such as rodents, are most frequently used in chronic hypoxia models. There is, however, strain variability, and rodent models do not exactly recapitulate the human newborn disease. In utero small animal hypoxia models have also been used to explore the mechanisms underlying PPHN associated with placental malperfusion, but these models exhibit modest vascular remodeling along with impaired alveolar development and growth retardation.[41,42] Murine models, however, have the advantage of providing a targeted approach for studying genes and having a shorter gestation. For example, mice with *S52 F Foxf1* mutation have provided invaluable insight into the pathogenesis of alveolar capillary dysplasia and provided new therapeutic targets.[43]

CONGENITAL DIAPHRAGMATIC HERNIA

Congenital diaphragmatic hernia (CDH) is a developmental defect of the diaphragm that occurs in approximately 2.6 per 10,000 total births worldwide, with a high mortality rate of about 40%.[44] The disorder is characterized by 4 distinct pathologies: diaphragmatic defect; lung hypoplasia of the ipsilateral and contralateral lungs; pulmonary hypertension (PH); and biventricular cardiac dysfunction. High PVR in CDH patients leads to decreased pulmonary venous return and leftward bowing of the interventricular septum, resulting in decreased left ventricular preload and systemic hypoxemia, predisposing to reduced coronary perfusion and myocardial ischemia. The cardiac dysfunction resulting from these events decreases cardiac contractility further reducing pulmonary blood flow, perpetuating a vicious cycle of increasing PVR and systemic hypotension.

The authors have summarized diaphragm and lung development across different species in **Fig. 2**. The primary embryologic defect leading to CDH is still a subject of debate. Currently, CDH is attributed to abnormal formation of pleuroperitoneal folds

Table 1
Summary of PPHN animal models

Model	Species	Features	Clinical Correlate	Biochemical Alterations
Antenatal Ductal Constriction[36,40]	Fetal lambs	• Increased medial and adventitial thickening • Extension of muscularization into peripheral pulmonary arteries • Increased pulmonary vascular smooth muscle reactivity • Right ventricular hypertrophy and dysfunction	Idiopathic PPHN	• Downregulated eNOS • Decreased soluble guanyl cyclase • Increased phosphodiestase-5 activity • Increased oxidative stress • Elevated endothelin-1
Group B β-hemolytic streptococci Sepsis[92]	Piglets	• Sustained elevation of pulmonary artery pressure • Reduction in cardiac output • Metabolic acidosis	PPHN secondary to pneumonia	• Early phase mediated by increased thromboxane • Late phase characterized by increased leukotrienes and platelet activating factor • Elevated endothelin-1 • Increased NO production
Postnatal Hypoxia[93,94,95]	Rodents Piglets Calves	• Rodents: strain dependent responses, remodeling is modest • Piglets: retain the fetal shape, position, overlap and interdigitation of pulmonary vascular endothelial and smooth muscle cells, and exhibit increased medial thickening and pulmonary vascular tone, cardiac dysfunction • Calves: pulmonary vascular remodeling in proximal and distal pulmonary vasculature, infiltration of inflammatory cells and mesenchymal progenitors	PPHN secondary to abnormal transition	• Downregulated eNOS • Increased oxidative stress • Increased Rho A and Rho-kinase • Elevated endothelin-1

(continued on next page)

Table 1
(continued)

Model	Species	Features	Clinical Correlate	Biochemical Alterations
Meconium Instillation[96]	Piglets, dogs, cats, rabbits, lambs, rodents, baboons	• Pulmonary vascular response variable • Degree of PH not related to concurrent perinatal asphyxia	PPHN secondary to meconium aspiration	• Increased lung inflammation • Increased oxidative stress • Inhibition of surfactant function
Aorto-pulmonary shunts[97]	Piglets lambs	• Heart failure • Elevated pulmonary artery pressure • Increased medial wall thickness Extension of muscularization into peripheral arteries	PH associated with congenital heart disease	• Altered angiopoietin-1/bone morphogenetic receptor-2 (BMP2), nitric oxide, and endothelin-1 signaling

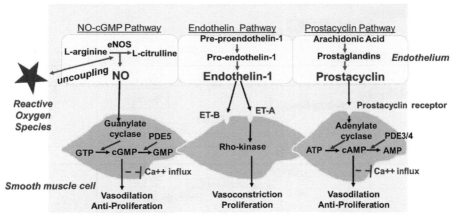

Fig. 1. Key signaling pathways involved in the pathogenesis of persistent pulmonary hypertension of the newborn (PPHN). Endothelin-1 (ET) is a potent vasoconstrictor which acts through 2 receptor proteins, ET-A and ET-B. ET-A mediates vasoconstriction and ET-B mediates vasodilation through nitric oxide (NO) and prostacyclin pathways. NO and prostacyclin stimulate the release of cGMP and cAMP respectively in pulmonary vascular smooth muscle cells leading to decreased calcium influx and pulmonary vascular smooth muscle relaxation. NO signaling is inactivated by reactive active species such as superoxide, hydrogen peroxide and peroxynitrite. Phosphodiesterase 5 (PDE5) and PDE3 limit vasodilation by breaking down cGMP and cAMP respectively. Activation of the Rho-kinase pathway by calcium ions and ET-1 induces pulmonary vasoconstriction by phosphorylation of myosin light chain.

with failure of formation in the mesenchymal structure that provides the scaffold for diaphragm muscularization and innervation[45] leading to a defect in the diaphragm and allowing herniation of abdominal contents into the thorax. The diaphragmatic defect would lead to growth of abdominal organs into the thoracic cavity and impairment of lung development.[46] Overall, these processes result in severe lung hypoplasia and pulmonary hypertension. The ideal preclinical model of CDH would allow researchers to understand the contribution of all processes leading to pulmonary hypoplasia and hypertension and investigation of potential therapies for CDH. The animal models of CDH, their contributions to our understanding of the disease, advantages, and disadvantages are summarized in **Table 2**.

BRONCHOPULMONARY DYSPLASIA COMPLICATED BY PULMONARY HYPERTENSION

Bronchopulmonary dysplasia (BPD) is a chronic lung disorder frequently occurring in extremely low gestational age newborns.[47] The disease has several phenotypes, with PH representing the most severe form of the vascular phenotype associated with BPD and affecting up to 43% of infants with moderate-to-severe BPD.[48] Although complementary clinical and preclinical studies have shed light on the multifactorial and diverse pathobiology of BPD-associated PH (BPD-PH), there are no effective strategies to manage PH and substantially decrease its associated mortality[49] and morbidities in BPD infants.

Pathogenesis of Bronchopulmonary Dysplasia-Pulmonary Hypertension

Most infants who develop BPD-PH have more than 1 risk factor in antenatal, natal, or postnatal periods (**Fig. 3**). There is a substantial overlap of risk factors between BPD

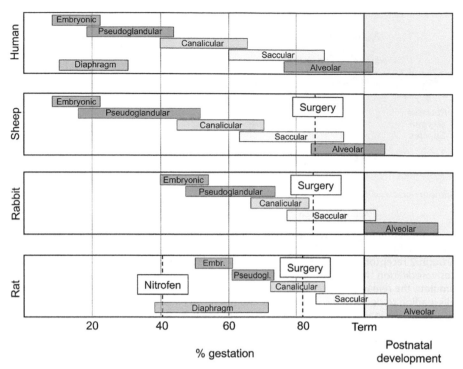

Fig. 2. Overview of diaphragm and lung development across different species. The dashed vertical line refers to the time when surgery is conducted to create the congenital diaphragmatic hernia (CDH) model.

and BPD-PH. Preclinical and clinical studies strongly suggest that fetal growth restriction (FGR) is a major antenatal risk factor associated with BPD-PH.[50] The mechanisms through which FGR causes BPD-PH include dysfunction and remodeling of pulmonary vasculature,[51] and placenta.[52] The second major antenatal risk factor strongly associated with BPD-PH is placental vascular abnormalities,[52] which can disrupt the equilibrium between pro-angiogenic and anti-angiogenic factors[53,54] and negatively affect overall lung health.[55] Genetic anomalies,[56] hypertensive pregnancy disorders,[52] oligohydramnios,[50,57,58] and maternal diabetes[59] can also predispose a neonate to develop BPD-PH. The natal risk factors, prematurity and low birthweight, are the strongest predictors of BPD-PH. A low 5-min Apgar score is another natal risk factor associated with the disorder.[58] The common postnatal risk factors related to BPD-PH include severe BPD,[57,60] early pulmonary vascular disease,[61] prolonged positive pressure respiratory support,[57] sepsis,[57] ventilator-associated pneumonia,[62] left atrial hypertension,[63] persistence of hemodynamically significant patent ductus arteriosus[64] and other cardiac shunt lesions,[65] and severe intermittent hypoxemic events.[66] Pulmonary vein stenosis, a fatal condition associated with prolonged mechanical ventilation[67] and necrotizing enterocolitis,[68] can also contribute to and worsen pulmonary vascular disease in BPD-PH.[69]

Pathophysiology of Bronchopulmonary Dysplasia-Pulmonary Hypertension

The pathophysiology of BPD-PH is based mainly on the concept of vascular hypothesis[55,70] of lung development, injury, and repair that states alveolarization and lung

Table 2
Summary of CDH models

	Species	Contributions of Model	Advantages	Disadvantages
Vitamin A deficiency[98]	Rats	• First animal model of CDH • Role of retinoids in the etiology of CDH	• Low cost	• Only a third of the pups develop CDH • Other concurrent congenital defects • Can only assess up to saccular stage of lung development
Nitrofen[45,99]	Rats	• Most used model • Identification of the defect of the pleuroperitoneal folds • Relationship between timing of insult and laterality	• Reproducibility • Low cost	• Only 40% of the pups develop CDH • Need for timed pregnancy • Multisystem effects of nitrofen on development • Can only assess up to saccular stage of lung development • Primary lung hypoplasia from nitrofen
Surgical	Rats[100]	• Teratogen-free model • Assess effect of mechanical compression alone	• Low cost • Teratogen-free	• Requires skilled surgeon • Can only assess up to saccular stage of lung development
	Rabbits[101]	• First teratogen-free model • Assess effect of mechanical compression alone	• Lung assessment up to alveolarization • Large enough to study surgical interventions • Singleton pregnancies • Large size • Study of fetal interventions	• Requires skilled surgeon • Limited availability of antibodies
	Lambs[102,103]	• Tracheal occlusion for lung growth		• High cost • Limited availability of antibodies • Alveolarization completed at term
Genetic[104,105]	Mice	• Identification of genes associated with CDH development • Mechanisms of normal and abnormal diaphragm development	• Reproducibility	• Development of new models require expertise and high cost
Ex vivo[106]	Human cells	• Identification of cell intrinsic abnormalities and effects of mechanical compression	• High translational relevance	• Technically labor intensive • Requires access to human samples

CDH, Congenital diaphragmatic hernia

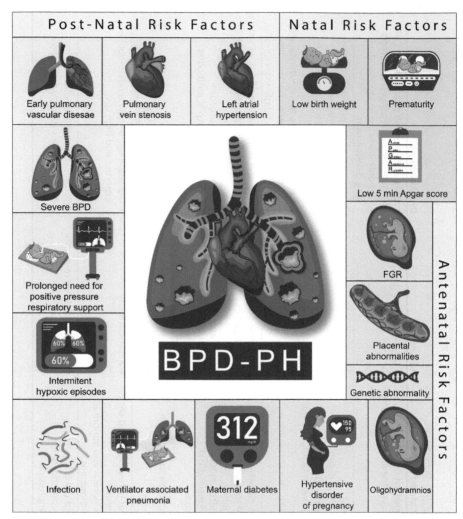

Fig. 3. Illustration of risk factors for BPD-PH. AT2: alveolar type II epithelial cells; BPD: bronchopulmonary dysplasia; PH: pulmonary hypertension; PVR: pulmonary vascular resistance; RV: right ventricle.

vascularization are highly coordinated and interdependent processes; therefore, conditions affecting the homeostasis of one process are highly likely to affect that of the other. The overarching histopathological traits of BPD-PH include lung inflammation, alveolar simplification, and decreased cross-sectional area and extracellular matrix of lung vasculature.[55,71] The functional consequences of these traits include altered vasoreactivity, decreased compliance, and increased resistance of the pulmonary vasculature leading to hypertrophy, dysfunction, and failure of the right ventricle.[72] Further, BPD-PH infants have lung dysfunction associated with inflammation and alveolar simplification. The additional pathologic hallmarks of BPD-PH infants include the persistence of fetal connections between pulmonary vessels and the presence of airway hemosiderin-laden macrophages. The pathologic persistence of fetal vessels between pulmonary arteries and veins usually occurs in infants with severe BPD.[73] By shunting blood away from the lungs and bypassing the normal oxygenation process, these fetal vessels cause hypoxemic episodes and worsen pulmonary vascular disease in BPD-PH patients.[73] Increased airway hemosiderin-laden macrophages were recently observed in BPD-PH infants.[74] The mechanisms behind this finding need to be clarified. The presence of simplified and dysfunctional capillaries predisposes BPD-PH infants to pulmonary hemorrhage from increased vascular pressure and leakiness when exposed to positive pressure and oxygen therapies. Hemosiderin-laden macrophages may be a consequence of pulmonary hemorrhage-mediated lung inflammation.[74]

Animal Models of Bronchopulmonary Dysplasia-Pulmonary Hypertension

Animal models are crucial for understanding disease pathophysiology and evaluating novel therapies. Several experimental models of BPD-PH have been developed over the past decades, many of which have improved our understanding of the disease pathogenesis. While small animals such as rats and mice are the predominant experimental animals used to model BPD-PH, larger animals such as lambs, rabbits, and piglets have also been used to model the disease. For designing the experiments and interpreting the results, it is essential to understand the variability of the timing of the lung developmental stages among humans and the animal species[2,8] (**Table 3**) and the advantages and disadvantages of the animal species used to model BPD-PH (**Table 4**).

To determine the molecular mechanisms and discover therapeutic targets for BPD-PH, several animal models have been generated and used based on the risk factors of the disease in infants and the technical feasibility of exposing the animals to these risk factors. Hyperoxia exposure during the postnatal period is the most common risk factor used to model the disease. There are several advantages to using hyperoxia as an injurious insult. Oxygen is readily available and cheap, its effects can be easily reproduced, and its concentration can be easily titrated. With an improved understanding of the antenatal origins of BPD-PH as described in the pathogenesis section, several recent studies have efficiently used antenatal insults to model the disease. Additionally, keeping up with the multifactorial etiology of BPD-PH, there is an increasing emphasis on developing 2-hit models to discover meaningful therapies for the disease. A summary of the clinical risk-factor-based BPD-PH animal models with references is shown in **Table 5**. Phenotyping of BPD-PH in preclinical studies typically includes quantifying alveolarization, lung angiogenesis, pulmonary vascular remodeling, echocardiography indices of PH such as pulmonary acceleration time (PAT) and PAT/ejection time ratio, indirect estimation of right ventricular systolic pressure, and

Table 3
Timeline of lung developmental stages in humans and experimental BPD-PH animals

Species	Embryonic Phase	Pseudoglandular Phase	Canalicular Phase	Saccular Phase	Alveolar Phase
Mouse	E9.2-E12	E12-E16.5	E16.5-E17.5	E17.5-P5	P5-P36
Rat	E11-E13	E13-E18.5	E18.5-E20	E21-P4	P4-P60
Sheep	E17-E30	E30-E85	E80-E120	E110-E140	E120-n.d.
Rabbit	Up to E18	E18-E24	E23-E27	E27-E30	E30-n.d.
Monkey	Up to E55	E55-E85	E75-E115	E105-Term	E125-8 y
Human	3-7 wk (p.c.)	5-17 wk (p.c.)	16-26 wk (p.c.)	26-36 wk (p.c.)	36 wk (p.c.)-21 y

Abbreviations: E: embryonic day; n.d., not determined; p.c., post coitum; P, postnatal day; wks, weeks; yrs, years.

Table 4
Summary of the advantages and disadvantages of various animal species used to model BPD-PH

Species	Advantages	Disadvantages	References

Mouse	• Comparable anatomic lung developmental stage to humans
	• Reproducible disease phenotype
	• Short gestation and lung maturation times
	• Larger litter size
	• Feasible long-term studies
	• Conducive to genetic engineering methods and deciphering cause and effect relationship
	• Cost-effective
		• Discrepancy in lung function compared to human lungs: rat are surfactant sufficient despite being born in the saccular stage of lung development and don't require respiratory support for survival
		• Lack of a robust pulmonary vascular remodeling response on exposure to various insults
		• Strain-specific variability in responses to noxious stimuli
		• Practical difficulties with:
		  ○ Providing mechanical ventilation
		  ○ Administrating short-acting medications
		  ○ Providing parenteral nutrition
		  ○ Performing precise and high-value cardiopulmonary function tests
			Whitehead[107] 2006

Rat	• Comparable anatomic lung developmental stage to humans
	• Reproducible disease phenotype
	• Short gestation and lung maturation times
	• Larger litter size
	• Feasible long-term studies
	• Better pulmonary vascular remodeling response on exposure to various insults compared to mice
	• More conducive than mice for performing hemodynamic and other functional tests because of their size
	• Cost-effective
		• Discrepancy in lung function compared to human lungs: Mouse are surfactant sufficient despite being born in the saccular stage of lung development and don't require respiratory support for survival
		• Not as conducive to genetic engineering methods as mice
		• Strain-specific variability in responses to noxious stimuli
		• Practical difficulties with:
		  ○ Providing mechanical ventilation
		  ○ Administrating short-acting medications
		  ○ Providing parenteral nutrition
		  ○ Performing precise and high-value cardiopulmonary function tests
			O'Reilly[108] 2014

Model	Advantages	Disadvantages	References
Rabbit	• Larger lung capacity than rodents • Better suited than rodents to provide mechanical ventilation and perform precise and high-value cardiopulmonary function tests • Short life cycle • Large litter size • Alternative choice to more expensive and high-maintenance larger animals such as sheep and non-human primates	• Unlike rodents, the alveolar stage of lung development starts in utero • Expensive than rodents • Higher mortality rate • Not as conducive to genetic engineering methods as mice • Strict regulations for maintenance, handling, and interventions	D'Angio[109] 2014

Sheep and Monkey	• Feasibility of preterm delivery
	• Comparable anatomic and functional lung developmental stage
	• Ability to recreate NICU environment:
	  o Administration of antenatal steroids and parenteral and enteral nutrition
	  o Conducive to instrumentation, mechanical ventilation, hemodynamic monitoring, and performing precise and high-value cardiopulmonary function tests
	• Ease of administration of short-acting medications
		• Expensive
		• Slower turnover times
		• Not as conducive to genetic engineering methods as mice
		• Ethical considerations
			Albertine[110] 2015; Yoder and Coalson[111] 2014

Table 5
Summary of clinical risk factor-based animal models of BPD-PH

Species	Exposure Antenatal Period	Exposure Postnatal Period	Single-Hit Model	Multiple-Hit Model	References
Mouse	None	Hyperoxia	+	-	Reynolds et al,[112] 2016, Leary et al,[113] 2019
Mouse	None	Hypoxia	+	-	Ambalavanan et al,[114] 2008
Mouse	LPS	Hyperoxia	-	+	Bui et al,[81] 2019; Syed et al,[115] 2017
Mouse	None	Hyperoxia and LPS	-	+	Shrestha et al,[116] 2020
Rat	None	Hyperoxia	+	-	Sharma et al,[117] 2020
Rat	Endogenous VEGF antagonist, sFlt-1	None	+	-	Wallace et al,[78] 2018
Rat	Endotoxin	None	+	-	Wallace et al,[78] 2018; Seedorf et al,[118] 2020
Rat	None	Monocrotaline	+	-	Lesage et al,[119] 2021
Rat	LPS	Hyperoxia	-	+	Chen[120] 2017
Rat	None	Hyperoxia followed by intermittent hypoxia	-	+	Mankouski et al,[121] 2017
Rat	None	Hyperoxia and growth restriction	-	+	Wedgwood et al,[122] 2016
Rabbit	None	Hyperoxia	+	-	Jiménez et al,[123] 2016; Mühlfeld et al,[124] 2021
Sheep	None	Prolonged MV and oxygen exposure	-	+	Albertine[110] 2015; Albertine[125] 2013
Monkey	None	Prolonged MV and oxygen exposure	-	+	Yoder and Coalson[111] 2014; Albertine[125] 2013

Abbreviations: LPS, lipopolysaccharide; MV, mechanical ventilation; sFlt-1, soluble Fms-like tyrosine kinase-1; VEGF, vascular endothelial growth factor.

lung function tests. In larger animals, PH is better quantified by invasive hemodynamic monitoring and a more accurate assessment of pulmonary arterial pressure.

FUTURE DIRECTIONS AND RESEARCH GAPS

Lessons learnt from animal models have provided fundamental knowledge to guide the development of novel therapies. For example, intratracheal antioxidant administration with or without inhaled NO improves oxygenation in the ductal ligation PPHN model.[75] L-citrulline improves NO production by recoupling eNOS and decreases hypoxia-induced PH in piglets.[76] Some of the promising therapeutic targets for BPD-PH based on preclinical studies include connective tissue growth factor,[77] endogenous VEGF inhibitors such as soluble fms-like tyrosine kinase 1,[78] exosomes,[79,80] interleukin-1 receptor antagonist,[81] microbiome,[82] mesenchymal stem cells,[83–85] and endothelial colony-forming cells.[86]

Despite the strengths of preclinical studies for innovation and discovery of specific therapies, several weaknesses must be addressed to advance the field. The models need to be standardized for meaningful comparison of results and outcomes of the studies. For instance, wide variation in the concentration and duration of oxygen used in the BPD-PH rodent studies makes it difficult to draw meaningful conclusions. While standardizing the concentration and duration of oxygen exposure in rodents, it is also important to realize that creating a robust rodent model of hyperoxia-induced BPD-PH using lower concentration and short duration of oxygen exposure as observed in neonatal intensive care units is challenging. Infants are usually exposed to more insults in addition to oxygen exposure; therefore, developing multiple-hit mouse models based on the significant clinical risk factors is needed for meaningful discoveries. It is also necessary to consider strain-specific differences while standardizing rodent disease models. Further, the accuracy and specificity of our results can be improved by implementing rigorous methodology. Preventing distortion of the preserved lung tissues,[87,88] using 3-dimensional and design-based stereology models to visualize and analyze alveolarization and pulmonary vascularization,[87] and using ex vivo approaches to study pulmonary vascular reactivity to various interventions[81] are some approaches to improve the rigor of preliminary studies. Finally, the rigor of phenotyping PH can be increased by accurately measuring and quantifying additional echocardiography parameters such as tricuspid annular plane systolic excursion, right ventricular strain, and right ventricular fractional area of contraction[89] and complementing echocardiography with cardiac magnetic resonance imaging studies.[90,91] Therapeutic targets identified by high-quality small animal studies should also undergo robust testing for safety and efficacy in larger animal models before human studies.

Best Practice Box

Determining PH pathogenesis and pathophysiology using preclinical models

What is the Current Practice?

- Using different
  - Animal species
  - Type and duration of insults to model PH
  - Time points and methods to assess pathology and pathophysiology

What changes in current practice are likely to improve scientific output?

- Develop standardized preclinical models of PH tailored to the lung anatomy and physiology of each animal species

- Use unbiased and highly reproducible methods to robustly examine and quantify the pathophysiology of PH in preclinical models
- Include a multidisciplinary and multi-institutional team with complementary expertise to increase the accuracy and precision of the study findings

Major Recommendations:

- Standardization of the duration and severity of insults to model preclinical PH
- Use multiple insults based on the clinical risk factors for neonatal PH to develop a clinically meaningful preclinical PH model
- Incorporate precise and reproducible methods to evaluate and quantify PH and its underlying pathology based on the animal species. For instance, use hemodynamic indices in larger animal species or older small animal species and use less operator dependent methodologies such as cardiac magnetic resonance imaging in smaller animal species
- Establish normal indices of pulmonary vascular pressure and other relevant hemodynamic indices based on the age and species of experimental animals
- To be cost-effective, validate mechanistic and therapeutic studies of neonatal PH in smaller animal species, if feasible, before studying in larger animal species

DISCLOSURE

The authors have nothing to disclose.

FUNDING

BS is funded by NHLBI - R01HL139594. KY, AS and AT are funded by Batchelor Research Foundation and Project Newborn. Lourenco Sbragia is supported by the State of Sao Paulo Research Foundation (FAPESP); Grant Number : 2022/12021-1. Augusto Schmidt is supported by National Institute of Health (5K08HD102718).

REFERENCES

1. Peng T, Morrisey EE. Development of the pulmonary vasculature: current understanding and concepts for the future. Pulm Circ 2013;3(1):176–8.
2. Mammoto A, Mammoto T. Vascular niche in lung alveolar development, homeostasis, and regeneration. Front Bioeng Biotechnol 2019;7:318.
3. Gebb SA, Shannon JM. Tissue interactions mediate early events in pulmonary vasculogenesis. Dev Dynam 2000;217(2):159–69.
4. Parera MC, van Dooren M, van Kempen M, et al. Distal angiogenesis: a new concept for lung vascular morphogenesis. Am J Physiol Lung Cell Mol Physiol 2005;288(1):L141–9.
5. White AC, Lavine KJ, Ornitz DM. FGF9 and SHH regulate mesenchymal Vegfa expression and development of the pulmonary capillary network. Development 2007;134(20):3743–52.
6. Karaman S, Leppänen VM, Alitalo K. Vascular endothelial growth factor signaling in development and disease. Development 2018;145(14). dev151019.
7. Apte RS, Chen DS, Ferrara N. VEGF in signaling and disease: beyond discovery and development. Cell 2019;176(6):1248–64.
8. Schittny JC. Development of the lung. Cell Tissue Res 2017;367(3):427–44.
9. Caduff JH, Fischer LC, Burri PH. Scanning electron microscope study of the developing microvasculature in the postnatal rat lung. Anat Rec 1986;216(2):154–64.

10. Yamamoto H, Yun EJ, Gerber HP, et al. Epithelial-vascular cross talk mediated by VEGF-A and HGF signaling directs primary septae formation during distal lung morphogenesis. Dev Biol 2007;308(1):44–53.

11. Willem M, Miosge N, Halfter W, et al. Specific ablation of the nidogen-binding site in the laminin gamma1 chain interferes with kidney and lung development. Development 2002;129(11):2711–22.

12. Kaner RJ, Crystal RG. Compartmentalization of vascular endothelial growth factor to the epithelial surface of the human lung. Mol Med 2001;7(4):240–6.

13. Kool H, Mous D, Tibboel D, et al. Pulmonary vascular development goes awry in congenital lung abnormalities. Birth Defects Res C Embryo Today 2014;102(4): 343–58.

14. Guo M, Du Y, Gokey JJ, et al. Single cell RNA analysis identifies cellular heterogeneity and adaptive responses of the lung at birth. Nat Commun 2019;10(1):37.

15. Goss K. Long-term pulmonary vascular consequences of perinatal insults. J Physiol 2019;597(4):1175–84.

16. Robinet A, Fahem A, Cauchard JH, et al. Elastin-derived peptides enhance angiogenesis by promoting endothelial cell migration and tubulogenesis through upregulation of MT1-MMP. J Cell Sci 2005;118(Pt 2):343–56.

17. Yun EJ, Lorizio W, Seedorf G, et al. VEGF and endothelium-derived retinoic acid regulate lung vascular and alveolar development. Am J Physiol Lung Cell Mol Physiol 2016;310(4):L287–98.

18. Mammoto T, Jiang E, Jiang A, et al. Extracellular matrix structure and tissue stiffness control postnatal lung development through the lipoprotein receptor-related protein 5/Tie2 signaling system. Am J Respir Cell Mol Biol 2013;49(6): 1009–18.

19. Lakshminrusimha SJCip. The pulmonary circulation in neonatal respiratory failure. Clin Perinatol 2012;39(3):655–83.

20. Hooper SB, Te Pas AB, Lang J, et al. Cardiovascular transition at birth: a physiological sequence. Pediatr Res 2015;77(5):608–14.

21. Lang JA, Pearson JT, Binder-Heschl C, et al. Increase in pulmonary blood flow at birth: role of oxygen and lung aeration. J Physiol 2016;594(5):1389–98.

22. Konduri GG, Theodorou AA, Mukhopadhyay A, et al. Adenosine triphosphate and adenosine increase the pulmonary blood flow to postnatal levels in fetal lambs. Pediatr Res 1992;31(5):451–7.

23. Abman SH, Chatfield BA, Hall S, et al. Role of endothelium-derived relaxing factor during transition of pulmonary circulation at birth. Am J Physiol 1990;259(6): H1921–7.

24. Velvis H, Moore P, Heymann MAJPr. Prostaglandin inhibition prevents the fall in pulmonary vascular resistance as a result of rhythmic distension of the lungs in fetal lambs. Pediatr Res 1991;30(1):62–8.

25. Leffler CW, Hessler JR, Green RSJPr. The onset of breathing at birth stimulates pulmonary vascular prostacyclin synthesis. Pediatr Res 1984;18(10):938–42.

26. Gersony WJCl. "PFC" syndrome (persistence of the fetal circulation). Circulation 1969;87–94.

27. Lakshminrusimha S, Keszler M. Persistent pulmonary hypertension of the newborn. NeoReviews 2015;16(12):e680–92.

28. Simonneau G, Gatzoulis MA, Adatia I, et al. Updated clinical classification of pulmonary hypertension. J Am Coll Cardiol 2013;62(25 Suppl):D34–41.

29. Murphy JD, Rabinovitch M, Goldstein JD, et al. The structural basis of persistent pulmonary hypertension of the newborn infant. J Pediatr 1981;98(6):962–7.

30. Haworth SG, Reid L. Persistent fetal circulation: newly recognized structural features. J Pediatr 1976;88(4 Pt 1):614–20.
31. Chambers CD, Hernandez-Diaz S, Van Marter LJ, et al. Selective serotonin-reuptake inhibitors and risk of persistent pulmonary hypertension of the newborn. N Engl J Med 2006;354(6):579–87.
32. Alano MA, Ngougmna E, Ostrea EM Jr, et al. Analysis of nonsteroidal antiinflammatory drugs in meconium and its relation to persistent pulmonary hypertension of the newborn. Pediatrics 2001;107(3):519–23.
33. Levin DL, Mills LJ, Parkey M, et al. Constriction of the fetal ductus arteriosus after administration of indomethacin to the pregnant Ewe. J Pediatr 1979;94(4): 647–50.
34. Fornaro E, Li D, Pan J, et al. Prenatal exposure to fluoxetine induces fetal pulmonary hypertension in the rat. Am J Respir Crit Care Med 2007;176(10):1035–40.
35. Shaul PW, Yuhanna IS, German Z, et al. Pulmonary endothelial NO synthase gene expression is decreased in fetal lambs with pulmonary hypertension. Am J Physiol 1997;272(5):L1005–12.
36. Ivy DD, Ziegler JW, Dubus MF, et al. Chronic intrauterine pulmonary hypertension alters endothelin receptor activity in the ovine fetal lung. Pediatr Res 1996;39(3):435–42.
37. Ivy DD, Parker TA, Ziegler JW, et al. Prolonged endothelin A receptor blockade attenuates chronic pulmonary hypertension in the ovine fetus. J Clin Invest 1997;99(6):1179–86.
38. Rosenberg AA, Kennaugh J, Koppenhafer SL, et al. Elevated immunoreactive endothelin-1 levels in newborn infants with persistent pulmonary hypertension. J Pediatr 1993;123(1):109–14.
39. Gien J, Seedorf GJ, Balasubramaniam V, et al. Chronic intrauterine pulmonary hypertension increases endothelial cell Rho kinase activity and impairs angiogenesis in vitro. Am J Physiol Lung Cell Mol Physiol 2008;295(4):L680–7.
40. Abman SH, Shanley PF, Accurso FJ. Failure of postnatal adaptation of the pulmonary circulation after chronic intrauterine pulmonary hypertension in fetal lambs. J Clin Invest 1989;83(6):1849–58.
41. Massaro GD, Olivier J, Dzikowski C, et al. Postnatal development of lung alveoli: suppression by 13% O2 and a critical period. Am J Physiol 1990;258(6 Pt 1): L321–7.
42. Goldberg SJ, Levy RA, Siassi B, et al. The effects of maternal hypoxia and hyperoxia upon the neonatal pulmonary vasculature. Pediatrics 1971;48(4):528–33.
43. Sun F, Wang G, Pradhan A, et al. Nanoparticle delivery of STAT3 alleviates pulmonary hypertension in a mouse model of alveolar capillary dysplasia. Circulation 2021;144(7):539–55.
44. Politis MD, Bermejo-Sanchez E, Canfield MA, et al. Prevalence and mortality in children with congenital diaphragmatic hernia: a multicountry study. Ann Epidemiol 2021;56:61–69 e63.
45. Kluth D, Tenbrinck R, von Ekesparre M, et al. The natural history of congenital diaphragmatic hernia and pulmonary hypoplasia in the embryo. J Pediatr Surg 1993;28(3):456–62, discussion 462-453.
46. Nagai A, Thurlbeck WM, Jansen AH, et al. The effect of chronic biphrenectomy on lung growth and maturation in fetal lambs. morphologic and morphometric studies. Am Rev Respir Dis 1988;137(1):167–72.
47. Cuevas Guaman M, Dahm PH, Welty SE. The challenge of accurately describing the epidemiology of bronchopulmonary dysplasia (BPD) based on the various current definitions of BPD. Pediatr Pulmonol 2021;56(11):3527–32.

48. Khemani E, McElhinney DB, Rhein L, et al. Pulmonary artery hypertension in formerly premature infants with bronchopulmonary dysplasia: clinical features and outcomes in the surfactant era. Pediatrics 2007;120(6):1260–9.

49. Mourani PM, Abman SH. Pulmonary hypertension and vascular abnormalities in bronchopulmonary dysplasia. Clin Perinatol 2015;42(4):839–55.

50. Kim YJ, Shin SH, Park HW, et al. Risk factors of early pulmonary hypertension and its clinical outcomes in preterm infants: a systematic review and meta-analysis. Sci Rep 2022;12(1):14186.

51. Rozance PJ, Seedorf GJ, Brown A, et al. Intrauterine growth restriction decreases pulmonary alveolar and vessel growth and causes pulmonary artery endothelial cell dysfunction in vitro in fetal sheep. Am J Physiol Lung Cell Mol Physiol 2011;301(6):L860–71.

52. Pierro M, Villamor-Martinez E, van Westering-Kroon E, et al. Association of the dysfunctional placentation endotype of prematurity with bronchopulmonary dysplasia: a systematic review, meta-analysis and meta-regression. Thorax 2022; 77(3):268–75.

53. Mestan KK, Gotteiner N, Porta N, et al. Cord blood biomarkers of placental maternal vascular underperfusion predict bronchopulmonary dysplasia-associated pulmonary hypertension. J Pediatr 2017;185:33–41.

54. Korzeniewski SJ, Romero R, Chaiworapongsa T, et al. Maternal plasma angiogenic index-1 (placental growth factor/soluble vascular endothelial growth factor receptor-1) is a biomarker for the burden of placental lesions consistent with uteroplacental underperfusion: a longitudinal case-cohort study. Am J Obstet Gynecol 2016;214(5):621 9.e617.

55. Thébaud B, Abman SH. Bronchopulmonary dysplasia: where have all the vessels gone? Roles of angiogenic growth factors in chronic lung disease. Am J Respir Crit Care Med 2007;175(10):978–85.

56. Trittmann JK, Bartenschlag A, Zmuda EJ, et al. Using clinical and genetic data to predict pulmonary hypertension in bronchopulmonary dysplasia. Acta Paediatr 2018;107(12):2158–64.

57. Nagiub M, Kanaan U, Simon D, et al. Risk factors for development of pulmonary hypertension in infants with bronchopulmonary dysplasia: systematic review and meta-analysis. Paediatr Respir Rev 2017;23:27–32.

58. Kim DH, Kim HS, Choi CW, et al. Risk factors for pulmonary artery hypertension in preterm infants with moderate or severe bronchopulmonary dysplasia. Neonatology 2012;101(1):40–6.

59. Sheth S, Goto L, Bhandari V, et al. Factors associated with development of early and late pulmonary hypertension in preterm infants with bronchopulmonary dysplasia. J Perinatol 2020;40(1):138–48.

60. Arjaans S, Zwart EAH, Ploegstra MJ, et al. Identification of gaps in the current knowledge on pulmonary hypertension in extremely preterm infants: a systematic review and meta-analysis. Paediatr Perinat Epidemiol 2018;32(3):258–67.

61. Mourani PM, Sontag MK, Younoszai A, et al. Early pulmonary vascular disease in preterm infants at risk for bronchopulmonary dysplasia. Am J Respir Crit Care Med 2015;191(1):87–95.

62. Vayalthrikkovil S, Vorhies E, Stritzke A, et al. Prospective study of pulmonary hypertension in preterm infants with bronchopulmonary dysplasia. Pediatr Pulmonol 2019;54(2):171–8.

63. Mourani PM, Ivy DD, Rosenberg AA, et al. Left ventricular diastolic dysfunction in bronchopulmonary dysplasia. J Pediatr 2008;152(2):291–3.

64. Gentle SJ, Travers CP, Clark M, et al. Patent ductus arteriosus and development of bronchopulmonary dysplasia-associated pulmonary hypertension. Am J Respir Crit Care Med 2023;207(7):921–8.

65. Madden BA, Conaway MR, Zanelli SA, et al. Screening echocardiography identifies risk factors for pulmonary hypertension at discharge in premature infants with bronchopulmonary dysplasia. Pediatr Cardiol 2022;43(8):1743–51.

66. Gentle SJ, Travers CP, Nakhmani A, et al. Intermittent hypoxemia and bronchopulmonary dysplasia with pulmonary hypertension in preterm infants. Am J Respir Crit Care Med 2023;207(7):899–907.

67. Vyas-Read S, Varghese NP, Suthar D, et al. Prematurity and pulmonary vein stenosis: the role of parenchymal lung disease and pulmonary vascular disease. Children 2022;9(5):713.

68. Heching HJ, Turner M, Farkouh-Karoleski C, et al. Pulmonary vein stenosis and necrotising enterocolitis: is there a possible link with necrotising enterocolitis? Arch Dis Child Fetal Neonatal Ed 2014;99(4):F282–5.

69. del Cerro MJ, Sabaté Rotés A, Cartón A, et al. Pulmonary hypertension in bronchopulmonary dysplasia: clinical findings, cardiovascular anomalies and outcomes. Pediatr Pulmonol 2014;49(1):49–59.

70. Abman SH. Bronchopulmonary dysplasia: "a vascular hypothesis". Am J Respir Crit Care Med 2001;164(10 Pt 1):1755–6.

71. Cornfield DN. Developmental regulation of oxygen sensing and ion channels in the pulmonary vasculature. Adv Exp Med Biol 2010;661:201–20.

72. Malloy KW, Austin ED. Pulmonary hypertension in the child with bronchopulmonary dysplasia. Pediatr Pulmonol 2021;56(11):3546–56.

73. Galambos C, Sims-Lucas S, Abman SH. Histologic evidence of intrapulmonary anastomoses by three-dimensional reconstruction in severe bronchopulmonary dysplasia. Ann Am Thorac Soc 2013;10(5):474–81.

74. Franklin SD, Fierro J, Hysinger EB, et al. Hemosiderin-laden macrophages in bronchoalveolar lavage samples of children with bronchopulmonary dysplasia. J Pediatr 2023;253:79–85.

75. Lakshminrusimha S, Russell JA, Wedgwood S, et al. Superoxide dismutase improves oxygenation and reduces oxidation in neonatal pulmonary hypertension. Am J Respir Crit Care Med 2006;174(12):1370–7.

76. Fike CD, Dikalova A, Kaplowitz MR, et al. Rescue treatment with l-citrulline inhibits hypoxia-induced pulmonary hypertension in newborn pigs. Am J Respir Cell Mol Biol 2015;53(2):255–64.

77. Alapati D, Rong M, Chen S, et al. Connective tissue growth factor antibody therapy attenuates hyperoxia-induced lung injury in neonatal rats. Am J Physiol Lung Cell Mol Physiol 2011;45(6):1169–77.

78. Wallace B, Peisl A, Seedorf G, et al. Anti-sFlt-1 therapy preserves lung alveolar and vascular growth in antenatal models of bronchopulmonary dysplasia. Am J Respir Crit Care Med 2018;197(6):776–87.

79. Willis GR, Fernandez-Gonzalez A, Reis M, et al. Macrophage immunomodulation: the gatekeeper for mesenchymal stem cell derived-exosomes in pulmonary arterial hypertension? Int J Mol Sci 2018;19(9):2534.

80. Willis GR, Fernandez-Gonzalez A, Anastas J, et al. Mesenchymal stromal cell exosomes ameliorate experimental bronchopulmonary dysplasia and restore lung function through macrophage immunomodulation. Am J Respir Crit Care Med 2018;197(1):104–16.

81. Bui CB, Kolodziej M, Lamanna E, et al. Interleukin-1 receptor antagonist protects newborn mice against pulmonary hypertension. Front Immunol 2019;10: 1480.
82. Wedgwood S, Warford C, Agvatisiri SR, et al. The developing gut-lung axis: postnatal growth restriction, intestinal dysbiosis, and pulmonary hypertension in a rodent model. Pediatr Res 2020;87(3):472-9.
83. Augustine S, Avey MT, Harrison B, et al. Mesenchymal stromal cell therapy in bronchopulmonary dysplasia: systematic review and meta-analysis of preclinical studies. Stem Cells Transl Med 2017;6(12):2079-93.
84. Benny M, Courchia B, Shrager S, et al. Comparative effects of bone marrow-derived versus umbilical cord tissue mesenchymal stem cells in an experimental model of bronchopulmonary dysplasia. Stem Cells Transl Med 2022;11(2): 189-99.
85. Moreira A, Winter C, Joy J, et al. Intranasal delivery of human umbilical cord Wharton's jelly mesenchymal stromal cells restores lung alveolarization and vascularization in experimental bronchopulmonary dysplasia. Stem Cells Transl Med 2020;9(2):221-34.
86. Durlak W, Thébaud B. The vascular phenotype of BPD: new basic science insights-new precision medicine approaches. Pediatr Res 2022. https://doi.org/10.1038/s41390-022-02428-7.
87. Ochs M, Mühlfeld C. Quantitative microscopy of the lung: a problem-based approach. Part 1: basic principles of lung stereology. Am J Physiol Lung Cell Mol Physiol 2013;305(1):L15-22.
88. Mühlfeld C, Knudsen L, Ochs M. Stereology and morphometry of lung tissue. Methods Mol Biol 2013;931:367-90.
89. Kohut A, Patel N, Singh H. Comprehensive echocardiographic assessment of the right ventricle in murine models. J Cardiovasc Ultrasound 2016;24(3): 229-38.
90. Urboniene D, Haber I, Fang YH, et al. Validation of high-resolution echocardiography and magnetic resonance imaging vs. high-fidelity catheterization in experimental pulmonary hypertension. Am J Physiol Lung Cell Mol Physiol 2010;299(3):L401-12.
91. Menon RT, Shrestha AK, Reynolds CL, et al. Long-term pulmonary and cardiovascular morbidities of neonatal hyperoxia exposure in mice. Int J Biochem Cell Biol 2018;94:119-24.
92. Navarrete CT, Devia C, Lessa AC, et al. The role of endothelin converting enzyme inhibition during group b streptococcus–induced pulmonary hypertension in newborn piglets. Pediatr Res 2003;54(3):387-92.
93. Nicola T, Ambalavanan N, Zhang W, et al. Hypoxia-induced inhibition of lung development is attenuated by the peroxisome proliferator-activated receptor-γ agonist rosiglitazone. Am J Physiol Lung Cell Mol Physiol 2011;301(1):L125-34.
94. Fike CD, Slaughter JC, Kaplowitz MR, et al. Reactive oxygen species from NADPH oxidase contribute to altered pulmonary vascular responses in piglets with chronic hypoxia-induced pulmonary hypertension. Am J Physiol Lung Cell Mol Physiol 2008;295(5):L881-8.
95. Davie NJ, Crossno JT Jr, Frid MG, et al. Hypoxia-induced pulmonary artery adventitial remodeling and neovascularization: contribution of progenitor cells. Am J Physiol Lung Cell Mol Physiol 2004;286(4):L668-78.
96. Davey AM, Becker JD, Davis JM. Meconium aspiration syndrome: physiological and inflammatory changes in a newborn piglet model. Pediatr Pulmonol 1993; 16(2):101-8.

97. Rondelet B, Kerbaul F, Beneden RV, et al. Signaling molecules in overcirculation-induced pulmonary hypertension in piglets. Circulation 2004;110(15):2220–5.

98. Andersen DH. Effect of diet during pregnancy upon the incidence of congenital hereditary diaphragmatic hernia in the rat; failure to produce cystic fibrosis of the pancreas by maternal vitamin A deficiency. Am J Pathol 1949;25(1):163–85.

99. Kluth D, Kangah R, Reich P, et al. Nitrofen-induced diaphragmatic hernias in rats: an animal model. J Pediatr Surg 1990;25(8):850–4.

100. Sbragia L, Oria M, Scorletti F, et al. A novel surgical toxicological-free model of diaphragmatic hernia in fetal rats. Pediatr Res 2022;92(1):118–24.

101. Fauza DO, Tannuri U, Ayoub AA, et al. Surgically produced congenital diaphragmatic hernia in fetal rabbits. J Pediatr Surg 1994;29(7):882–6.

102. Pringle KC, Turner JW, Schofield JC, et al. Creation and repair of diaphragmatic hernia in the fetal lamb: lung development and morphology. J Pediatr Surg 1984;19(2):131–40.

103. Soper RT, Pringle KC, Scofield JC. Creation and repair of diaphragmatic hernia in the fetal lamb: techniques and survival. J Pediatr Surg 1984;19(1):33–40.

104. Clugston RD, Klattig J, Englert C, et al. Teratogen-induced, dietary and genetic models of congenital diaphragmatic hernia share a common mechanism of pathogenesis. Am J Pathol 2006;169(5):1541–9.

105. Nakamura H, Doi T, Puri P, et al. Transgenic animal models of congenital diaphragmatic hernia: a comprehensive overview of candidate genes and signaling pathways. Pediatr Surg Int 2020;36(9):991–7.

106. Kunisaki SM, Jiang G, Biancotti JC, et al. Human induced pluripotent stem cell-derived lung organoids in an ex vivo model of the congenital diaphragmatic hernia fetal lung. Stem Cells Transl Med 2021;10(1):98–114.

107. Whitehead GS, Burch LH, Berman KG, et al. Genetic basis of murine responses to hyperoxia-induced lung injury. Immunogenetics 2006;58(10):793–804.

108. O'Reilly M, Thébaud B. Animal models of bronchopulmonary dysplasia. The term rat models. Am J Physiol Lung Cell Mol Physiol 2014;307(12):L948–58.

109. D'Angio CT, Ryan RM. Animal models of bronchopulmonary dysplasia. The preterm and term rabbit models. Am J Physiol Lung Cell Mol Physiol 2014;307(12):L959–69.

110. Albertine KH. Utility of large-animal models of BPD: chronically ventilated preterm lambs. Am J Physiol Lung Cell Mol Physiol 2015;308(10):L983–1001.

111. Yoder BA, Coalson JJ. Animal models of bronchopulmonary dysplasia. The preterm baboon models. Am J Physiol Lung Cell Mol Physiol 2014;307(12):L970–7.

112. Reynolds CL, Zhang S, Shrestha AK, et al. Phenotypic assessment of pulmonary hypertension using high-resolution echocardiography is feasible in neonatal mice with experimental bronchopulmonary dysplasia and pulmonary hypertension: a step toward preventing chronic obstructive pulmonary disease. Int J Chron Obstruct Pulmon Dis 2016;11:1597–605.

113. Leary S, Das P, Ponnalagu D, et al. Genetic strain and sex differences in a hyperoxia-induced mouse model of varying severity of bronchopulmonary dysplasia. Am J Pathol 2019;189(5):999–1014.

114. Ambalavanan N, Nicola T, Hagood J, et al. Transforming growth factor-beta signaling mediates hypoxia-induced pulmonary arterial remodeling and inhibition of alveolar development in newborn mouse lung. Am J Physiol Lung Cell Mol Physiol 2008;295(1):L86–95.

115. Syed M, Das P, Pawar A, et al. Hyperoxia causes miR-34a-mediated injury via angiopoietin-1 in neonatal lungs. Nat Commun 2017;8(1):1173.

116. Shrestha AK, Menon RT, El-Saie A, et al. Interactive and independent effects of early lipopolysaccharide and hyperoxia exposure on developing murine lungs. Am J Physiol Lung Cell Mol Physiol 2020;319(6):L981–96.
117. Sharma M, Bellio MA, Benny M, et al. Mesenchymal stem cell-derived extracellular vesicles prevent experimental bronchopulmonary dysplasia complicated by pulmonary hypertension. Stem Cells Transl Med 2022;11(8):828–40.
118. Seedorf G, Kim C, Wallace B, et al. rhIGF-1/BP3 preserves lung growth and prevents pulmonary hypertension in experimental bronchopulmonary dysplasia. Am J Respir Crit Care Med 2020;201(9):1120–34.
119. Lesage F, Deng Y, Renesme L, et al. Characterization of a new monocrotaline rat model to study chronic neonatal pulmonary hypertension. Am J Respir Cell Mol Biol 2021;65(3):331–4.
120. Chen CM, Lin W, Huang LT, et al. Human mesenchymal stem cells ameliorate experimental pulmonary hypertension induced by maternal inflammation and neonatal hyperoxia in rats. Oncotarget 2017;8(47):82366–75.
121. Mankouski A, Kantores C, Wong MJ, et al. Intermittent hypoxia during recovery from neonatal hyperoxic lung injury causes long-term impairment of alveolar development: a new rat model of BPD. Am J Physiol Lung Cell Mol Physiol 2017;312(2):L208–16.
122. Wedgwood S, Warford C, Agvateesiri SC, et al. Postnatal growth restriction augments oxygen-induced pulmonary hypertension in a neonatal rat model of bronchopulmonary dysplasia. Pediatr Res 2016;80(6):894–902.
123. Jiménez J, Richter J, Nagatomo T, et al. Progressive vascular functional and structural damage in a bronchopulmonary dysplasia model in preterm rabbits exposed to hyperoxia. Int J Mol Sci 2016,17(10):1776.
124. Mühlfeld C, Schulte H, Jansing JC, et al. Design-based stereology of the lung in the hyperoxic preterm rabbit model of bronchopulmonary dysplasia. Oxid Med Cell Longev 2021;2021:4293279.
125. Albertine KH. Progress in understanding the pathogenesis of BPD using the baboon and sheep models. Semin Perinatol 2013;37(2):60–8.

Targeted Neonatal Echocardiography in the Management of Neonatal Pulmonary Hypertension

Stephanie M. Boyd, MBBS (Hons), BSc (Med), MPHTM, FRACP, CCPU[a,b],
Martin Kluckow, MBBS, FRACP, PhD, CCPU[b,c],
Patrick J. McNamara, MB, BCh, MRCPCH, FASE[d,*]

KEYWORDS

- Neonate • Pulmonary hypertension • Targeted neonatal echocardiography
- Hemodynamics

KEY POINTS

- The pathophysiology of pulmonary hypertension (PH) involves a complex interplay between arterial and venous pressure, flow, resistance, and the effects of hemodynamic changes on the unique cardiovascular system of the newborn infant.
- Several distinct pathophysiological phenotypes exist in both acute and chronic neonatal PH.
- Targeted neonatal echocardiography (TNE) is useful in the appraisal of individual patient physiology in PH and facilitates rational targeting of therapy.
- A standard TNE includes the assessment of pulmonary artery pressure, pulmonary vascular resistance, cardiac function (systolic and diastolic), pulmonary and systemic blood flow, and extrapulmonary shunts.
- Echocardiography markers have been shown to correlate with important outcomes in neonatal PH; however, the impact of TNE-guided care on clinically important outcomes represents a knowledge gap.

INTRODUCTION

Neonatal pulmonary hypertension (PH) is a serious cardiopulmonary condition affecting term and preterm infants with a range of underlying disease processes,

[a] Grace Centre for Newborn Intensive Care, The Children's Hospital at Westmead, Corner Hawkesbury Road, Hainsworth Street, Westmead, Sydney 2145, Australia; [b] The University of Sydney, Sydney, Australia; [c] Department of Neonatology, Royal North Shore Hospital, Reserve Road, St Leonards 2065, Sydney, Australia; [d] Division of Neonatology, The University of Iowa, 200 Hawkins Drive, Iowa City, IA 52242, USA
* Corresponding author.
E-mail address: patrick-mcnamara@uiowa.edu

Clin Perinatol 51 (2024) 45–76
https://doi.org/10.1016/j.clp.2023.11.006
0095-5108/24/© 2023 Elsevier Inc. All rights reserved.
perinatology.theclinics.com

the hallmark of which is elevated mean pulmonary artery pressure (mPAP). There is associated dysregulation of the pulmonary vascular bed and exposure of the right ventricle to a sustained increase in afterload. The pathophysiology of the disorder involves a complex interplay between pulmonary arterial and venous pressure, flow, resistance, and the effects of hemodynamic changes on the unique cardiovascular system of the newborn infant. There is increasing recognition that under the singular clinical umbrella of hypoxemia, there exists a range of underlying pathophysiological drivers of disease. Therefore, the concept of multiple hemodynamic phenotypes of neonatal PH[1,2] has significant implications for both treatment approaches and clinical trial design in modern neonatology.

The mPAP, governed by pulmonary vascular resistance (PVR), cardiac output (CO), and left atrial pressure (LAP), may be calculated according to the following equation, using pulmonary capillary wedge pressure (PCWP) as a proxy for LAP:

$$mPAP = [PVR \times CO] + PCWP$$

Although elevated mPAP in newborns is frequently considered to be primarily a resistance-driven disorder due to increased PVR, excessive pulmonary blood flow (flow-driven PH) and increased LAP in the setting of left ventricular (LV) dysfunction (postcapillary PH or pulmonary venous hypertension) are alternative and important causes of neonatal PH.[3-5] Irrespective of the underlying cause, elevated mPAP and the effects of high afterload on the right ventricle (RV) may result in progressive hypoxemia and reduced LV output, leading to systemic arterial hypotension and worsening RV dysfunction. Clinical features of elevated PH range from mildly reduced oxygen saturations with varying degrees of respiratory distress, to severe hypoxemia with cardiopulmonary instability and markers of poor tissue perfusion necessitating advanced intensive care therapies. Understanding the degree of the pulmonary parenchymal contribution to hypoxemia, hypercarbia, and lung volume versus the cardiovascular drivers of increased RV afterload may be challenging clinically; therefore, a detailed understanding of real-time pathophysiology is critical for providing optimal supportive care to affected infants.

Targeted neonatal echocardiography (TNE), performed by a neonatologist with advanced training in neonatal hemodynamics and echocardiography, is a highly useful modality in the setting of neonatal PH; both acute pulmonary hypertension (aPH) and chronic pulmonary hypertension (cPH).[1,2,5,6] The specific goals of TNE in the assessment of neonatal PH include (1) confirming the diagnosis of PH and determining its severity; (2) adjudicating the underlying PH phenotype(s) and targeting treatment, including pulmonary vasodilator therapy and cardiotropic medications, according to pathophysiology; (3) monitoring response to therapy over time as hemodynamic conditions change; and (4) appropriately weaning therapy. Exclusion of significant structural cardiac disease should ideally occur as part of the initial TNE assessment[7] or as soon as practicable. If there is clinical suspicion of congenital heart disease (CHD), the first echocardiography evaluation should be a comprehensive anatomic assessment, ideally performed by a pediatric cardiologist. If the first evaluation is a TNE assessment, due to lack of on-site pediatric cardiology services or where there is low risk of CHD, the study should include the necessary views and sweeps to exclude major CHD. The study may be reviewed by a pediatric cardiologist in a timely manner, wherever feasible. Concerns regarding missed major congenital heart lesions on TNE assessment have not been borne out in the literature,[8-11] and strong agreement with cardiologist-performed echocardiography has been documented.[8,12]

A limited cardiac point-of-care ultrasound should not be used as the primary mode of initial evaluation for either acute or chronic PH. Neonatal hemodynamics training programs facilitating high-level skill development in TNE and neonatal cardiovascular physiology exist throughout multiple countries, although training pathways and assessment requirements vary significantly.[13,14] There is an increasing focus on a competency-based framework[14] and a neonatologist "hemodynamic consultation" model has been adopted successfully in North America as part of establishment of TNE services in that region.[8,14]

PATHOPHYSIOLOGY

Elevations in mPAP reduce the pressure gradient between the RV cavity and the pulmonary vascular bed. In response to the initial increase in RV afterload, there is compensatory RV hypertrophy and increased contractility (referred to as "coupling" or *homeometric adaptation*) (**Fig. 1**).[15] To maintain CO despite the increased afterload, RV dilation and an increase in heart rate occur. These changes serve to maintain stroke volume initially by way of the increase in stroke volume associated with increased preload—via the Frank-Starling mechanism, with a larger ventricle emptying proportionally less blood—as well as an intact force-frequency response. With excessive and sustained increases in pulmonary arterial pressure (PAP), ischemia, hypoxemia, and myocardial stretching cause progressive RV dysfunction and uncoupling.[15,16] This is referred to as *heterotopic maladaptation* (see **Fig. 1**).[17]

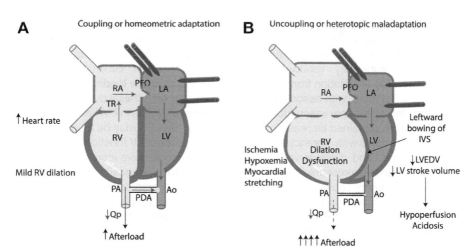

Fig. 1. Relationship between right ventricle (RV) and pulmonary arterial dynamics in pulmonary hypertension. (*A*) With mild to moderate elevations in RV afterload, there is a coupled right ventricular hypertrophy with mild RV dilation (homeometric adaptation). (*B*) With severe increase in RV afterload, the RV decompensates leading to dilation and dysfunction resulting in uncoupling of RV function and afterload (heterotopic maladaptation). Ventricular interactions lead to left ventricular dysfunction. RA – right atrium, LA – left atrium; LV – left ventricle, PFO – patent foramen ovale, PDA – patent ductus arteriosus, Qp – pulmonary blood flow, PA – pulmonary artery, Ao – aorta, LVEDV – left ventricular end diastolic volume, IVS – interventricular septum. Image courtesy of Dr. Satyan Lakshminrusimha.

High PAP is further associated with leftward bowing of the interventricular septum (IVS) due to prolonged contraction of the RV free wall compared with the septum or LV free wall, impairing diastolic LV filling.[18] This is referred to as *ventricular interdependence*, whereby the function of one ventricle is affected by dysfunction of the other, in this case due to the shared IVS. Together with RV dilation, septal flattening further compromises RV function and pulmonary blood flow (PBF).[2] The leftward shift in IVS position also reduces LV end-diastolic volume (LVEDV), LV stroke volume,[19] and RV systolic contractile force,[20,21] causing systemic hypoperfusion, acidosis, and a further reduction in PBF. This is sometimes referred to as *ventriculo-ventricular interaction* (VVI). In some infants with aPH, this results in a cycle of reduced PBF, worsening acidosis, progressive hypoxemia, ventilation-perfusion mismatch, and cardiac dysfunction, with a clinical phenotype of hypoxemic respiratory failure with circulatory compromise.

Acute Pulmonary Hypertension Phenotypes

Arterial (classic) aPH due to failure of the usual postnatal decline in PVR leading to extrapulmonary right-to-left (R-L) shunting and hypoxemia (traditionally referred to as persistent pulmonary hypertension of the newborn [PPHN]) is sometimes erroneously considered to be synonymous with neonatal PH. Hypoxemia and cardiovascular instability may occur irrespective of the underlying cause of elevated PAP because adaptive responses to high RV afterload fail. It may be challenging clinically to differentiate resistance-mediated PH from that caused by excessive PBF (flow-driven PH) or LV dysfunction (postcapillary PH), and the implications for management are significant. In congenital diaphragmatic hernia (CDH), for example, LV hypoplasia and dysfunction may coexist with abnormalities of the pulmonary vasculature and altered vasoreactivity[22]; therefore, understanding the presence and relative contributions of these pathologic conditions is important for guiding management. Treatment with selective pulmonary vasodilators in the setting of primary or severe LV diseases is likely to be deleterious, whereas, in the setting of normal or mildly impaired LV function and predominant RV dysfunction, reduction in RV afterload is one of the cornerstones of treatment.

Infants with high volume left-to-right (L-R) shunts, such as those caused by large systemic to pulmonary venous connections (eg, vein of Galen malformation [VGAM]), develop RV dilation from chronic volume and pressure loading. A marked increase in PBF occurs, with associated shear stress and endothelial dysfunction.[23] Alterations in the pulmonary vasculature with secondary elevation in PVR also develop in response to the sustained increase in PBF,[24,25] such that aPH may be multifactorial in this group. In infants with a postcapillary PH phenotype, poor LV function leads to inefficient ejection of end-diastolic volume, resulting in a progressive increase in left ventricular end-diastolic pressure (LVEDP). Pulmonary venous congestion develops, with increased pulmonary capillary pressure and a hydrostatic gradient across the interstitium, resulting in transudation of fluid into alveolar spaces; that is, pulmonary edema. Similar to flow-mediated PH, endothelial dysfunction is also implicated in the pathogenesis of PH in pulmonary venous hypertension.[26]

Chronic Pulmonary Hypertension Phenotypes

In chronic PH associated with bronchopulmonary dysplasia (BPD), maldevelopment of the pulmonary vasculature with abnormal lung parenchyma and elevated PVR is typical. However, in addition to pulmonary vascular remodeling,[27,28] the contribution of LV disease to the symptomatology of BPD is increasingly recognized.[29–32] High rates of systemic hypertension have been observed in association with LV diastolic impairment among infants with BPD.[33–35] The increased afterload imposed by aortic stiffness associated with systemic hypertension (loss of Windkessel effect) is hypothesized to result in

Table 1
Pulmonary hypertension phenotypes—pathophysiology and echocardiography features

PH Phenotype	Pathophysiology	Echocardiography Features
Acute PH		
Arterial (classic)	Hypoxic pulmonary vasoconstriction and V/Q mismatch	Dilated (possibly hypertrophied) RV, septal flattening in systole, predominantly R→L PDA and atrial shunts, ↑PVRi (RVET:PAAT) > 4 and/or PA Doppler notching, ↓ PV Vmax < 0.25 m/s, ↓ LVO
Flow mediated (eg, VGAM)	High volume of blood in a circuit with limited capacitance, endothelial dysfunction, and oxidative stress	Dilated RV and/or LV, discordant ventricular outputs with either ↑RVO, ↑LVO or both, septal flattening in diastole if ASD/VSD
Left heart dysfunction (postcapillary)	Poor LV compliance and high LVEDP resulting in impaired flow through pulmonary circuit	Dilated LA and/or LV, LV systolic and diastolic dysfunction [↓MVE, ↑IVRT or E:e', ↓ PV S/D ratio, PV a wave], MR and/or AI, ↓LVO
Chronic PH		
Arterial (classic) for example, associated with BPD	Pulmonary vascular remodeling, impaired angiogenesis, and alveolar hypoxia/hyperoxia	Dilated and hypertrophied RV, septal flattening in systole, predominantly R→L PDA and atrial shunts, ↑↑PVRi (RVET:PAAT) > 4 and/or PA Doppler notching, ↓ LVO
Flow mediated (eg, ASD shunt)	High volume of blood in a circuit with limited capacitance, interstitial edema, and pulmonary vascular remodeling	Dilated RV or LV, discordant ventricular outputs with either ↑RVO, ↑LVO or both, septal flattening in diastole if ASD/VSD
Systemic hypertension	High LV afterload causing ↑LVEDP, LA hypertension, and pulmonary venous congestion	Dilated LA, LV, LV diastolic dysfunction [↓MVE, ↑IVRT or E:e', ↓ PV S/D ratio, PV a wave], MR, and/or AI

Abbreviations: AI, aortic insufficiency; ASD, atrial septal defect; BPD, bronchopulmonary dysplasia; D, d wave; IVRT, isovolumetric relaxation time; LA, left atrium; LV, left ventricle; LVEDP, left ventricular end-diastolic pressure; LVO, left ventricular output; MR, mitral regurgitation; MVE, mitral valve early wave; PA, pulmonary artery; PAAT, pulmonary artery acceleration time; PDA, patent ductus arteriosus; PV, pulmonary vein; PVRi, pulmonary vascular resistance index; R-L, right-to-left; RV, right ventricle; RVET, right ventricular ejection time; RVO, right ventricular output; S, s wave; V/Q, ventilation/perfusion; VGAM, vein of Galen malformation; VSD, ventricular septal defect.

Adapted from: Giesinger R, Kinsella JP, Abman SH, McNamara PJ. Pulmonary hypertension phenotypes in the newborn. In: Dakshinamurti S, ed. *Hypoxic Respiratory Failure in the Newborn: From Origins to Clinical Management.* Boca Raton: Taylor & Francis Group; 2021.

sufficient back pressure over time to cause disturbances of left heart function and resultant pulmonary venous hypertension.[31] Flow-driven cPH may originate from the excessive PBF associated with prolonged exposure to L-R shunts, such as a PDA or atrial septal defect (ASD). Left untreated, pulmonary vascular remodeling may ensue,[36,37] with secondary elevations in PVR, resulting in a mixed phenotype. Infants with multilevel shunts, such as at both ductal and atrial level, are at a higher risk of developing pulmonary vascular sequelae.[1] A comparison of the pathophysiology and echocardiographic features of underlying PH phenotypes is presented in **Table 1**.

MANAGEMENT APPROACH

Comprehensive TNE assessment in suspected neonatal PH encompasses confirmation of elevated PAP; assessment of PVR and right ventricular (RV) performance; exclusion of major structural CHD that may mimic primary PH; and appraisal of LV function, systemic blood flow, and the presence, magnitude, and direction of intracardiac shunts. Delineation of the underlying hemodynamic phenotype(s) of PH is important for determining therapeutic goals and instituting appropriate cardiorespiratory management, and most importantly decision-making around the utility of pulmonary vasodilators, for the individual infant (**Fig. 2**). Several congenital cardiac lesions, including transposition of the great arteries and total anomalous pulmonary venous drainage (TAPVD) may present with marked hypoxemia and mimic PH. Lability in oxygenation, such as with handling, and/or presence of systemic arterial hypotension are important clinical findings that may make primary PH more likely.[38] This distinction is, however, not absolute, and the possibility of CHD should be borne in mind for any neonate presenting with significant hypoxemia.

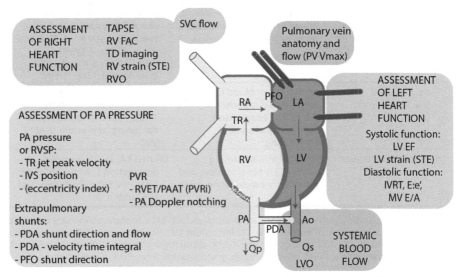

Fig. 2. Echocardiographic parameters to assess acute pulmonary hypertension in neonates. The factors to assess right heart function, left heart function, pulmonary flow, aortic flow and assessment of pulmonary arterial (PA) pressure are shown. TAPSE – tricuspid annular plane systolic excursion; RV – right ventricle; FAC – fractional area change; TD – tissue Doppler; STE – speckle-tracking echocardiography; RVO – right ventricular output; RVSP – right ventricular systolic pressure; TR – tricuspid regurgitation; IVS – interventricular septum; PVR – pulmonary vascular resistance; RVET – right ventricular ejection time; PAAT – pulmonary arterial acceleration time; PDA – patent ductus arteriosus; PFO – patent foramen ovale; Qp – pulmonary blood flow; Ao – aorta; Qs – systemic blood flow; LVO – left ventricular output; PV – pulmonary vein; Vmax – peak velocity; EF – ejection fraction; IVRT – isovolumic relaxation time; E:e' – ratio of early diastolic mitral inflow velocity to early diastolic mitral annulus velocity; E/A – ratio of peak velocity of blood flow during left ventricular early diastole (E) to peak velocity in late diastole caused by atrial contraction (A). Image courtesy of Dr. Satyan Lakshminrusimha.

Assessment of Pulmonary Artery Pressure and Pulmonary Vascular Resistance

Several methods exist for the evaluation of PAP, including peak velocity of the tricuspid regurgitant (TR) jet, pulmonary regurgitation peak velocity, peak velocity of R-L flow across the patent ductus arteriosus (PDA), proportion of R-L flow by time and velocity time integral (VTI) across the PDA, IVS configuration, and LV systolic eccentricity index (LV-sEI).[6] Benefits and limitations of the various TNE tools used in the evaluation of PAP are outlined in **Table 2**.

A TR jet is identifiable in approximately 70% of newborns with PH[39] but the absence of a TR jet does not imply the absence of PH.[40] The following modified Bernoulli equation is used to calculate an estimated right ventricular systolic pressure (RVSp, which approximates PAP), where P is pressure gradient (in mm Hg), and v is velocity (in m/s).

$$P = 4 \times v^2$$

Right atrial pressure (RAP), although not measured, is assumed to be 3 to 5 mm Hg[6] and is added to the pressure calculated by the TR jet to obtain an estimate of RVSp. RAP may be higher in the setting of significant RA dilatation due to RV failure or excessive venous return (such as in hepatic or cerebral arteriovenous malformations [AVMs]), or lower in healthy newborn infants, although the approximation is generally used. Estimation of PAP using the TR jet is unreliable in the presence of either RV outflow tract obstruction or RV failure.[6] When assessing PAP using the TR jet, the angle of insonation should be less than 20° to avoid underestimating the true PAP. A full Doppler spectral envelope should be used for an accurate measurement, with good correlation reported with invasive catheter measures of PAP.[41]

In the presence of pulmonary valve regurgitation, it is possible to estimate mPAP using the following equation, where VMaxPR is the peak velocity of pulmonary valve regurgitation (in m/s) and RVDP is the RV diastolic pressure (in mm Hg). The RVDP is generally assumed to be 2 to 5 mm Hg.

$$mPAP = 4 \times (VMaxPR)^2 + RVDP$$

Although PAP may be estimated using R-L transductal flow peak velocity where R-L shunting occurs for 30% or greater of the cardiac cycle, this is often unreliable, and assessment of direction of the transductal shunt is probably more useful for understanding the relationship between systemic and pulmonary pressures.[6]

RV systolic time intervals have been validated for the estimation of PVR in newborns.[42] A pulmonary artery acceleration time (PAAT), also referred to as time to peak velocity, of less than 90 milliseconds is 97% sensitive and 95% specific for PH.[43] Because PAAT depends on heart rate, other investigators have studied the value of indexed PAAT. A PAAT to RV ejection time (RVET) ratio of less than 0.31 suggests PH, and a value of less than 0.23 is consistent with markedly elevated PAP.[43] Lower values have been observed in preterm infants with BPD-associated PH compared with infants with BPD and no PH.[44] Use of a "PVR index" has also been described[45,46] using the inverse relationship RVET:PAAT, where a value of 4 or greater is indicative of elevated PVR. Additional measures of PVR, such as the tricuspid regurgitation velocity to RV outflow time-velocity integral (TRV/VTI[RVOT]) and pulmonary artery compliance may also be used, although are less commonly reported.

PAP may also be estimated using interventricular septal configuration either qualitatively, or by using the LV-sEI. Normal ventricular geometry consists of an "O"-shaped LV, when the RVSp is less than 50% of LV pressure (LVP). As PAP increases,

Table 2
Echocardiographic markers used in the assessment of pulmonary hypertension

Hemodynamic Parameter	Clinical Application	Normal Range	Advantages	Limitations
Assessment of PAP				
RVSp using TR jet (mm Hg)	Direct measure of RVSp	<35 mm Hg[126,127]	Moderate correlation with invasive measures of RVSp[41]	• TR jet may not be present despite significant PH • Angle-dependent and requires complete envelope
Septal curvature: subjective assessment	Assessment of RV vs LV pressure	Round	Easily measured and universally present	• Subjective measure • Low interobserver reliability • Affected by ventricular function (VI and VVI) • May underestimate RVSp in systemic hypertension
LV eccentricity index (EI)	Assessment of RV vs LV pressure	1 ± 0.06[50] LV EI > 1.3 consistent with PH	Reproducible, validated in newborns	• Pressure relative to LVSp; may underestimate RVSp in systemic hypertension
PAAT PVRi (RVET:PAAT) (ms) Midsystolic notching of PA Doppler waveform	Serial assessment to monitor PVR over time or with treatment	55 ± 7 ms[45] 4 ± 0.5[45]	Easily measured	• PAAT affected by HR • Underestimated by RV dysfunction • Unreliable in presence of shunts • Single time-point measures • Limited evidence in neonates
Assessment of right heart function				
RVO (mL/kg/min)	Marker of PBF and RV function	219 ± 93.8 mL/kg/min[128]	• Well-studied in neonates across a range of physiologic and disease states • Serial evaluations useful for following disease progression and treatment response	• Accuracy dependent on Doppler angle and precise measurement • Affected by atrial shunt • May be overestimated if RVOT dilated

Parameter	Measure	Normative value	Advantages	Limitations
TAPSE (mm)	Measure of RV systolic function	9 ± 1 mm[129]	• Normative data exist for newborns[51] • Provides information about longitudinal RV contractility; good correlation with estimations of RV global function • Independent of HR and shunts • Easily measured	• Angle dependent and load dependent • Exaggerated by severe TR • May overestimate global function if regional wall dysfunction (rare in the neonatal population)
RV FAC	Measure of global RV systolic function	38 ± 6%[129]	Normative data exist for newborns[70]	• Requires high-quality imaging • Affected by septal motion in apical 4-chamber view
TDI of IVS and RV free wall	Assessment of systolic and diastolic function	RV S′ 6.8 ± 2.1 cm/s[130]	May be useful for monitoring response to treatment	• Requires high-quality imaging • Dependent on angle of insonation
RV strain using STE	Assessment of global RV systolic function	RV 3-chamber strain −21.4 ± 4.4 (day 1)[70]	• May be more sensitive in earlier stages of disease • Global measure of function	• Limited but increasing data in newborns, including in PH[55] and CDH[131] • Requires high-quality imaging
Assessment of systemic blood flow				
LVO (mL/kg/min)	Marker of systemic blood flow and LV function	222 ± 91.6 mL/kg/min[128]	• Well studied in neonates across a range of physiologic and disease states • Serial evaluations useful for following disease progression and treatment response • Comparison with RVO may provide useful information	• Affected by PDA shunt • Accuracy dependent on Doppler angle and precise measurement

(continued on next page)

Table 2
(continued)

Hemodynamic Parameter	Clinical Application	Normal Range	Advantages	Limitations
Assessment of left heart function				
LV EF (M-mode and Simpson's biplane methods)	Measure of LV systolic function	$55 \pm 7\%$[132] (day 1) by Simpson's biplane	Well-studied measure	• Affected by IVS configuration and may be unreliable in PH—Simpson's biplane preferred • Subjective measure
IVRT, E:e', MV E/A	Assessment of LV diastolic function	IVRT 52 ± 10 ms[132] E/e' 7.40–12.05[133] E/e' may be up to 14.6 ± 4.0 in preterm infants <30 wk[134] MV E/A 1 ± 0.3[135]	Useful for understanding LV diastolic function	• Limited but increasing evidence in term and preterm neonates • Affected by PDA and shunts
LV strain using STE	Measure of global LV systolic function	LS -20.8% to -25.9%[136,137]	• May be more sensitive in earlier stages of disease • Global measure of function	• Limited but increasing data in newborns, including in PH[55] and CDH[131] • Requires high-quality imaging
Assessment of shunts				
PDA: ratio of pulmonary artery to aortic pressure (PAP:AOP) based on shunt direction: Uses Doppler of ductus arteriosus	Direct comparison of pulmonary to systemic arterial pressure	R-L for ≥30% of cardiac cycle suggests elevated PAP[73] R-L for ≥60% of systole suggests suprasystemic PH[73]	Useful for qualifying RVSp as subsystemic, systemic or suprasystemic	• PDA may not be present • May be unreliable depending on PDA morphology (eg, tortuous, S-shaped) • Dynamic: varies with ambient conditions (eg, pH, SpO_2)

| Atrial communication: shunt direction | • Predominantly R-L shunt suggestive of ↑RVSp; pure R-L shunt requires exclusion of TAPVD
• L-R shunt in setting of other features of ↑PAP requires assessment for ↑LA pressure, pulmonary venous hypertension and LV dysfunction | Predominantly R-L shunt suggestive of ↑RVSp Shunt may be L-R in postcapillary PH | • Important in understanding drivers of flow-mediated PH (PDA, ASD)
• May provide clues as to etiology of ↑PAP | • Atrial communication not universally present |

Abbreviations: AOP, aortic pressure; ASD, atrial septal defect; CDH, congenital diaphragmatic hernia; E, e', early, mitral inflow velocity (E-wave) and mitral annular early diastolic velocity (e') ratio; EF, ejection fraction; EI, eccentricity index; FAC, fractional area change; GLS, global longitudinal strain; HR, heart rate; IVRT, isovolumic relaxation time; IVS, interventricular septum; L, left; LA, left atrial; LV, left ventricle; LVSp, left ventricular systolic pressure; mitral, valve E-wave to A-wave ratio; MV, E/A; PA, pulmonary artery; PAAT, pulmonary artery acceleration time; PAP, pulmonary artery pressure; PDA, patent ductus arteriosus; PH, pulmonary hypertension; PVR, pulmonary vascular resistance; PVRi, pulmonary vascular resistance index; R, right; RV, right ventricle; RVET, right ventricular ejection time; RVO, right ventricular output; RVOT, right ventricular outflow tract; RVSp, right ventricular systolic pressure; STE, speckle tracking echocardiography; TAPSE, tricuspid annular plane systolic excursion; TAPVD, total anomalous pulmonary venous drainage; TDI, tissue Doppler imaging; TR, tricuspid regurgitant/regurgitation; VI, ventricular interdependence; VVI, ventricular–ventricular interaction.

Adapted from: Jain A, Giesinger RE, Dakshinamurti S, ElSayed Y, Jankov RP, Weisz DE, et al. Care of the critically ill neonate with hypoxemic respiratory failure and acute pulmonary hypertension: framework for practice based on consensus opinion of neonatal hemodynamics working group. *J Perinatol* 2022; 42:3–13.

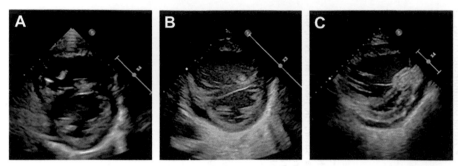

Fig. 3. (*A*) Normal, round IVS. (*B*) Flat, D-shaped IVS. (*C*) IVS bowing into left ventricle.

there is flattening of the IVS, resulting in a loss of circularity and a D-shaped LV (estimated RVSp 50%–100% of LVP) (**Fig. 3**). As RV afterload increases further, the RV eventually curves into the LV, resulting in a crescent-shaped LV, and an estimated RVSp that is systemic or suprasystemic ($\geq$100% of LVP).[6,47] Qualitative assessment of RV size and function, including septal flattening, has been shown to be unreliable however, even in the setting of expert assessors.[48] The LV-sEI provides a more objective estimate of IVS flattening/bowing[6] and uses the end-systolic ratio of the anterior-inferior and septal-posterolateral dimensions of the LV cavity, respectively (**Fig. 4**). LV-sEI shows higher interobserver agreement than subjective assessment of septal configuration[49] and values of 1.3 or greater are well-correlated with catheterization laboratory measurements with high sensitivity and specificity.[50] The normal value for LV-sEI is 1, and greater than 50% systemic RV pressure has been demonstrated for values 1.3 or greater in an echocardiographic study of 216 newborns at risk of PH.[49]

Assessment of Right Ventricular Performance

Evaluation of RV function is a crucial aspect of hemodynamic assessment in neonatal PH. Although often used in practice, the reliability of qualitative appraisal of RV function in neonates has not been established[48] and is not recommended in isolation. Both tricuspid annular plane systolic excursion (TAPSE) and RV fractional area change (RV-FAC) have published normative values for term and preterm infants[51,52] and show

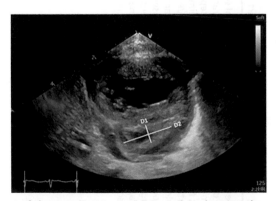

Fig. 4. Measurement of the systolic LV eccentricity index, showing the end-systolic ratio of the anterior-inferior (D2) and septal-posterolateral (D1) dimensions of the LV cavity.

good correlation with cardiac MRI-derived RV ejection fraction (EF).[53] Markers of RV dysfunction, including TAPSE and RV global longitudinal peak strain, have been associated with poor outcome in infants with PH,[54,55] with TAPSE values of less than 4 mm shown to be predictive of extracorporeal membrane oxygenation (ECMO) or death.[54] Limitations of TAPSE include its angle-dependency and load-dependency.[6] In infants with aPH and hypoxic-ischemic encephalopathy (HIE) undergoing therapeutic hypothermia, reductions in RV and LV systolic and RV diastolic performance have been demonstrated,[55] with a clear correlation between RV function and cerebral function and oxygenation.[56] Impairments in RV performance have been associated with adverse outcomes in this patient group,[57] including an independent association between TAPSE less than 6 mm and the composite outcome of death, diagnosis of cerebral palsy, or low developmental assessment scores.[58]

Although right ventricular output (RVO) is a measure of PBF and is affected by RV function, RVO also represents systemic venous return along with the net effects of any atrial level shunt. As such, in resistance-mediated PH, RVO is typically low due to the combined effects of reduced systemic blood flow secondary to LV preload compromise and any R-L atrial shunting. In flow-mediated PH, RVO is increased, especially in patients with large systemic to pulmonary venous connections. Pulmonary vein (PV) velocity may also provide an indication as to the likely cause of PH. In resistance-driven PH, PV velocity is typically low due to the reduction in PBF. This contrasts with flow-driven and postcapillary PH. In flow-driven PH, PV velocity is typically increased due to high PBF, although PV dilation may occur with chronicity, offsetting this finding. In postcapillary PH, secondary to elevated LA pressure, the amplitude of the diastolic D wave increases and that of the systolic S wave decreases, resulting in reversal of the PV S/D ratio to less than 1, with filling occurring predominantly in diastole. Presence of an atrial "a" wave may also be evident, consistent with elevated left heart filling pressures.

RV-FAC is a quantitative measure of RV function with published normative values in term and preterm neonates (25%–45%).[52] An RV-FAC of 19% has been associated with death or a requirement for ECMO in a cohort of term and near-term infants with aPH attributed to PPHN.[54] In infants with CDH and aPH, early echocardiographic evidence of RV dysfunction has been associated with death and adverse outcomes, including a requirement for ECMO.[50] Lower FAC has also been correlated with duration of respiratory support in preterm infants with BPD[60] and has been shown to persist in infants with BPD and severe PH to the age of 6 months.[61]

RV longitudinal strain using speckle tracking echocardiography (STE) shows strong correlation with cardiac MRI-derived RV EF and may be more sensitive in detecting myocardial dysfunction at earlier disease stages.[62] Reductions in both RV and LV global longitudinal strain have been documented in neonatal aPH[55] and RV function in response to treatment with inhaled nitric oxide (iNO) has been monitored serially using STE.[63] In term infants with PPHN that are nonresponsive to iNO, RV strain and strain rates improved during a 24-hour period following treatment with milrinone,[64] highlighting the utility of strain imaging in identifying and longitudinally follow-up of PH-related cardiac dysfunction. Diastolic function may be assessed using tissue Doppler imaging (TDI), by measuring the tricuspid inflow velocities (Early [E], Late [A], and ratio [E/A]) during diastole from the apical 4-chamber view using pulse wave (PW) Doppler. Peak systolic (s'), early diastolic (e'), and late diastolic (a') myocardial velocities may be measured using TDI, as well as the systolic to diastolic (S/D) ratio and isovolumic relaxation time (IVRT). Both systolic and diastolic TDI-derived velocities have been shown to be reduced in aPH, including in infants with CDH.[65]

Assessment of Left Ventricular Function and Systemic Blood Flow

In the setting of PH, LV dysfunction most often results from a combination of reduced PBF and decreased LV preload, RV impairment through altered ventricular–ventricular interactions and/or ventricular interdependence, and myocardial ischemia due to low coronary perfusion pressure. In postcapillary PH, LV dysfunction may instead represent the primary pathologic condition. In term and near-term infants with resistance-driven aPH, a low LV output (LVO) and diminished LV stroke volume with a normal or mildly reduced LV-EF secondary to R-L ductal shunting (reduced preload) and altered septal configuration are common findings.[6] Reduced LV size and output correlate with markers of disease severity, such as a requirement for ECMO and prolonged mechanical ventilation.[66] The important role of the LV in the pathophysiology of cardiopulmonary instability in CDH is also increasingly recognized.[67,68] Early-onset LV dysfunction and severe aPH are independent predictors of adverse outcome in infants with CDH otherwise considered to be "low risk."[69] PH in this group may be multifactorial, with LV dysfunction causing postcapillary aPH secondary to pulmonary venous hypertension occurring alongside classic arterial resistance-mediated aPH. The presence of near exclusive left–right shunting across the atrial septum should raise suspicion that the primary contributor to PH is a left heart (postcapillary) phenotype.

In a CDH registry study of infants assessed with echocardiography in the first 48 hours after birth, with varying degrees of pretreatment with cardiovascular medications and pulmonary vasodilators, the rate of isolated LV impairment was low (5%), with normal cardiac function, isolated RV dysfunction, or biventricular dysfunction more commonly observed.[68] Although biventricular function in aPH is typically RV dysfunction with secondary LV impairment, evaluation for features of primary or predominant LV dysfunction should occur before initiating pharmacotherapy. This is particularly important when considering the use of pulmonary vasodilators. Elevated PAP with an L-R atrial shunt and/or other evidence of left atrial hypertension, suggestive of LV impairment, may be considered a contraindication to pulmonary vasodilators including iNO. Echocardiography markers suggestive of LV diastolic impairment include prolonged IVRT (>55 milliseconds), reduction in the ratio of passive to active transmitral flow (E/A ratio; due to reliance of the poorly compliant LV on the atrial "kick" for filling; <0.8 in a term infant), elevation in LV E:e' greater than 12, and LV dilatation.

In aPH, LVO measurement is useful as a surrogate marker of LV preload (PBF), LV function, and systemic perfusion.[5] The myocardial performance index (MPI) may be used to estimate global LV function, although RV function may also be assessed using MPI.[6,7] Normative values have been published for the neonatal population.[70] Ventricular dysfunction results in elevated MPI via increased isovolumic contraction and relaxation times, although as with several echocardiographic measures, the MPI is load dependent. Both LV and RV MPI values have been shown to be elevated in neonatal aPH.[71] Additional measures of LV function are recommended for a comprehensive assessment, such as EF, TDI of the IVS and LV free wall, and STE.[6] The geometry of the LV and contraction is a combination of longitudinal, circumferential, and radial shortening. Hence, although there may be advantages to using M-mode measurements for calculation of EF and shortening fraction in some circumstances (eg, poor acoustic windows due to lung interference), use of the Simpson's biplane method is preferable over M-mode in the setting of abnormal LV shape or septal wall motion,[7] such as occurs in PH.

Appraisal of Shunts

R-L shunting at the ductal and atrial levels has been associated with adverse outcomes in neonatal PH.[54,72] It is important to be cognizant of the fact that the magnitude of the pulmonary-systemic shunt is a marker of disease severity in PH, rather than the precipitant of adverse outcomes. R-L ductal shunting may be advantageous in patients with PH and moderate–severe RV dysfunction, both as a popoff mechanism for the RV exposed to high afterload and to augment systemic perfusion. R-L PDA shunting for 30% or greater of the cardiac cycle is suggestive of elevated PAP and R-L shunting for 60% or greater of systole is consistent with suprasystemic pulmonary pressures.[73] In addition to measuring both the duration and VTI of R-L flow, the ratio to the L-R component may provide additional insights into the relative pressures in the systemic and pulmonary circulations. A retrospective study of infants with CDH demonstrated that infants with a VTI ratio of L-R to R-L PDA flow less than 1.0 were 4.7 times more likely to require ECMO and had a mortality rate 3.3 times greater.[74] Similar findings of a greater risk of progression to death or ECMO have been observed in term and near-term infants with PPHN.[54] Proportion of R-L flow through the PDA by time and VTI are measured using either PW Doppler, or continuous wave Doppler if there is a high velocity PDA shunt.

A degree of R-L atrial shunting is one of the hallmarks of resistance-mediated PH and contributes to a reduction in RV preload.[75] Exclusive R-L atrial shunting should prompt anatomic cardiac assessment to exclude TAPVD, in which there is an obligate R-L atrial shunt. In the context of features of significantly elevated mPAP, findings of an L-R shunt via the atrial communication should raise concern regarding the possibility of LV dysfunction, pulmonary venous hypertension, and elevated LAP. In PH due to either high PVR or excessive PBF, the elevated right-sided pressures result in an R-L atrial shunt, which may be exacerbated by the reduction in venous return to the left heart. In contrast, in the setting of primary or severe LV disease, LAP is elevated above RAP and the result is an L-R atrial shunt. Infants with CDH, where there is LV maldevelopment and dysfunction alongside abnormalities of the pulmonary vascular bed, may present with this hemodynamic phenotype. Assessment of the atrial shunt direction before initiating pulmonary vasodilator therapy has been proposed as an efficient means of determining the dominant pathologic condition in CDH.[22]

Echocardiography findings differ according to the underlying drivers of PH, adaptive responses of the cardiovascular system to adverse loading conditions, presence of extrapulmonary shunts, and the effects of cardiotropic medications and supportive care strategies. Typical findings in resistance-driven PH include RV systolic and diastolic failure in response to a sustained increase in afterload, reduced RV stroke volume and filling, decreased PBF with V/Q mismatch, RV dilatation resulting in a D-shaped left ventricle with reduced LV preload and stroke volume, and R-L shunting through the PDA and/or PFO.[6] Changes in IVS morphology throughout the cardiac cycle may also provide insight as to the likely underlying pathophysiology. In resistance-mediated PH, bowing of the IVS occurs a result of prolonged contraction of the RV free wall (against the increased afterload) compared with the LV free wall or septum.[18] Flattening or bowing of the IVS therefore tends to predominantly occur during systole, with impairment of LV diastolic filling.[18] Conversely, in the setting of flow-driven PH, the RV pressure relative to the LV is typically higher in diastole due to increased filling from L-R shunting.

PHENOTYPE-SPECIFIC FRAMEWORK FOR MANAGEMENT
Acute Pulmonary Hypertension

Resistance-mediated pulmonary hypertension

1. PVR reduction

In resistance-driven aPH, where LV function is preserved and the RV remains coupled, pulmonary vasodilatation using iNO may produce a sufficient reduction in PVR and thereby PAP[76] to augment RV performance and facilitate recovery of PBF.[17,77] Treatment goals in resistance-mediated aPH include: reduction of PVR, augmentation of RV performance as needed, restoration of systemic blood flow, ensuring adequate RV perfusion pressure, supportive care of the underlying condition(s), and correction of associated metabolic and hematologic derangements. Factors related to either the underlying disease process (eg, sepsis and hypoxia-ischemia) or medical therapies (eg, high-dose dopamine)[17] may drive further increases in PVR, perpetuating hypoxic vasoconstriction and hypoxemia. Overly aggressive attempts at lung recruitment in the setting of minimal parenchymal disease (eg, HIE) may further compromise PBF[78] and systemic perfusion from reduced LV stroke volume and LVEDV.[79] Care should be taken to exclude significant LV dysfunction before the initiation of therapy with selective pulmonary vasodilators in PH. A suggested algorithm for hemodynamic management in aPH is outlined in **Fig. 5**. Specific physiologic goals and recommendations according to the underlying PH phenotype are outlined in **Table 3**.

2. Support of RV performance

Where there is echocardiographic evidence of cardiac dysfunction and/or low systolic arterial pressure (SAP), inotropic support should be considered. Milrinone is a good first-line agent in the absence of systemic hypotension. Evidence for efficacy of *milrinone* in neonatal PH is currently limited to case series,[80,81] and the results of randomized trials are awaited.[82,83] Where milrinone may be less desirable (eg, significant prematurity, HIE requiring therapeutic hypothermia, and renal impairment), *dobutamine* and *low-dose epinephrine* (eg, 0.03–0.05 mcg/kg/min) represent suitable second-line options. Dobutamine is not associated with increases in PVR and, although epinephrine increases PVR, there is a proportionate increase in SVR.[84]

The neonatal RV myocardium is exquisitely sensitive to increased afterload, more so than the LV.[85] R-L ductal shunting may offload the failing RV and support systemic perfusion, although this occurs at the expense of postductal oxygenation.[2] Nevertheless, maintaining patency of the ductus with a low-dose prostaglandin infusion represents a therapeutic option in the setting of severe aPH, impaired RV performance, and a restrictive PDA in infants with a classic arterial aPH phenotype or in the setting of CDH.

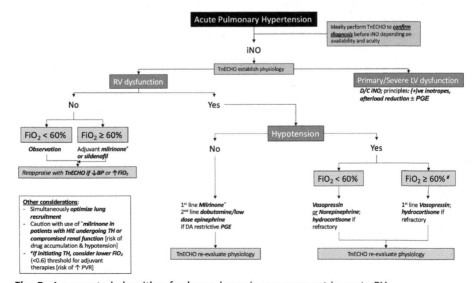

Fig. 5. A suggested algorithm for hemodynamic management in acute PH.

Table 3
Physiologic goals and therapeutic recommendations by pulmonary hypertension phenotype

PH Phenotype	Physiologic Goals	Suggested Treatment Approach
Acute PH		
Arterial (classic)	Reduce PVR	Optimize lung recruitment and supportive care
	Augment RV performance	Offload RV with pulmonary vasodilators
		Augment RV function with inotropes if required
	Support SAP and maintain coronary perfusion pressure	Support SAP with vasoconstrictors which do not ↑PVR
		Consider maintaining ductal patency with PGE
Flow mediated	Shunt control	Specific shunt management
	Maintain ↑PVR	Avoid selective pulmonary vasodilators
		Consider permissive hypercapnia (pCO_2 50–60 mmHg, pH > 7.25)
		Avoid hyperoxia (goal preductal SpO_2 91%–95%* and preductal pCO_2 50–80 mm Hg[138])
		*higher SpO_2 may be needed if undergoing TH
Left heart dysfunction (postcapillary)	LV afterload reduction	LV afterload reduction if SAP adequate, for example, inodilator
	Positive inotropy	Positive inotropy
	Maintain ↑PVR	Avoid selective pulmonary vasodilators
	Maintain R→L ductal shunt if ↓SBF	Diuretics for pulmonary edema
Chronic PH		
Arterial (classic) for example, associated with BPD	Reduce PVR	Optimize lung recruitment and supportive care
		Offload RV with pulmonary vasodilators
		Consider diuretics if RV dilation
		Avoid hypoxia and hyperoxia (target oxygen saturations 92%–95%[106])
Flow mediated	Shunt control	Specific shunt management (reduction in or closure of L-R shunt if feasible and appropriate)
	Maintain ↑PVR	Avoid selective pulmonary vasodilators
		Diuretics for ASD/VSD
		Positive end expiratory pressure
Systemic hypertension	LV afterload reduction	Antihypertensive therapy role for ACE inhibitors/ARB
	Maintain ↑PVR	Avoid pulmonary vasodilators

Abbreviations: ACE, angiotensin converting enzyme; ARB, angiotensin II receptor blocker; ASD, atrial septal defect; L, left; PGE, prostaglandin E, PH; pulmonary hypertension, PVR; pulmonary vascular resistance, R; right, RV; right ventricle, SAP; systolic arterial pressure, SBF; systemic blood flow, TH; therapeutic hypothermia, VSD; ventricular septal defect.

Adapted from: Giesinger R, Kinsella JP, Abman SH, McNamara PJ. Pulmonary hypertension phenotypes in the newborn. In: Dakshinamurti S, ed. *Hypoxic Respiratory Failure in the Newborn: From Origins to Clinical Management.* Boca Raton: Taylor & Francis Group; 2021.

3. Use of vasopressors

Adequate SAP is essential for maintaining coronary perfusion pressure and myocardial oxygen delivery, and ameliorating RV ischemia, which contributes to the cascade of hemodynamic sequelae in PH. Low SAP in infants with aPH may require *vasopressor therapy* once RV afterload reduction and support of RV performance have been optimized. Dopamine, although frequently used in neonatology, produces nonspecific pulmonary and systemic vasoconstriction and may adversely affect physiology in aPH.[17] In the presence of aPH, dopamine results in marked elevation of PAP without improving oxygenation in animal models and is therefore not recommended.[86,87]

Vasopressin, a systemic vasoconstrictor acting via V1 receptors on vascular smooth muscle cells, is increasingly being considered the preferred agent for augmentation of systemic blood pressure in aPH where oxygen requirement remains high despite pulmonary vasodilator treatment. Vasodilation with vasopressin treatment has been observed in the pulmonary vascular bed in an animal model,[88] occurring via endothelial cell V1 receptor-mediated release of nitric oxide.[88] Vasopressin has been shown to positively influence hemodynamics in a range of shock states in children and adults,[89,90] and there are case series demonstrating improved oxygenation[91,92] and SAP[91,93] in neonatal aPH. Careful attention must be provided to sodium and water balance with vasopressin use due to the risk of hyponatremia, which occurs due to several factors, including marked natriuresis in some infants as renal perfusion is restored.[93] *Norepinephrine* is an alternative vasopressor option; however, there is limited evidence for its use. Increased PVR with norepinephrine use has been documented in an animal model,[94] particularly with coadministration of a high concentration of inspired oxygen, and in the adult population.[95,96] This may be poorly tolerated by infants with significant RV impairment and/or significant labile hypoxemia. Increased LVO and SAP and a minor improvement in oxygenation has been demonstrated in an observational study of term infants with aPH[97]; however, further evidence is awaited. It is important to highlight that there is no randomized clinical trial evidence for either vasopressin or norepinephrine in neonates with aPH and systemic hypotension. A single randomized controlled trial in a catheterization laboratory setting in adults with PH demonstrated reversal of systemic hypotension with terlipressin (a vasopressin analog), without the increase in PAP that was observed with norepinephrine.[96] *Corticosteroids* such as hydrocortisone potentiate the vasoactive response to catecholamines[98] and may be a useful adjunctive therapy for refractory hypotension.

Flow-mediated pulmonary hypertension

In the setting of VGAM or similar high volume systemic to venous connections, postductal perfusion is compromised due to intracranial vascular "steal" through the AVM. This is reflected on TNE as retrograde diastolic flow in the aorta and markedly increased superior vena caval flow in the case of a cerebral AVM.[99] Pulmonary pressures may be suprasystemic,[99] with R-L shunting at atrial and ductal levels.[99,100] Although RV coronary perfusion usually occurs throughout the cardiac cycle, coronary perfusion is limited to diastole by the increase in RV pressure associated with a maladaptive, dilated, and hypertrophied RV.[101] Vascular steal through the AVM may further compromise coronary perfusion pressure by lowering coronary root pressure, leading to a "pseudocoarctation" physiology.[101] In these infants, maintaining ductal patency may be essential to avert critical postductal hypoperfusion. Although there are circumstances whereby RV afterload reduction with pulmonary vasodilation is needed, inappropriate use of pulmonary vasodilators in this setting may result in critically low postductal perfusion through modulation of the supportive R-L ductal shunt. Achieving AVM shunt control, which is often via interventional neurosurgical means, is a cornerstone of management.

Postcapillary pulmonary hypertension

Determining the relative contribution of LV disease is an important consideration in the rational selection of therapy. Where there is primary LV disease, RV afterload reduction with selective pulmonary vasodilators (eg, iNO) may worsen LV diastolic dysfunction and perpetuate hypoxemia. Increases in LV afterload through aggressive vasopressor use may also be poorly tolerated. An alternative therapeutic approach is necessary in this instance, including positive inotropy, avoidance of pulmonary vasodilators, and consideration of LV afterload reduction and lusitropy if systemic artery pressure is adequate.

Chronic Pulmonary Hypertension

In terms of cPH, TNE evidence of PH identified within the first 7 to 14 days after birth may help predict subsequent moderate–severe BPD or death at 36 weeks postmenstrual age.[102,103] Although many units in North America routinely assess preterm infants considered to be at high-risk for BPD-cPH, use of standardized screening protocols for at-risk infants occurs in a minority.[104] Elevated levels of the biomarker, brain natriuretic peptide (BNP), at the time of diagnosis of BPD may be useful in predicting patients at risk of late PH when used alongside echocardiographic markers including RA dilatation, RV hypertrophy, RV FAC, and main pulmonary artery diameter z-score.[105] Guidelines for BPD-cPH screening in at-risk preterm infants have been published and advocate for screening with echocardiography at 36 weeks corrected age for infants with moderate or severe BPD.[27,106] Use of N-Terminal pro-BNP is incorporated into some published guidelines,[27] may be elevated as early as 14 days in infants who go on to develop BPD,[107] and can detect BPD-PH at 28 weeks corrected age.[108] Lung ultrasound has also been described as an adjunct to echocardiography assessment in BPD-cPH,[109] although it requires further validation.

Resistance-mediated pulmonary hypertension

As part of cPH assessment, in addition to estimation of mPAP using the TR jet, the PAAT:RVET may be used in the evaluation of PVR, including in the assessment of pulmonary vasodilator responsiveness over time.[1] A ratio of less than 0.31 is considered low and consistent with elevated PAP.[110] TAPSE z-score less than -3 and RV/LV end-systolic ratio greater than 1.5 are additional TNE markers of risk for cPH in BPD.[27] Lung optimization is an important priority, alongside treatment with pulmonary vasodilators. Sildenafil therapy has been associated with improvement in both clinical and echocardiographic markers of raised pulmonary pressures.[111] Diuretics may be considered for optimizing RV configuration when RV dilatation is identified on echocardiography.[1] Although long-term benefits have not been demonstrated with diuretic treatment in infants with BPD, improvements in both oxygenation and pulmonary mechanics have been demonstrated.[112] A standardized management approach using diuretics has been associated with high rates of symptomatic improvement in cPH associated with BPD where RV dilatation was used as the treatment threshold.[113]

Cardiac catheterization should be strongly considered when assessment of PH severity using echocardiography is not possible, to quantify PH severity, determine the contribution of shunts, exclude alternative causes of pulmonary vascular disease, and in the setting of a poor response to PH therapy[2] or need for multiple pulmonary vasodilators.[27] PV stenosis, a potential cause of cPH in preterm infants with chronic lung disease,[114] develops over time,[114] is often diagnosed late and is associated with poor survival in this patient group.[115] Limited data exist to guide management of BPD-PH.[113] Treatment goals include reducing PVR, offloading the RV, avoiding coronary ischemia and cardiac failure, and optimizing cardiorespiratory symptomatology, thus minimizing aggravation of PH.[27] Avoidance of V/Q mismatch and localized hypoxic vasoconstriction, secondary to atelectasis, through appropriate noninvasive respiratory support is advised.[27] Sildenafil is generally considered first-line therapy for pulmonary vasodilation in BPD-PH, particularly in infants responsive to iNO. Endothelin receptor antagonists such as bosentan or inhaled epoprostenol are additional second-line options, with limited evidence of efficacy. A recent case series also showed efficacy of the oral-soluble guanylate cyclase stimulator, riociguat, in 10 infants with cPH, with improvements in respiratory status, right heart dilation, cardiac function, and chronic PH observed in the majority of infants,[116] warranting further study in newborns.

Flow-mediated pulmonary hypertension

Chronic L-R shunting results in cardiac dilatation, and alterations in CO, which are measurable using RVO and LVO. Atrial level shunting causes RA/RV dilation and an increase in RVO relative to LVO, whereas chronic PDA shunting leads to LA/LV dilation and increased LVO (typically >300 mL/kg/min). The reliability of the RVO to LVO ratio has not been formally validated and represents a knowledge gap. Increased transductal flow also eventually tends to result in stretching of the atrial communication, which in turn increases both ventricular outputs.[1] The increased LAP associated with large L-R ductal shunting results in earlier mitral valve opening and increased early passive filling, which shortens the IVRT (<40 milliseconds) and results in "pseudonormalization" of the E/A ratio to greater than 1. In longstanding PDA, both elevated PVR and chronic excessive PBF may contribute to cPH. Evidence of left heart volume loading tends to persist in most patients with flow-mediated PH, including dilated left heart structures and elevated PV and mitral valve flow velocities.[1,117]

In flow-mediated PH, shunt control is the mainstay of therapy. In the case of PDA, choice of pharmacologic or interventional (surgical or transcatheter) management is made according to individual patient factors, including postnatal age, presence of comorbidities and prior pharmacologic treatment. Although fluid management should be judicious, aggressive fluid restriction tends to precipitate a reduction in overall circulating fluid volume without any effect on the proportion of CO directed toward the lungs and may exacerbate existing postductal hypoperfusion from a hemodynamically significant PDA.[118] Although diuretics are often used as part of symptomatic management, an increased incidence of PDA[119] and prostaglandin-mediated dilation of the ductus arteriosus in an animal model[120] have been observed historically with the use of furosemide. Diuretics are, however, a key aspect of supportive management in ASD, with device closure reported in infants as small as 2 to 2.5 kg.[121] Pulmonary vasodilator use may be harmful due to the drop in PVR resulting in increased SVR:PVR ratio and the risk of worsening oxidative stress.[1] It is important to note that although PDA closure may ameliorate pulmonary overcirculation and improve symptomatology in flow-driven cPH, once secondary elevation of PVR develops, closure of the ductus risks precipitating a PH crisis and significant RV impairment.[1]

Postcapillary pulmonary hypertension

Postcapillary PH with LV diastolic dysfunction is a more recently recognized driver of cPH-CLD,[31] and chest x-ray may be unable to differentiate between cardiac diastolic and respiratory pathophysiology.[122] Assessment of features of high LA pressure seem to be useful for differentiating patients with similar clinical features into those with and without LV disease.[122] Findings may include decreased transmitral E/A ratio, prolonged IVRT,[31] higher E/e' ratio,[29,31] and abnormal MPI.[29,31] An elevated E:e' at 28 days postnatal age is associated with a prolonged requirement for respiratory support.[123] A multiparametric approach for the assessment of LV diastolic function in preterm infants has been advocated, using a combination of left atrial volume, E/A ratio, e' velocity, E/e' ratio, the presence of PH and peak left atrial strain.[122] Angiotensin converting enzyme (ACE) inhibition as a strategy for LV afterload reduction in infants with severe BPD, systemic hypertension, and LV diastolic dysfunction is an emerging therapeutic option warranting further study.[124,125] The role of lung ultrasound in phenotypic triaging is another knowledge gap.

To illustrate the use of TNE in the management of neonatal PH, the following 2 case studies describe 2 different phenotypic presentations of aPH and provide example management approaches based on assessment of clinical and echocardiographic parameters.

CASE STUDY 1: ACUTE PULMONARY HYPERTENSION OF ARTERIAL (CLASSIC) ORIGIN

Case presentation: A female infant was born via a forceps delivery at 41 weeks gestation, complicated by Group B Streptococcus-positive maternal screening, meconium-stained amniotic fluid, and prolonged rupture of membranes for 39 hours. Intrapartum antibiotics were administered. Apgar scores were 4, 6, and 8 at 1, 5, and 10 minutes, respectively, managed with mask ventilation. The infant was initially admitted to the Special Care Nursery on continuous positive airway pressure (CPAP) 6 cmH_2O, requiring FiO_2 0.5 initially, which subsequently increased to 7 cmH_2O. Progressive hypoxemia developed requiring an FiO_2 of 1.0 with an associated respiratory acidosis (pCO_2 89 mmHg). The patient was intubated, ventilated, and commenced on in iNO at 20 ppm based on a presumptive clinical diagnosis of hypoxemic respiratory failure. The chest x-ray was consistent with meconium aspiration syndrome. Two boluses of 0.9% saline were given, and vasoactive support was with intravenous infusions of epinephrine (0.2 mcg/kg/min) and norepinephrine (0.24 mcg/kg/min). The infant was retrieved to the tertiary neonatal intensive care unit. Preductal oxygen saturations were 85%, with heart rate 160/min and preductal noninvasive (cuff) blood pressure 43/30 mm Hg (mean arterial pressure [MAP] 35 mm Hg). Serum lactate was 3.7 mmol/L. TNE assessment demonstrated suprasystemic PAP (68 mm Hg + RAP) with flattening of the IVS in systole, mild to moderate TR, LV sEI 2.1, PVR index 6.5, a small patent foramen ovale (PFO) with bidirectional shunt, and a moderate PDA with bidirectional shunt (R-L for 82% of systole). There was moderate RV dilation (RV to LV ratio 1.4), moderate impairment in RV systolic function (RV S' 3.4 cm/s, TAPSE 6.2 mm, RV FAC 21%, and RVO 97 mL/kg/min), and mild impairment in LV systolic function (LV EF 53% by Simpson's biplane).

Lung recruitment was optimized, and an intravenous vasopressin infusion (0.3 mU/kg/min) was added for augmentation of systemic arterial pressure without adversely affecting PVR. Epinephrine was reduced to an inotropic dose (0.08 mcg/kg/min), and an intravenous milrinone infusion (0.33 mcg/kg/min) was added to maximize pulmonary vasodilation and further support RV function. Norepinephrine was weaned to 0.15 mcg/kg/min, with hydrocortisone given to optimize response to catecholamines. An intravenous infusion of sildenafil was added for further RV afterload reduction and iNO was continued. Oxygenation, systemic blood pressure, and serum lactate showed sustained improvement. Follow-up TNE after 4 hours showed improvement in RV systolic function, normal LV systolic function, improved RVO and LVO, and ongoing evidence of suprasystemic PH. The infant stabilized thereafter, and vasoactive medications were able to be weaned, followed by extubation to room air on day 9.

CASE STUDY 2: ACUTE PULMONARY HYPERTENSION RELATED TO EXCESSIVE PULMONARY BLOOD FLOW

A male infant was born at 36 weeks gestation via emergency cesarean section (C/S) for abnormal umbilical Dopplers and nonreassuring fetal heart rate on a background of fetal anomaly. Third trimester growth scan demonstrated bilateral ventriculomegaly and a fetal MRI had indicated presence of a dural venous malformation. Initial

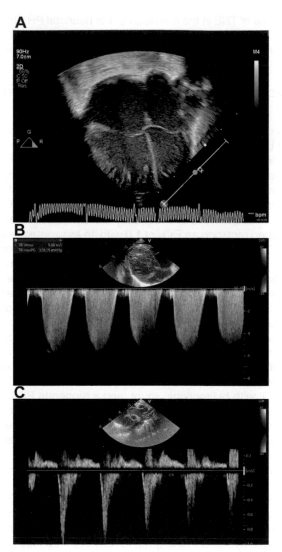

Fig. 6. (*A*) Apical 4-chamber view showing right heart volume and pressure loading. (*B*) RVSp by TR jet, measuring 128 mm Hg + RAP. (*C*) PW Doppler of the descending aorta showing holodiastolic flow reversal.

respiratory management had been with CPAP. There was persistent hypoxemia after birth (FiO$_2$ 0.6) with a postductal arterial blood gas showing pH 7.27, pCO$_2$ 56 mm Hg, pO$_2$ 45 mm Hg, BE −2.0, and lactate 2.9 mmol/L, prompting endotracheal intubation and administration of surfactant (Curosurf® [poractant alpha]) for suspected respiratory distress syndrome. The heart rate was 146/min, respiratory rate 70/min, with postductal invasive blood pressure 61/30 mmHg (MAP 45 mmHg). There was a hyperdynamic precordium and an audible cranial bruit. TNE demonstrated high-output cardiac failure with a moderately dilated RV (**Fig. 6**A; RV to LV ratio 1.6), moderate-to-severe TR with RVSp 128 mmHg + RAP (**Fig. 4**B) and paradoxic septal wall motion, RVO 612 mL/kg/min, LVO 436 mL/kg/min, dilation of the superior vena cava, mild-moderate RV systolic impairment, a small PDA shunting R-L, and holodiastolic flow reversal in the descending aorta (**Fig. 4**C), consistent with a large preductal systemic to venous connection. Brain MRI confirmed an extensive dural sinus malformation. Therapy included (1) Shunt modulation with serial interventional neurosurgical procedures and (2) Maintenance of an R-L ductal shunt to preserve postductal systemic perfusion. Pulmonary vasodilator support was not provided because the patient had high PBF. Support of PDA patency with an infusion of prostaglandin was considered; however, the ductus remained patent on serial assessment. Gentle diuresis was also given. Improvements in cardiorespiratory status were observed.

Despite similar presentations with hypoxemic respiratory failure, these 2 cases highlight the variability in underlying pathophysiology in neonatal PH, utility of TNE evaluation, and implications for clinical management.

SUMMARY

Comprehensive TNE evaluation is an invaluable tool for adjudicating underlying pathophysiology and guiding clinical management in acute and chronic neonatal PH. An assumption that all PH is mediated by elevated PVR may lead to inappropriate treatment pathways and patient harm, and differentiating drivers of disease clinically can be challenging even for experienced clinicians. PH may be resistance-mediated; however, it also develops secondary to increased PBF associated with L-R shunt lesions and in the setting of LV dysfunction with elevated LA pressure and pulmonary venous hypertension. Treatment goals in resistance-driven PH include RV afterload reduction, augmentation of RV performance, and maintenance of adequate systemic blood flow and coronary perfusion pressure. In flow-driven PH, shunt control is the primary treatment aim, although secondary elevations in PVR also occur. Due to the obligate nature of the shunt, in the setting of high-volume shunting due to large systemic to venous connections, increases in PVR do not offset the pulmonary overcirculation as occurs with atrial, ductal, and/or ventricular shunts, contributing to the severity of cardiac failure in affected infants.

The role of primary LV disease in contributing to neonatal PH is increasingly recognized, particularly in preterm infants with BPD-PH and in the setting of CDH. Positive inotropy, avoidance of pulmonary vasodilators, and consideration of LV afterload reduction where systemic arterial pressure is adequate are the mainstays of treatment in this patient group; recognition of the problem is an essential first step. Neonatal hemodynamic research has failed to provide definitive answers to several important questions in neonatology, in part due to the unrecognized physiologic heterogeneity of enrolled patients. Identification of distinct hemodynamic phenotypes is an important step in the provision of appropriate, individualized neonatal intensive care for some of our most vulnerable patients, and prospectively investigating this approach is a neonatology research imperative. In the interim, clinicians should not always interpret nonresponse or negative response to selective pulmonary vasodilators as an indication that the patient is worsening; rather consideration of an alternative phenotype and the need to wean the pulmonary vasodilators is warranted.

Best Practice Box

- In infants with hypoxemic respiratory failure, echocardiography can estimate PAP and assess the presence of PH. The precise physiologic phenotype of PH determines therapy.
- Elevated PAP can be associated with increased peak velocity of the tricuspid regurgitation jet, R-L or bidirectional shunt across the PDA and PFO, and change in the configuration of IVS and LV-sEI.

- Resistance-driven PH is characterized by elevated RVET/PAAT and is typically managed with pulmonary vasodilators such as iNO.
- Flow-driven PH such as VGAM is associated with high PBF, increased vena caval flow, and retrograde diastolic flow in the aorta. Use of iNO can further increase PBF and should be avoided.
- Postcapillary PH is often secondary to LV dysfunction. In infants with LV dysfunction and PH, R-L shunt at the PDA may be seen but an L-R shunt may occur at the PFO due to high LAP, and is associated with low LV output and low EF. Use of iNO is contraindicated and can worsen pulmonary edema in the presence of primary, severe LV dysfunction.

ACKNOWLEDGMENTS

Thank you to Dr Nilarni Jayakumar, for her assistance in preparation of the case studies.

DISCLOSURE

The authors have nothing to disclose.

REFERENCES

1. Giesinger R, Kinsella JP, Abman SH, et al. Pulmonary hypertension phenotypes in the newborn. In: Dakshinamurti S, editor. Hypoxic respiratory failure in the newborn: from Origins to clinical management. Boca Raton: Taylor & Francis Group; 2021.
2. Ruoss J, Rios DR, Levy PT. Updates on management for acute and chronic phenotypes of neonatal pulmonary hypertension. Clin Perinatol 2020;47:593–615.
3. Boyd S, Chatmethakul T, McNamara PJ. How to diagnose and treat acute pulmonary hypertension when you have no cardiology support. Early Hum Dev 2022;174:105668.
4. Jones C, Crossland DS. The interplay between pressure, flow, and resistance in neonatal pulmonary hypertension. Semin Fetal Neonatal Med 2022;27:101371.
5. Jain A, Giesinger RE, Dakshinamurti S, et al. Care of the critically ill neonate with hypoxemic respiratory failure and acute pulmonary hypertension: framework for practice based on consensus opinion of neonatal hemodynamics working group. J Perinatol 2022;42:3–13.
6. De Boode W, Singh Y, Molnar Z, et al, European Special Interest Group 'Neonatologist Performed Echocardiography' NPE. Application of Neonatologist Performed Echocardiography in the assessment and management of persistent pulmonary hypertension of the newborn. Pediatr Res 2018;84:68–77.
7. Mertens L, Seri I, Marek J, et al, Writing Group of the American Society of Echocardiography ASE, European Association of Echocardiography EAE, Association for European Pediatric Cardiologists AEPC. Targeted neonatal echocardiography in the neonatal intensive care unit: practice guidelines and recommendations for training. Eur J Echocardiogr 2011;12(10):715–36.
8. Papadhima I, Louis D, Purna J, et al. Targeted neonatal echocardiography (TNE) consult service in a large tertiary perinatal center in Canada. J Perinatol 2018;38:1039–45.
9. Nguyen J, Cascione M, Noori S. Analysis of lawsuits related to point-of-care ultrasonography in neonatology and pediatric subspecialties. J Perinatol 2016; 36(9):784–6.

10. Moss S, Kitchiner DJ, Yoxall CW, et al. Evaluation of echocardiography on the neonatal unit. Arch Dis Child Fetal Neonatal Ed 2003;88:287F–91F.
11. Mukerji A, Diambomba Y, Lee S, et al. Use of targeted neonatal echocardiography and focused cardiac sonography in tertiary neonatal intensive care units: time to embrace it? J Ultrasound Med 2016;35:1579–91.
12. Rahde Bischoff A, Giesinger RE, Rios DR, et al. Anatomic concordance of neonatologist-performed echocardiography as part of hemodynamics consultation and pediatric cardiology. J Am Soc Echocardiogr 2021;34(3):301–7.
13. Boyd S, Kluckow M. Point of care ultrasound in the neonatal unit: applications, training and accreditation. Early Hum Dev 2019;138.
14. Hébert ALP, Giesinger RE, Ting YT, et al. Evolution of training guidelines for echocardiography performed by the neonatologist: toward hemodynamic consultation. J Am Soc Echocardiogr 2019;32(6):785–90.
15. Noordegraaf A, Westerhof BE, Westerhof N. The relationship between the right ventricle and its load in pulmonary hypertension. J Am Coll Cardiol 2017;69(2):236–43.
16. Arrigo M, Huber LC, Winnik S, et al. Right ventricular failure: pathophysiology, diagnosis and treatment. Card Fail Rev 2019;5(3):140–6.
17. McNamara P, Giesinger RE, Lakshminrusimha S. Dopamine and neonatal pulmonary hypertension - pressing need for a better pressor? J Pediatr 2022;246:242–50.
18. Sanz J, Sánchez-Quintana D, Bossone E, et al. Anatomy, function, and dysfunction of the right ventricle: JACC state-of-the-art review. Cardiol 2019;73(12):1463–82.
19. Oishi P, Fineman JR. Pulmonary hypertension. Pediatr Crit Care Med 2016;17:S140–5.
20. Bronicki R, Anas NG. Cardiopulmonary interaction. Pediatr Crit Care Med 2009;10:313–22.
21. Ren X, Johns RA, Gao WD. Right heart in pulmonary hypertension: from adaptation to failure. Pulm Circ 2019;9(3):1–20.
22. Kinsella J, Steinhorn RH, Mullen MP, et al, Pediatric Pulmonary Hypertension Network PPHNet. The left ventricle in congenital diaphragmatic hernia: implications for the management of pulmonary hypertension. J Pediatr 2018;197(17–22).
23. Hamrick S, Sallmon H, Rose AT, et al. Patent ductus arteriosus of the preterm infant. Pediatrics 2020;146(5):e20201209.
24. Dahdah N, Alesseh H, Dahms B, et al. Severe pulmonary hypertensive vascular disease in two newborns with aneurysmal vein of Galen. Pediatr Cardiol 2001;22(6):538–41.
25. Reddy V, Meyrick B, Wong J, et al. In utero placement of aortopulmonary shunts. a model of postnatal pulmonary hypertension with increased pulmonary blood flow in lambs. Circulation 1995;92(3):606–13.
26. Serraf A, Hervé P, Labat C, et al. Endothelial dysfunction in venous pulmonary hypertension in the neonatal piglet. Ann Thorac Surg 1995;59(5):1155–61.
27. Hansmann G, Sallmon H, Roehr CC, et al, European Pediatric Pulmonary Vascular Disease Network EPPVDN. Koestenberger, for the european pediatric pulmonary vascular disease network (EPPVDN). pulmonary hypertension in bronchopulmonary dysplasia. Pediatr Res 2020;89:446–55.
28. Lignelli E, Palumbo F, Myti D, et al. Recent advances in our understanding of the mechanisms of lung alveolarization and bronchopulmonary dysplasia. Am J Physiol Lung Cell Mol Physiol 2019;317:L832–87.

29. Yates A, Welty SE, Gest AL, et al. Changes in patients with bronchopulmonary dysplasia. J Pediatr 2008;152:766–70.
30. Mourani P, Ivy DD, Rosenberg AA, et al. Left ventricular diastolic dysfunction in bronchopulmonary dysplasia. J Pediatr 2008;152:291–3.
31. Seghal A, Malikiwi A, Paul E, et al. A new look at bronchopulmonary dysplasia: postcapillary pathophysiology and cardiac dysfunction. Pulm Circ 2016;6(4): 508–15.
32. Bokiniec R, Właskienko P, Borszewska-Kornacka, et al. Evaluation of left ventricular function in preterm infants with bronchopulmonary dysplasia using various echocardiographic techniques. Echocardiography 2017;34(4):567–76.
33. Abman S, Warady BA, Lum GM, et al. Systemic hypertension in infants with bronchopulmonary dysplasia. J Pediatr 1984;104:928–31.
34. Anderson A, Warady BA, Daily DK, et al. Systemic hypertension in infants with severe bronchopulmonary dysplasia: associated clinical factors. Am J Perinatol 1993;10:190–3.
35. Alagappan A, Malloy MH. Systemic hypertension in very low birth weight infants with bronchopulmonary dysplasia: incidence and risk factors. Am J Perinatol 1998;15:3–8.
36. Philip R, Nathaniel Johnson J, Naik R, et al. Effect of patent ductus arteriosus on pulmonary vascular disease. Congenit Heart Dis 2019;14:37–41.
37. Philip R, Lamba V, Talati A, et al. Pulmonary hypertension with prolonged patency of the ductus arteriosus in preterm infants. Children 2020;7:139.
38. Gupta N, Kamlin CO, Cheung M, et al. Improving diagnostic accuracy in the transport of infants with suspected duct-dependent congenital heart disease. J Paediatr Child Health 2014;50:64–70.
39. Skinner J, Hunter S, Hey EN. Haemodynamic features at presentation in persistent pulmonary hypertension of the newborn and outcome. Arch Dis Child Fetal Neonatal Ed 1996;74:F26–32.
40. O'Leary M, Assad TR, Xu M, et al. Lack of a tricuspid regurgitation Doppler signal and pulmonary hypertension by invasive measurement. J Am Heart Assoc 2018;7:e009362.
41. D'Alto M, Romeo E, Argiento P, et al. Accuracy and precision of echocardiography versus right heart catheterization for the assessment of pulmonary hypertension. Cardiology 2017;168:4058–62.
42. Patel M, Breatnach CR, James AT, et al. Echocardiographic assessment of right ventricular afterload in preterm infants: maturational patterns of pulmonary artery accleration time over the first year of age and implications for pulmonary hypertension. J Am Soc Echocardiogr 2019;32(7):884–94.e884.
43. Levy P, Patel MD, Groh G, et al. Pulmonary artery acceration time provides a reliable estimate of invasive pulmonary hemodynamics in children. J Am Soc Echocardiogr 2016;29(11):1056–65.
44. Savoia M, Morassutti FR, Castriotta L, et al. Pulmonary hypertension in a neonatologist-performed echocardiographic follow-up of bronchopulmonary dysplasia. Eur J Pediatr 2021;180:1711–20.
45. Jain A, Mohamed A, Kavanagh B, et al. Cardiopulmonary adaptation during first day of life in human neonates. J Pediatr 2018;200:50–7.e52.
46. Bhattacharya S, McNamara P, Jain A, et al. Validating the use of pulmonary artery acceleration time in estimating pulmonary pressure in neonates. Paediatr Child Health 2018;23:e25–6.
47. Bendapudi P, Rao GG, Greenough A. Diagnosis and management of persistent pulmonary hypertension of the newborn. Pediatr Respir Rev 2015;16:157–61.

48. Smith A, Purna JR, Castaldo MP, et al. Accuracy and reliability of qualitative echocardiography assessment of right ventricular size and function in neonates. Echocardiography 2019;36(7):1346–52.

49. Abraham S, Weismann CG. Left ventricular end-systolic eccentricity index for assessment of pulmonary hypertension in infants. Echocardiography 2016; 33(6):910–5.

50. Burkett D, Patel SS, Mertens L, et al. Relationship between left ventricular geometry and invasive hemodynamics in pediatric pulmonary hypertension. Circ Cardiovasc Imaging 2020;13(5):e009825.

51. Koestenberger M, Nagel B, Ravekes W, et al. Systolic right ventricular function in preterm and term neonates: reference values of the tricuspid annular plane systolic excursion (TAPSE) in 258 patients and calculation of Z-score values. Neonatology 2011;100(1):85–92.

52. Levy P, Dioneda B, Holland MR, et al. Right ventricular function in preterm and term neonates: reference values for right ventricle areas and fractional area of change. J Am Soc Echocardiogr 2015;28(5):559–69.

53. Shiran H, Zamanian RT, McConnell MV, et al. Relationship between echocardiographic and magnetic resonance derived measures of right ventricular size and function in patients with pulmonary hypertension. J Am Soc Echocardiogr 2014; 27(4):405–12.

54. Malowitz J, Forsha DE, Smith PB, et al. Right ventricular echocardiographic indices predict poor outcomes in infants with persistent pulmonary hypertension of the newborn. Eur Heart J 2015;16:1224–31.

55. Jain A, El-Khuffash AF, van Herpen CH, et al. Cardiac function and ventricular interactions in persistent pulmonary hypertension of the newborn. Pediatr Crit Care Med 2021;22(2):e145–3157.

56. Rodriguez M, Coredera A, Martinez-Orgado J, et al. Cerebral blood flow velocity and oxygenation correlate predominantly with right ventricular function in cooled neonates with moderate-severe hypoxic-ischemic encephalopathy. Eur J Pediatr 2020;179(10):1609–18.

57. Giesinger R, El Shahed AI, Castaldo MP, et al. Impaired right ventricular performance is associated with adverse outcome after hypoxic ischemic encephalopathy. Am J Respir Crit Care Med 2019;200(10):1294–305.

58. Giesinger R, Elsayed YN, Castaldo MP, et al. Neurodevelopmental outcome following hypoxic ischaemic encephalopathy and therapeutic hypothermia is related to right ventricular performance at 24-hour postnatal age. Arch Dis Child Fetal Neonatal Ed 2022;107(1):70–5.

59. Aggarwal S, Shanti C, Lelli J, et al. Prognostic utility of noninvasive estimates of pulmonary vascular compliance in neonates with congenital diaphragmatic hernia. J Pediatr Surg 2019;54(3):439–44.

60. Seghal A, Malikiwi A, Paul E, et al. Right ventricular function in infants with bronchopulmonary dysplasia: association with respiratory sequelae. Neonatology 2016;109(4):289–96.

61. Blanca A, Duijts L, van Mastrigt E, et al. Right ventricular function in infants with bronchopulmonary dysplasia and pulmonary hypertension: a pilot study. Pulm Circ 2019;9(1). 2045894018816063.

62. Smolarek D, Gruchala M, Sobiczewski W. Echocardiographic evaluation of right ventricular systolic function: the traditional and innovative approach. Cardiol J 2018;24(5):563–72.

63. Sehgal A, Ibrahim M, Tan K. Cardiac function and its evolution with pulmonary vasodilator therapy: a myocardial deformation study. Echocardiography 2014; 31:E185–8.

64. James A, Corcoran JD, McNamara PJ, et al. The effect of milrinone on right and left ventricular function when used as a rescue therapy for term infants with pulmonary hypertension. Cardiol Young 2015;26:1–10.

65. Patel N, Mills JF, Cheung MMH. Assessment of right ventricular function using tissue Doppler imaging in infants with pulmonary hypertension. Neonatology 2009;96(3):193–9.

66. Peterson A, Deatsman S, Frommelt MA, et al. Correlation of echocardiographic markers and therapy in persistent pulmonary hypertension of the newborn. Pediatr Cardiol 2009;30(2):160–5.

67. Tingay D, Kinsella JP. Heart of the matter? Early ventricular dysfunction in congenital diaphragmatic hernia. Am J Respir Crit Care Med 2019;200(12): 1462–4.

68. Patel N, Lally PA, Kipfmueller F, et al. Ventricular dysfunction is a critical determinant of mortality in congenital diaphragmatic hernia. Am J Respir Crit Care Med 2019;200(12):1522–30.

69. Dao D, Patel N, Harting MT, et al. Early left ventricular dysfunction and severe pulmonary hypertension predict adverse outcomes in "low-risk" congenital diaphragmatic hernia. Pediatr Crit Care Med 2020;21(7):637–46.

70. Jain A, Mohamed A, El-Khuffash A, et al. A comprehensive echocardiographic protocol for assessing neonatal right ventricular dimensions and function in the transitional period: normative data and z scores. J Am Soc Echocardiogr 2014; 27(12):1293–304.

71. Aggarwal S, Natarajan G. Echocardiographic correlates of persistent pulmonary hypertension of the newborn. Early Hum Dev 2015;91:285–9.

72. Breinig S, Dicky O, Ehlinger V, et al. Echocardiographic parameters predictive of poor outcome in persistent pulmonary hypertension of the newborn (PPHN): preliminary results. Pediatr Cardiol 2021;42(8):1848–53.

73. Musewe N, Poppe D, Smallhorn JF, et al. Doppler echocardiographic measurement of pulmonary artery pressure from ductal Doppler velocities in the newborn. J Am Coll Cardiol 1990;15(2):446–56.

74. Bo B, Pugnaloni F, Licari A, et al. Ductus arteriosus flow predicts outcome in neonates with congenital diaphragmatic hernia. Pediatr Pulmonol 2023;58(6): 1711–8.

75. Siefkes H, Lakshminrusimha S. Management of systemic hypotension in term infants with persistent pulmonary hypertension of the newborn (PPHN) - an illustrated review. Arch Dis Child Fetal Neonatal Ed 2021;106(4):446–55.

76. Tworetzky W, Bristow J, Moore P, et al. Inhaled nitric oxide in neonates with persistent pulmonary hypertension. Lancet 2001;357:118–20.

77. Creagh-Brown B, Griffiths MJD, Evans TW. Bench-to-bedside review: inhaled nitric oxide therapy in adults. Crit Care 2009;13(3):221.

78. Polglase G, Morley CJ, Crossley KJ, et al. Positive end-expiratory pressure differentially alters pulmonary hemodynamics and oxygenation in ventilated, very premature lambs. J Appl Physiol 2005;99:1453–61.

79. Reller M, Donovan EF, Kotagal UR. Kotagal UR Influence of airway pressure waveform on cardiac output during positive pressure ventilation of healthy newborn dogs. Pediatr Res 1985;19:337–41.

80. McNamara P, Laique F, Muang-In S, et al. Milrinone improves oxygenation in neonates with severe persistent pulmonary hypertension of the newborn. J Crit Care 2006;21:217–22.
81. James A, Corcoran JD, McNamara PJ, et al. The effect of milrinone on right and left ventricular function when used as a rescue therapy for term infants with pulmonary hypertension. Cardiol Young 2016;26:90–9.
82. El-Khuffash A, McNamara PJ, Breatnach C, et al. The use of milrinone in neonates with persistent pulmonary hypertension of the newborn - a randomised controlled trial pilot study (MINT 1): study protocol and review of literature. Matern Health Neonatol Perinatol 2018;4:24.
83. Cochius-den Otter S, Schaible T, Greenough A, et al, CDH EURO Consortium. The CoDiNOS trial protocol: an international randomised controlled trial of intravenous sildenafil versus inhaled nitric oxide for the treatment of pulmonary hypertension in neonates with congenital diaphragmatic hernia. BMJ Open 2019;9(11):e032122.
84. Barrington K, Finer NN, Chan WK. A blind, randomized comparison of the circulatory effects of dopamine and epinephrine infusions in the newborn piglet during normoxia and hypoxia. Crit Care Med 1995;23(23):740–8.
85. Reller M, Morton MJ, Reid DL, et al. Fetal lamb ventricles respond differently to filling and arterial pressures and to in utero ventilation. Pediatr Res 1987;22(6): 621–6.
86. Cheung P-Y, Barrington KJ, Pearson RJ, et al. Systemic, pulmonary and mesenteric perfusion and oxygenation effects of dopamine and epinephrine. Am J Respir Crit Care Med 1997;155:32–7.
87. Cheung P-Y, Barrington KJ. The effects of dopamine and epinephrine on hemodynamics and oxygen metabolism in hypoxic anesthetized piglets. Crit Care 2001;5:158–66.
88. Evora P, Pearson PJ, Schaff HV. Arginine vasopressin induces endothelium-dependent vasodilatation of the pulmonary artery. V1-receptor-mediated production of nitric oxide. Chest 1993;103(4):1241–5.
89. Rosenzweig E, Starc TH, Chen JM, et al. Intravenous arginine-vasopressin in children with vasodilatatory shock after cardiac surgery. Circulation 1999;100: II182–6.
90. Patel B, Chittock DR, Russell JA, et al. Beneficial effects of short-term vasopressin infusion during severe septic shock. Anesthesiology 2002;96:576–82.
91. Mohamed A, Nasef N, Shah V, et al. Vasopressin as a rescue therapy for pulmonary hypertension in neonates: case series. Pediatr Crit Care Med 2014;15(2): 148–54.
92. Mohamed A, Louis D, Surak A, et al. Vasopressin for refractory persistent pulmonary hypertension of the newborn in preterm neonates - a case series. J Matern Fetal Neonatal Med 2022;35(8):1475–83.
93. Boyd S, Riley KL, Giesinger RE, et al. Use of vasopressin in neonatal hypertrophic cardiomyopathy: case series. J Perinatol 2021;41:126–33.
94. Lakshminrusimha S, Russell JA, Wedgwood S, et al. Superoxide dismutase improves oxygenation and reduces oxidation in neonatal pulmonary hypertension. Am J Respir Crit Care Med 2006;174:1370–7.
95. Jeon Y, Ryu JH, Lim YJ, et al. Comparative hemodynamic effects of vasopressin and norepinephrine after milrinone-induced hypotension in off-pump coronary artery bypass surgical patients. Eur J Cardio Thorac Surg 2006;29(6):952–6.

96. Abdelazziz M, Abdelhamid HM. Terlipressin versus norepinephrine to prevent milrinone-induced systemic vascular hypotension in cardiac surgery patient with pulmonary hypertension. Ann Card Anaesth 2019;22:136–42.

97. Tourneux P, Rakza T, Bouissou A, et al. Pulmonary circulatory effects of norepinephrine in newborn infants with persistent pulmonary hypertension. J Pediatr 2008;153:345–9.

98. Yang S, Zhang L. Glucocorticoids and vascular reactivity. Curr Vasc Pharmacol 2004;2(1):1–12.

99. Patel N, Mills JF, Cheung MMH, et al. Systemic haemodynamics in infants with vein of Galen malformation: assessment and basis for therapy. J Perinatol 2007; 27:460–3.

100. Frawley G, Dargaville PA, Mitchell PJ, et al. Clinical course and medical management of neonates with severe cardiac failure related to vein of Galen malformation. Arch Dis Child Fetal Neonatal Ed 2002;87:F144–9.

101. Van Wolferen S, Marcus JT, Westerhof N, et al. Right coronary artery flow impairment in patients with pulmonary hypertension. Eur Heart J 2008;29:120–7.

102. Mirza H, Ziegler J, Ford S, et al. Pulmonary hypertension in preterm infants: prevalence and association with bronchopulmonary dysplasia. J Pediatr 2014; 165(5):909–14.e901.

103. Mourani P, Sontag MK, Younoszai A, et al. Early pulmonary vascular disease in preterm infants at risk for bronchopulmonary dysplasia. Am J Respir Crit Care Med 2015;191(1):87–95.

104. Baczynski M, Bell EF, Finan E, et al. Survey of practices in relation to chronic pulmonary hypertension in neonates in the canadian neonatal network and the national institute of child health and human development neonatal research network. Pulm Circ 2020;10(3). 2045894020937126.

105. Behere S, Alapati D, McCulloch MA. Screening echocardiography and brain natriuretic peptide levels predict late pulmonary hypertension in infants with bronchopulmonary dysplasia. Pediatr Cardiol 2019;40:973–9.

106. Krishnan U, Feinstein JA, Adatia I, et al, Pediatric Pulmonary Hypertension Network PPHNet. Evaluation and management of pulmonary hypertension in children with bronchopulmonary dysplasia. J Pediatr 2017;188:24–34.e21.

107. Méndez-Abad P, Zafra-Rodríguez P, Lubián-López S, et al. NTproBNP is a useful early biomarker of bronchopulmonary dysplasia in very low birth weight infants. Eur J Pediatr 2019;178(5):755–61.

108. Dasgupta S, Aly AM, Malloy MH, et al. NTproBNP as a surrogate biomarker for early screening of pulmonary hypertension in preterm infants with bronchopulmonary dysplasia. J Perinatol 2018;38(9):1252–7.

109. Sánchez-Becerra JC G-TR, Becerra-Becerra R, Márquez-González H, et al. Targeted neonatal echocardiography and lung ultrasound in preterm infants with chronic lung disease with and without pulmonary hypertension, screened using a standardized algorithm. Front Pediatr 2023;11:1104940.

110. Fitzgerald D, Evans N, Van Asperen P, et al. Subclinical persisting pulmonary hypertension in chronic neonatal lung disease. Arch Dis Child Fetal Neonatal Ed 1994;70:F118–22.

111. Cohen J, Nees SN, Valencia GA, et al. Sildenafil use in children with pulmonary hypertension. J Pediatr 2019;205:29–34.e21.

112. Stewart A, Brion LP. Intravenous or enteral loop diuretics for preterm infants with (or developing) chronic lung disease. Cochrane Database Syst Rev 2011;9: CD001453.

113. Baczynski M, Kelly E, McNamara PJ, et al. Short and long-term outcomes of chronic pulmonary hypertension in preterm infants managed using a standardized algorithm. Pediatr Pulmonol 2020;56:1155–64.

114. Laux D, Rocchisani M-A, Boudjemline Y, et al. Pulmonary hypertension in the preterm infant with chronic lung disease can be caused by pulmonary vein stenosis: a must-know entity. Pediatr Cardiol 2016;37(2):313–21.

115. Mahgoub L, Kaddoura T, Kameny AR, et al. Pulmonary vein stenosis of ex-premature infants with pulmonary hypertension and bronchopulmonary dysplasia, epidemiology, and survival from a multicenter cohort. Pediatr Pulmonol 2017;52(8):1063–70.

116. Giesinger R, Stanford AH, Thomas B, et al. Safety and feasibility of riociguat therapy for the treatment of chronic pulmonary arterial hypertension in infancy. J Pediatr 2023;255:224–9.e221.

117. de Freitas Martins F, Ibarra Rios D, MH FR, et al. Relationship of patent ductus arteriosus size to echocardiographic markers of shunt volume. J Pediatr 2018;202:50–5.e53.

118. De Buyst J, Rakza T, Pennaforte T, et al. Hemodynamic effects of fluid restriction in preterm infants with significant patent ductus arteriosus. J Pediatr 2012;161(3):404–8.

119. Green T, Thompson TR, Johnson DE, et al. Furosemide promotes patent ductus arteriosus in premature infants with the respiratory distress syndrome. N Engl J Med 1983;308:743–8.

120. Toyoshima K, Momma K, Nakanishi T. In vivo dilatation of the ductus arteriosus induced by furosemide in the rat. Pediatr Res 2010;67:173–6.

121. Bishnoi R, Everett AD, Ringel RE, et al. Device closure of secundum atrial septal defects in infants weighing less than 8 kg. Pediatr Cardiol 2014;35(7):1124–31.

122. de Waal K, Crendal E, Poon AC-Y, et al. The association between patterns of early respiratory disease and diastolic dysfunction in preterm infants. J Perinatol 2023;43(10):1268–73.

123. Rigotti C, Doni D, Zannin E, et al. Left ventricular diastolic function and respiratory outcomes in preterm infants: a retrospective study. Pediatr Res 2023;93(4):1010–6.

124. Seghal A, Krishnamurthy MB, Clark M, et al. ACE inhibition for severe broncho-pulmonary dysplasia – an approach based on physiology. Phys Rep 2018;6(17):e13821.

125. Stanford A, Reyes M, Rios DR, et al. Safety, feasibility, and impact of enalapril on cardiorespiratory physiology and health in preterm infants with systemic hypertension and left ventricular diastolic dysfunction. J Clin Med 2021;10:4519.

126. Galie N, Torbicki A, Barst R, et al. Guidelines on diagnosis and treatment of pulmonary arterial hypertension. the task force on diagnosis and treatment of pulmonary arterial hypertension of the european society of cardiology. Eur Heart J 2004;25(24):2243–78.

127. Shiraishi H, Yanagisawa M. Pulsed Doppler echocardiographic evaluation of neonatal circulatory changes. Br Heart J 1987;57(2):161–7.

128. Groves A, Chiesa G, Durighel G, et al. Functional cardiac MRI in preterm and term newborns. Arch Dis Child Fetal Neonatal Ed 2011;96:F86–91.

129. Koestenberger M, Ravekes W, Everett AD, et al. Right ventricular function in infants, children and adolescents: reference values of the tricuspid annular plane systolic excursion (TAPSE) in 640 healthy patients and calculation of z score values. J Am Soc Echocardiogr 2009;22(6):715–9.

130. Koestenberger M, Nagel B, Ravekes W, et al. Right ventricular performance in preterm and term neonates: reference values of the tricuspid annular peak systolic velocity measured by tissue Doppler imaging. Neonatology 2013;103(4): 281–6.
131. Patel NMA, Paria A, Stenhous EJ, et al. Early postnatal ventricular dysfunction is associated with disease severity in patients with congenital diaphragmatic hernia. J Pediatr 2018;203:400–7.
132. Jain A, El-Khuffash AF, Kuipers BCW, et al. Left ventricular function in healthy term neonates during the transitional period. J Pediatr 2017;182:197–203.e192.
133. Ha KSCB, Lee EH, Shin J, et al. Chronological echocardiographic changes in healthy term neonates within postnatal 72 hours using Doppler studies. J Korean Med Sci 2018;33(22):e155.
134. de Waal K, Costley N, Phad N, et al. Left ventricular diastolic dysfunction and diastolic heart failure in preterm infants. Pediatr Cardiol 2019;40:1709–15.
135. Rios DR, Martins FF, El-Khuffash A, et al. Early role of the atrial-level communication in premature infants with patent ductus arteriosus. J Am Soc Echocardiogr 2021;34(4):423–432 e421.
136. Pena JLB, Faria SCC, Salemi VMC, et al. Quantification of regional left and right ventricular deformation indices in healthy neonates by using strain rate and strain imaging. J Am Soc Echocardiogr 2009;22(4):369–75.
137. Bulbul Z, Issa Z, Siblini G, et al. Normal range of left ventricular strain, dimensions and ejection fraction using three-dimensional spechkle-tracking echocardiography in neonates. J Cardiovasc Echogr 2015;25(3):57–71.
138. Chandrasekharan P, Rawat M, Lakshminrusimha S. How do we monitor oxygenation during the management of PPHN? Alveolar, arterial, mixed venous oxygen tension or peripheral saturation? Children 2020;7(10):180.

Oxygen Targets in Neonatal Pulmonary Hypertension

Individualized, "Precision-Medicine" Approach

Satyan Lakshminrusimha, MD[a],*, Steven H. Abman, MD[b]

KEYWORDS

- Oxygen saturation • Alveolar oxygen • Pulmonary vascular resistance
- Superoxide anions

KEY POINTS

- Alveolar oxygen tension is the primary determinant of pulmonary vascular resistance.
- Hypoxemia (preductal $Pao_2 \leq 49$ mm Hg or $SpO_2 \leq 89\%$) is associated with hypoxic pulmonary vasoconstriction.
- Hyperoxemia (preductal $Pao_2 > 100$ mm Hg or $SpO_2 \geq 99\%$) can lead to oxidative stress.
- Maintaining preductal SpO_2 between 90% and 97% and Pao_2 between 50 and 80 mm Hg results in low pulmonary vascular resistance in most patients with pulmonary hypertension.
- Every patient is unique, and optimal oxygen targets may vary between one patient to another and within a given patient based on changing pathophysiology.

INTRODUCTION

Oxygen is a specific and potent pulmonary vasodilator. At the microvascular level, hypoxic pulmonary vasoconstriction (HPV) is physiologically protective mechanism that limits blood flow to a diseased alveolus, thereby preserving optimal ventilation–perfusion (V/Q) matching.[1,2] With global hypoxia or when several segments of the lung suffer from alveolar hypoxia due to heterogeneous parenchymal lung disease, pulmonary vascular resistance (PVR) increases, resulting in pulmonary hypertension (PH). Primary vascular pathology resulting in pulmonary vasoconstriction and remodeling can also lead to PH without parenchymal lung disease.[3]

The etiology of PH varies with age.[3] Persistent PH of the newborn (PPHN) or acute PH (aPH) among late preterm, term, and post-term infants is secondary to a variety of

---

[a] Department of Pediatrics, University of California, UC Davis Children's Hospital, 2516 Stockton Boulevard, Sacramento, CA 95817, USA; [b] Department of Pediatrics, The Pediatric Heart Lung Center, University of Colorado Anschutz Medical Campus, Mail Stop B395, 13123 East 16th Avenue, Aurora, CO 80045, USA
* Corresponding author.
E-mail address: slakshmi@ucdavis.edu

Clin Perinatol 51 (2024) 77–94
https://doi.org/10.1016/j.clp.2023.12.003   perinatology.theclinics.com
0095-5108/24/© 2023 Elsevier Inc. All rights reserved.

causes such as birth asphyxia, meconium aspiration syndrome (MAS), pneumonia, respiratory distress syndrome (RDS), and congenital diaphragmatic hernia (CDH).[4] Among preterm infants, it is secondary to delayed transition or RDS during the first week or due to bronchopulmonary dysplasia (BPD) in the postneonatal period.[5] The underlying cause of PH, gestational age, and critical antenatal and postnatal determinants play key roles in determining the optimal oxygen target range and likely contribute to intersubject variability regarding the pulmonary vascular response to hypoxia.

GOALS OF OXYGEN THERAPY

Supplemental oxygen is commonly used in diverse clinical settings, including intensive care units (ICUs), hospital wards and as chronic therapy in outpatients. The primary purpose of oxygen therapy is to optimize oxygen delivery to the tissues while minimizing concerns regarding oxidative stress due to excessive supplemental oxygen.[6] Inadequate tissue oxygen delivery promotes anaerobic metabolism leading to lactic acidosis and reduces adenosine triphosphate (ATP) production from glucose. In patients with PH, oxygen therapy increases alveolar P_{AO_2} and prevents HPV.[1] Reduction of PVR in these patients reduces right ventricular afterload. Among neonates, infants, and children, optimal oxygenation is necessary to promote growth. Supplemental oxygen and prevention of sleep-associated hypoxemia improve growth in infants with BPD.[7]

Although arterial Pao_2 is the gold standard for assessing oxygenation, it is invasive, requires arterial access, and can only be assessed intermittently. Oxygen saturation assessment by pulse oximetry (SpO_2) provides a continuous, noninvasive assessment of oxygenation but has limitations requiring periodic Pao_2 assessment, and these limitations will be discussed later in this article. In each individual patient, evaluation of Fio_2, Pao_2, SpO_2, and regional oxygenation (rSO_2) by near-infrared spectroscopy (NIRS) provides information assesses oxygenation from different angles.[8] In order to identify an optimal oxygen target, we have to determine the lower and upper limits using physiologic principles and clinical outcomes.

Lower Limit of Oxygen Target Range

Two physiologic factors determine the lower limit of oxygenation: oxygen delivery to tissues and increasing PVR due to HPV, with detrimental effects of high PVR on cardiac output.

Oxygen consumption versus delivery and the "critical point"

To maintain aerobic metabolism and generate ATP, cells need a constant supply of oxygen. Hypoxia (inadequate delivery of oxygen to tissues) should be differentiated from hypoxemia (low Pao_2 levels). For example, a normal fetus is relatively hypoxemic (by postnatal standards) but is not hypoxic. Oxygen delivery to the tissues (DO_2) can be mathematically calculated as follows:

DO_2 = Arterial oxygen content (CaO_2) × Cardiac output (typically, 231 ± 38 mL/kg/min in term neonates)[9]; Cardiac output = stroke volume × heart rate.

CaO_2 = Hemoglobin (Hb) × SaO_2 × 1.39 mL + (Pao_2 × 0.003); in term infants with Hb of 15 g/dL, SaO_2 of 95%, and Pao_2 of 60 mm Hg, CaO_2 = 15 × 0.95 × 1.39 + (60 × 0.003) = 19.8 + 0.18 = 19.98 mL O_2/100 mL of blood. These calculations suggest that DO_2 may be approximately 35 to 46 mL/kg/min (20 mL/100 mL × 230 mL/kg/min) in neonates. It is clear from this equation that Hb and SaO_2 along with blood flow play a more important role than Pao_2 in determining DO_2.[6]

Under physiologic circumstances, the DO_2 exceeds oxygen consumption by the tissues (Vo_2, typically ~4 mL/100 mL of blood) by four- to fivefold (**Fig. 1**). When DO_2 decreases (secondary to reduced heart rate, stroke volume, blood flow, Hb, or SaO_2), compensatory mechanisms such as changes in Hb affinity, capillary recruitment, and hypoxic systemic regional vasodilation try to support normal Vo_2.[6] The point at which these compensatory mechanisms fail to meet tissue oxygen requirements is termed critical oxygen delivery point (DO_2-crit). Below this point, a decrease in DO_2 results in a fall in Vo_2 and serum lactate increases with a rapid decrease in rSO_2 (see **Fig. 1**).[6] The precise DO_2-crit in humans is not known. In adult human volunteers, a reduction in Hb to 4.8 ± 0.2 g/dL and DO_2 from 14 ± 2.9 to 7.3 ± 0.1 mL/kg/min did not result in lactic acidosis suggesting that DO_2-crit is lower than this value.[10] In one postoperative adult patient with severe anemia, the investigators estimated the DO_2-crit to be approximately 4.9 mL/kg/min while fully ventilated, sedated, and paralyzed.[11,12] To our knowledge, there are no studies evaluating DO_2-crit in human neonates. Mathematical translation of DO_2-crit to a Pao_2 or SaO_2 value is difficult as cardiac output and Hb vary among patients.

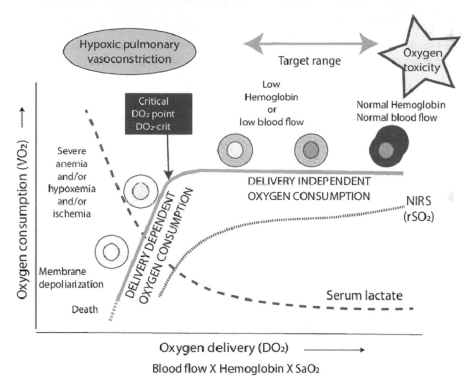

Fig. 1. The oxygen consumption (Vo_2) versus delivery (DO_2) curve. The horizontal portion of the curve depicts "delivery-independent oxygen consumption" as decrease in DO_2 does not impact Vo_2 and metabolism remains aerobic without lactic acidosis (*black hyphenated line*). However, during this phase with decreasing DO_2, regional oxygen saturation (rSO_2) measured by near-infrared spectroscopy (NIRS) decreases due to increased oxygen extraction with decreasing DO_2. Once oxygen delivery falls below the critical point (DO_2-crit), oxygen consumption decreases, and this sloped portion of the curve represents "delivery-dependent oxygen consumption." Lactic acid rapidly increases and rSO_2 markedly decreases during this phase. (Image Courtesy of Dr. Satyan Lakshminrusimha. Modified from references.[65,66])

Fetal hemoglobin and oxygen delivery

Newborn infants (both preterm and term) have high proportion of fetal hemoglobin (HbF). The oxygen dissociation curve of HbF is shifted to the left compared with hemoglobin A (HbA) (**Fig. 2**). HbF has higher affinity to oxygen compared with HbA. Hence, it is often assumed that oxygen delivery is decreased in newborns due to the presence of HbF.[13] However, during severe hypoxemia, HbF delivers more oxygen to the tissues (see **Fig. 2**).[13,14] Peripheral, but not cerebral fractional oxygen extraction, correlates with HbF in neonates.[15–17] Maintaining high HbF may be a protective factor against retinopathy of prematurity (ROP) in preterm infants.[18] Promoting placental transfusion at birth in infants at risk for PPHN or hypoxic ischemic encephalopathy (HIE) may potentially benefit tissue oxygen delivery by increasing HbF.[19] Although the presence of HbF significantly alters the relationship between Pao_2 and SpO_2, its impact on oxygen saturation targets in PPHN is not known.

Pulmonary vascular resistance, "change point" for hypoxic pulmonary vasoconstriction

The site of HPV is not clear but is considered to be the precapillary pulmonary arteriole (**Fig. 3**).[2] In neonatal animal models, pulmonary veins may also contribute to PVR and HPV.[20,21] The primary determinant of oxygen tension in these vessels is alveolar P_{AO_2} (see **Fig. 3**).[22] However, P_{AO_2} within each region of the lung cannot be measured and, in the absence of shunts, correlates well with preductal Pao_2. Hence, preductal Pao_2

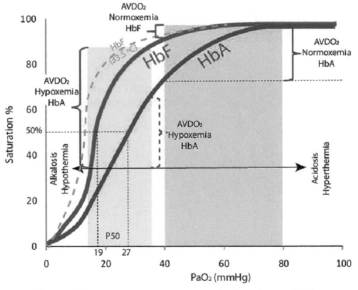

Fig. 2. Impact of hemoglobin type, temperature, and pH on hemoglobin–oxygen dissociation curve and arterio-venous oxygen difference ($AVDO_2$). Hemoglobin A (HbA) is shown by the red line, fetal hemoglobin (HbF) by the purple line, and HbF during whole body hypothermia by the purple-dashed line. The pink zone refers to the "normoxemic" arterial Pao_2 of 80 mm Hg and venous Po_2 of 40 mm Hg. The blue zone refers to hypoxemic arterial Pao_2 of 35 mm Hg and venous Po_2 of 15 mm Hg. P50 is the partial pressure of oxygen at 50% oxygen saturation and is 19 mm Hg for HbF and 27 mm Hg for HbA. (*Modified from* Polin R, Abman SH, Rowitch DH, Benitz WE. *Fetal and Neonatal Physiology, 2-Volume Set.* Vol 2: Elsevier; 2021, Chapter 109 – Developmental erythropoiesis by Timothy M. Bahr and Robin K. Ohls.)

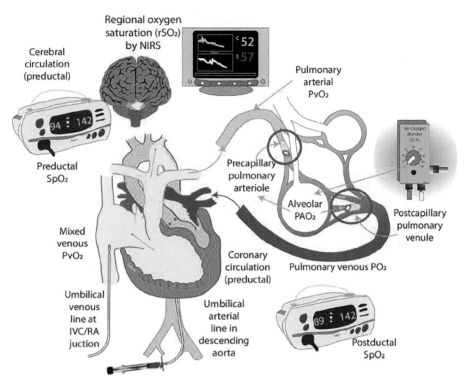

Fig. 3. Site of hypoxic pulmonary vasoconstriction (HPV) and different measures of oxygenation in neonates. The precapillary pulmonary arterioles and possibly the postcapillary venules are thought to be the sensing site for HPV (red circles). The oxygen tension in these vessels is determined mainly by alveolar PAO_2 and to a lesser extent by pulmonary arterial (or mixed venous) Po_2. Clinically, preductal and postductal Pao_2 and SpO_2 can be measured along with cerebral regional SO_2 (rSO_2). Of these values, preductal Po_2 (or SpO_2) correlates closely with alveolar PAO_2. (*Modified from* Chandrasekharan et al.[8] Image courtesy of Dr Satyan Lakshminrusimha.)

to PVR relationship is studied in translational studies. Pulmonary arterial Po_2 (similar to mixed venous Po_2) also plays a role in determining HPV.[22]

In 1966, Rudolph and Yuan instrumented newborn calves to measure PVR and ventilated them with different Fio_2 and plotted Pao_2 against PVR. When Pao_2 decreased below 45 to 50 mm Hg, there was an increase in PVR.[23] The Pao_2 (or SpO_2) value below which PVR increases is called the "change point" (**Fig. 4**). Studies in control lambs demonstrated a similar change point of 52.5 ± 1.7 mm Hg.[24,25] In lambs with PPHN induced by antenatal ductal ligation, the change point was higher at 59.6 ± 15.3 mm Hg (see **Fig. 4**).[24] Using preductal SpO_2 (instead of Pao_2), in lamb models of PPHN induced by asphyxia, and meconium aspiration or antenatal ductal ligation, the change point was approximately 90% (**Fig. 5A**). PVR was lowest with preductal SpO_2 between 90% and 97%.[26] Rawat and colleagues randomized term lambs with asphyxia induced by umbilical cord occlusion and meconium aspiration and PPHN into preductal SpO_2 target groups of 85% to 89%, 90% to 94%, 95% to 99% and inspired oxygen of 100%.[27] Pulmonary blood flow was significantly lower in the 85% to 89% SpO_2 target group. PVR was lowest in the 95% to 99% target group, but these lambs achieved median SpO_2 of 95% (IQR: 93%–97%). These

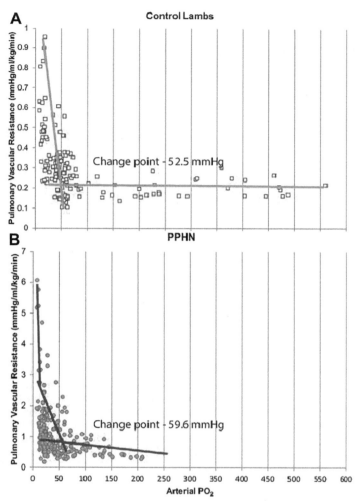

Fig. 4. Change point in the Pao$_2$ and PVR relationship. Data from control lambs (A) and lambs with PPHN induced by antenatal ductal ligation (B). Pao$_2$ values are low and PVR is high in lambs with PPHN. (*Modified from* Refs.[24,25])

results suggest that preductal SpO$_2$ in the low-to-mid 90s is associated with lowest PVR in animal models of PPHN.

Clinical observations

There are no clinical trials in newborn infants to determine the lower limit of oxygen target range in PPHN. However, among preterm infants, in the multinational NeOProM randomized controlled trials, targeting SpO$_2$ in the 85% to 89% range is associated with higher mortality compared with 91% to 95%.[28–30] Some of these trials excluded infants with PPHN and PH was not a prespecified outcome. Among centers that increased their SpO$_2$ target range from 88% to 92% to 90% to 95% or from 85% to 94% to 88% to 94% and 90% to 95% in response to NeOProM study results showed a decline in the incidence of PH among preterm infants.[31,32] Cardiac catheterization studies among infants with BPD suggest that targeting SpO$_2$ in the 92% to 94% range reduces pulmonary arterial pressures.[33,34] These clinical observations suggest that

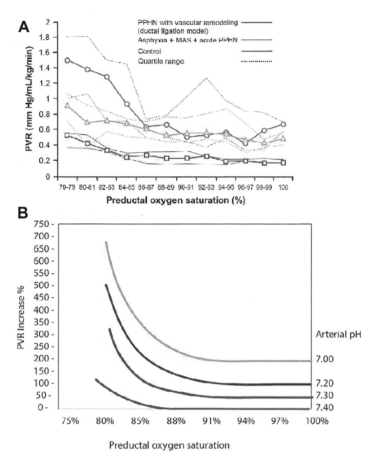

Fig. 5. Oxygen saturation and pulmonary vascular resistance (PVR). (*A*) Preductal SpO₂ plotted against PVR in three models of neonatal lambs. Red squares—control lambs delivered by elective cesarean section; green triangles—asphyxia by umbilical cord occlusion with meconium aspiration syndrome and PPHN; blue circles—PPHN induced by antenatal ductal ligation. In all three models, preductal SpO₂ between 90% and 97% is associated with low PVR. (*B*) Hypothetical figure showing the relationship between PVR, SpO₂ and pH. Acidosis exacerbates hypoxic pulmonary vasoconstriction (HPV). As pH decreases, the change point (SpO₂ below which PVR increases) increases and the degree of HPV markedly increases.[23,26,67]

the proposed target of 90% to 97% SpO₂ based on animal models of PPHN may be reasonable based on limited clinical data.

Arterial pH and lower limit of SpO₂/Pao₂ target. Acidosis exacerbates HPV (**Fig. 5B**). The degree of HPV and the Pao₂ change point both increase with lower pH.[23] Studies in newborn calves have shown that when pH less than 7.25, hypoxia induced by ventilation with 10% oxygen markedly increases PVR. However, when pH is greater than 7.3, 10% oxygen ventilation results in minimal increase in PVR compared with 100% oxygen ventilation (**Fig. 6**). A secondary analysis of data from studies in asphyxiated lambs with meconium aspiration shows that combination of hypoxemia (preductal Pao₂ < 50 mm Hg) and acidosis (pH < 7.25) results is marked exacerbation of HPV (**Fig. 7**). These studies show the importance of maintaining pH greater than 7.25 in the

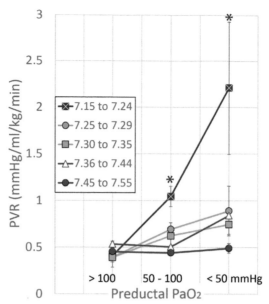

Fig. 6. Effect of ventilation with 10% (blue zones) and 100% oxygen (pink zones) on PVR (triangles plotted on primary vertical axis) and Pao_2 (circles plotted on secondary vertical axis) in newborn calves. Although Pao_2 levels with 10% oxygen ventilation are low (blue circles), the pulmonary vascular resistance (PVR) is low when pH is approximately 7.35 and high when it is < 7.25. (*Data from* Rawat et al.[27])

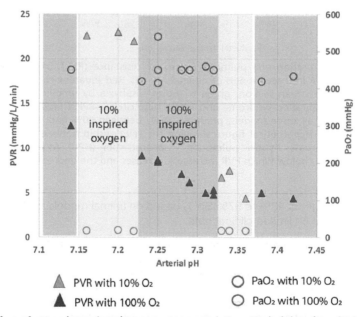

Fig. 7. Effect of pH on hypoxic pulmonary vasoconstriction. Pooled data from 30 lambs with acute MAS and asphyxia ventilated with varying Fio_2 from 0.21 to 1.0 sorted by pH and right carotid arterial Pao_2. Data are shown as mean ± SEM. Arterial pH < 7.25 markedly increases HPV. (*Data derived from* Rudolph et al.[23])

presence of hypoxemia in PPHN. The European Pediatric Pulmonary Vascular Disease Network recommends preductal SpO_2 between 91% and 95% and avoid hypoxemia (SpO_2 < 85%) or hyperoxemia (SpO_2 > 97%) with a pH greater than 7.25 during management of suspected or established PPHN.[35]

Other factors influencing the lower limit of oxygen target
Two key factors that determine the lower limit of oxygen target are the critical DO_2 point and the "change-point" for HPV (see **Figs. 1** and **4**). For most newborn infants, the change point for HPV is probably higher than the critical DO_2 point and is the main determinant of the lower limit of Pao_2 or SpO_2 target range. Based on the previous discussion with animal data, this limit seems to be a preductal SpO_2 of approximately 89% to 90% (see **Fig. 5A**) or a preductal Pao_2 of 45 to 50 mm Hg (slightly higher in PPHN). A couple of exceptions to this lower limit are explained as follows.

Fio_2 versus Pao_2 versus SpO_2. The limit for SpO_2 during the management of PPHN is partly dependent on Fio_2 and Pao_2. Infants showing signs of aPH on echocardiogram need adequate alveolar Pao_2 to minimize HPV.[2] Balancing the risk of pulmonary free radical injury with the risk of HPV may result in specific limits of SpO_2 in each patient and also at different times in a given patient (precision medicine approach). For example, in a patient with MAS and labile oxygenation due to PPHN, we recommend preductal SpO_2 range of 90% to 97%. If this patient is being ventilated with Fio_2 of 0.85 and has preductal SpO_2 of 90%, it may be better to tolerate the current settings to minimize the risk of free radical injury to the lung (the risk of free radical injury out-weighs the benefit of slightly higher Pao_2, Pao_2, or SpO_2 on pulmonary vasculature). In contrast, if this patient is on Fio_2 of 0.3 and experiencing severe PH and has preductal SpO_2 of 90%, it may be appropriate to increase Fio_2 to 0.4 to achieve SpO_2 in the 93% to 97% range to minimize the risk of HPV (the benefit of higher Pao_2, SpO_2, or Pao_2 on pulmonary vasculature outweighs the risk of oxidative stress). In this circumstance, increasing the lower limit of SpO_2 to 93% is justified.

Occult hypoxemia, skin pigmentation, and lower SpO_2 limit
During the COVID-19 pandemic, concerns were expressed on the accuracy of pulse oximetry among Black adults and individuals with dark skin pigmentation.[36] Occult hypoxemia defined as SpO_2 greater than 90% (or 92% in some studies) when arterial blood gas and SaO_2 by co-oximetry was below 88% (or 85% in some studies) was noted to be more common among Black adults compared with White adults. Similar concerns have been expressed among preterm infants[37] and children.[38] The incidence of occult hypoxemia was 56.3% among White and 69.8% among Black children when the SpO_2 values were 88% to 91%. At the current recommended SpO_2 range of 92% to 96%, occult hypoxemia was observed in 13.4% of White and 29.3% of Black children. Maintaining SpO_2 greater than 96% eliminated the difference in the incidence of occult hypoxemia between White and Black children (2.5% and 2.6%, respectively).[38] These findings suggest that the lower limit of SpO_2 target range may need to be higher in Black children.[39] Prospective trials evaluating the impact of skin pigmentation on pulse oximetry in the NICU are currently under investigation (Siefkes and colleagues, Racial disparities in accuracy of pulse oximetry, RO3HD106138). Evaluation of other factors associated with race that might influence SpO_2 in addition to skin pigmentation (such as hemoglobinopathies) will be required along with new technologies that can correct for variations in skin pigmentation. The higher incidence of neonatal conditions that are associated with hypoxemia (PPHN and necrotizing enterocolitis) among Black children and conditions associated

with hyperoxemia (ROP) among White children may potentially be due to impact of skin pigmentation on pulse oximetry.[39]

Anemia and hemoglobin type

Oxygen delivery to the tissues is based on arterial oxygen content (CaO_2) and both low Hb and low SaO_2 decrease CaO_2. Neonates with anemia may have less tolerance for a lower target SpO_2. In the SUPPORT trial, death before discharge in the lower SpO_2 target (85%–89%) arm was greater than the higher target (90%–94%), but this difference in survival was only evident after the first few postnatal weeks.[40] It has been speculated that decrease in Hb levels with time and switch from HbF to HbA with transfusions might have contributed to higher mortality after the first 2 weeks in the 85% to 89% target SpO_2 arm.[41] However, there was no difference in mortality or neurodevelopmental outcomes in a study on different transfusion thresholds among preterm infants.[42] We recommend maintaining Hb levels $\geq$ 12 g/dL during management of severe PPHN to optimize DO_2 and minimize lactic acidosis.

Upper Limit of Oxygen Target Range

Compared with physiologic factors determining the lower limit of oxygen target range (HPV and critical DO_2), the upper limit of oxygen target range is based on the risk of oxygen toxicity such as development of ROP and BPD in preterm infants. There are no similar conditions associated with oxygen toxicity in late-preterm and term infants. Evidence for oxygen toxicity at term gestation mainly comes from observational studies and animal models.

Oxygen toxicity and lung

We speculate that free radical formation is mainly mediated by partial pressure of oxygen as it creates a gradient for diffusion into mitochondria. The lung is exposed to the highest Po_2 among all the organs in the body and is subject to free radical injury. High inspired oxygen, especially $\sim$100% can increase free radical formation in the lungs,[43] increase pulmonary arterial contractility,[44] and impair inhaled nitric oxide (iNO)-mediated pulmonary vasodilation.[24] Interestingly, the inhibition of iNO-mediated decrease in PVR is related to high Fio_2 and not to hyperoxemia (high Pao_2), as lambs in this study had PPHN and low Pao_2 levels (40 $\pm$ 5 mm Hg) despite 100% inspired oxygen. The increased pulmonary arterial contractility was reversed by both in vitro[43] and in vivo treatment with superoxide dismutase[45] suggesting that it may be mediated by superoxide anion formation. The American Heart Association (AHA) and American Thoracic Society (ATS) caution that extreme hyperoxia (Fio_2 > 0.6) may be ineffective owing to extrapulmonary shunt in PPHN and aggravate lung injury.[46]

The use of higher SpO_2 targets (90%–94% vs 85%–89%) is associated with increased incidence of ROP among preterm infants.[28,30,47] Among preterm infants with pre-threshold ROP randomization to 96% to 99% SpO_2 (compared with 89%–94%) prolonged duration of oxygen need (46.8 vs 37%), hospitalization at 50 weeks postmenstrual age (12.7 vs 6.8%), and diuretic use (35.8 vs 24.4%). Pneumonia and exacerbations of BPD were more common in the supplemental oxygen arm (13.2 vs 8.5%).[48] Although these findings suggest that pulmonary toxicity of SpO_2 targets in the high 90s in preterm infants, we do not have similar data in late preterm and term infants.

Oxygen toxicity and the brain

Hypoxia causes cerebral vasodilation, and hyperoxia is associated with cerebral vasoconstriction.[49,50] Among term infants with perinatal acidosis, it is important to avoid high Pao_2 (especially >100 mm Hg) as it has been associated with increased incidence of HIE (58% vs 27%).[51] Among the neonates with signs suggestive of moderate-to-severe HIE during the first six postnatal hours, those with hyperoxemia (defined as $Pao_2 > 100$ mm Hg) had a higher incidence of abnormal brain MRI findings consistent with HIE (79% vs 33%) compared with those with $Pao_2 \leq 100$ mm Hg.[51] Although causation cannot be implied, this association suggests that perinatal asphyxia combined with postnatal hyperoxemia may potentially increase secondary free-radical mediated injury in HIE. Hence, high preductal SpO_2 ($\sim$99–100%) should be avoided, and periodic arterial blood gas evaluation may need to be conducted in infants with perinatal acidosis and HIE.

Additional factors influencing oxygen target range

a. Underlying lung disease: The phenotype of aPH secondary to pulmonary vasoconstriction is commonly managed with preductal SpO_2 range of 90% to 97% with a pH greater than 7.25. Management of PPHN associated with CDH and preterm PH (with RDS or BPD) may need different target SpO_2 levels.
   i. CDH: The European guidelines for management of PPHN in CDH recommend preductal SpO_2 of 80% to 95% in the delivery room, greater than 70% (if slowly improving) in the first two postnatal hours and 85% to 95% in the neonatal intensive care unit (NICU).[52] Postductal SpO_2 of greater than 70% is tolerated provided organs are well perfused as indicated by a pH greater than 7.2, lactate less than 5 mM/L, and urine output greater than 1 mL/kg/h. Several institutional protocols (personal communication with medical directors of multiple NICUs in the US and Canada) in the United States follow similar guidelines. However, these guidelines are not based on randomized controlled trials. The lungs in infants with CDH are hypoplastic and minimizing volutrauma and oxygen toxicity by gentle ventilation[53,54] and hence slightly lower SpO_2 targets are acceptable. However, each individual patient must be carefully evaluated before determining SpO_2 targets. A preductal SpO_2 of 88% may be acceptable in an infant with CDH with a pH greater than 7.30 but requiring high Fio_2 of greater than 0.8. However, the same SpO_2 of 88% is not acceptable if the CDH infant has lactic acidosis, pH less than 7.25, Fio_2 less than 0.5 and has echocardiographic evidence of severe PPHN. This infant needs a higher Fio_2 and preductal SpO_2 greater than 90%.
   ii. BPD: The AHA/ATS guidelines for PH management recommend SpO_2 of 92% to 94% during management of BPD-PH.[46] More recently, the European guidelines for management of PH associated with BPD recommend SpO_2 of $\geq$93% for suspected PH and $\geq$95% for confirmed PH associated with BPD.[55] There is no upper limit for SpO_2 target mentioned in these guidelines. Targeting very high SpO_2 (99%–100%) may be associated with lung toxicity. There are no clinical trials evaluating optimal SpO_2 targets in BPD-PH. We recommend SpO_2 of 92% to 95% in preterm infants with PH and BPD-PH.[56]
b. Therapeutic hypothermia (TH): Approximately 25% of infants undergoing TH for moderate to severe HIE are also diagnosed with PPHN.[57] The presence of lung disease such as MAS, severe birth asphyxia requiring chest compressions and epinephrine in the delivery room, and need for high Fio_2 greater than 0.5 before onset of TH increase the risk of PPHN.[58] Hypothermia and HbF shift the hemoglobin–oxygen dissociation curve to the left (see **Fig. 2**). In the presence of aPH during TH, a preductal Pao_2 corrected for body temperature of 60 to 80 mm Hg is recommended.[59] Achieving this Pao_2 might need higher preductal SpO_2 range of 93% to 98%. Based on the previous discussion, it is important to avoid SpO_2 of 99% to 100% and Pao_2 greater than 100 mm Hg in term infants with perinatal acidosis.[51]

c. Gestational age: Although several trials have evaluated optimal SpO$_2$ targets among preterm infants, there are no randomized trials in term infants. One single-center study (POST-IT trial) is currently recruiting patients.[39] The risk of ROP and lung toxicity with BPD exacerbations clearly set an upper limit among preterm infants that should be lower than late preterm and term infants.[56] Pending future trials, it may be prudent to recommend 92% to 95% targets for PH in preterm infants and 90% to 97% SpO$_2$ in late preterm/term infants. Among preterm infants greater than 6 weeks of age with associated BPD and PH, SpO$_2$ range of 92% to 95% is probably appropriate, although a range of 92% to 97% may be considered based on ROP status. A few exceptions to these general guidelines are listed in the summary section.

STUDIES IN OLDER INFANTS, CHILDREN, AND ADULTS

There are few trials evaluating optimal SpO$_2$ targets in postneonatal age groups (**Fig. 8**). These trials include infants with bronchiolitis,[60] pediatric ICU patients[61] requiring ventilation with supplemental oxygen or acute respiratory distress syndrome

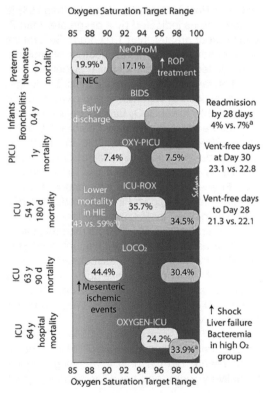

Fig. 8. Graphic representation of a few trials conducted in different age groups comparing low versus high SpO$_2$ target range. The blue ovals represent the range and mortality in the lower oxygen target group, and the pink ovals represent similar data from the higher target group. **Preterm neonatal data are** *from* **Askie and colleagues.**[28] **Data for infants with bronchiolitis are from Cunningham and colleagues.**[60] **PICU data are from the OXY-PICU trial by Peters and colleagues.**[68] **Adult studies included were ICU-ROX trial,**[69] **LOCO$_2$ trial,**[70] **and Oxy-ICU trial.**[71] [a]Significant difference between low and high SpO$_2$ target groups.

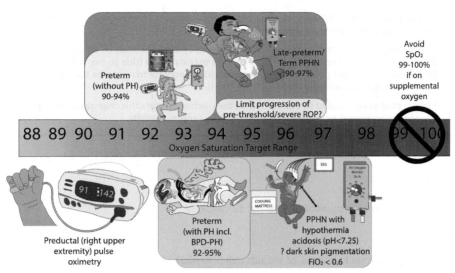

Fig. 9. Precision medicine approach to oxygen saturation targets in PPHN. Optimal preductal SpO$_2$ range based on gestational age and physiologic status is shown. BPD, bronchopulmonary dysplasia; PH, pulmonary hypertension; ROP, retinopathy of prematurity. (Image Courtesy of Dr. Satyan Lakshminrusimha.)

(ARDS) and adults admitted to ICU (see **Fig. 8**). For adult patients with ARDS, SpO$_2$ of 88% to 95% and a Pao$_2$ of 55 to 80 mm Hg are recommended.[62] At the peak of COVID-19, several pregnant women with SARS CoV-2 infection developed ARDS.[63] Societies recommended higher targets ($\geq$95%) in pregnant women with ARDS secondary to COVID-19 to optimize fetal oxygen delivery, although some investigators have suggested lower targets (92%–96%).[64]

SUMMARY

There are no randomized clinical trials guiding optimal SpO$_2$ targets in the management of PH in neonates. Based on available evidence from animal studies and expert opinion, we recommend preductal SpO$_2$ target of 90% to 97% in the management of acute PPHN in late preterm and term infants. Preterm infants without PH can be managed between 90% and 94% and those with PH between 92% and 95%. Targeting slightly higher range at 93% to 98% may be prudent in the following situations with acute severe PPHN: (1) when Fio$_2$ is less than 0.6 and risk of lung toxicity is low, (2) pH less than 7.25, (3) TH, (4) lactic acidosis, and (5) probably in patients with dark skin pigmentation. High SpO$_2$ (99%–100%) values should be avoided in most patients on supplemental oxygen (**Fig. 9**). In conclusion, every neonate with PPHN must be approached individually (precision medicine approach) and a SpO$_2$ target range determined based on current pathophysiological status. More translational studies and clinical trials are desperately needed to evaluate optimal SpO$_2$ and Pao$_2$ range in neonatal PH.

Best Practice Box

- In term infants with PPHN, preductal oxygen saturation between 90% and 97% is recommended based on its association with low PVR based on animal studies.

- In preterm infants (without pulmonary hypertension), saturation targets between 90% and 94% are associated with lower mortality but higher incidence of ROP in multicenter trials.

- Preterm infants with BPD-PH, slightly higher SpO_2 targets between 92% and 95%, are recommended to prevent episodes of hypoxemia.
- In the presence of acidosis (pH < 7.25), whole-body hypothermia, in infants with dark pigmentation and when the risk of lung oxygen toxicity is low (due to Fio_2 < 0.6), it may be prudent to consider preductal SpO_2 between 93% and 98% to minimize the risk of occult hypoxemia and hypoxic pulmonary vasoconstriction.
- Further studies are needed to evaluate short-term echocardiographic changes and long-term neurodevelopmental outcomes with various SpO_2 targets in PPHN.

DISCLOSURE

The authors have no conflict of interest to disclose.

FUNDING

Funded by National Institutes of Health (NIH) - HD072929 (SL).

REFERENCES

1. Sylvester JT, Shimoda LA, Aaronson PI, et al. Hypoxic pulmonary vasoconstriction. Physiol Rev 2012;92(1):367–520.
2. Moudgil R, Michelakis ED, Archer SL. Hypoxic pulmonary vasoconstriction. J Appl Physiol 2005;98(1):390–403.
3. Simonneau G, Montani D, Celermajer DS, et al. Haemodynamic definitions and updated clinical classification of pulmonary hypertension. Eur Respir J 2019;53(1).
4. Steurer MA, Jelliffe-Pawlowski LL, Baer RJ, et al. Persistent pulmonary hypertension of the newborn in late preterm and term infants in California. Pediatrics 2017; 139(1).
5. Mirza H, Mandell EW, Kinsella JP, et al. Pulmonary vascular phenotypes of prematurity: the path to precision medicine. J Pediatr 2023;259:113444.
6. Nichols D, Nielsen ND. Oxygen delivery and consumption: a macrocirculatory perspective. Crit Care Clin 2010;26(2):239–53, table of contents.
7. Moyer-Mileur LJ, Nielson DW, Pfeffer KD, et al. Eliminating sleep-associated hypoxemia improves growth in infants with bronchopulmonary dysplasia. Pediatrics 1996;98(4 Pt 1):779–83.
8. Chandrasekharan P, Rawat M, Lakshminrusimha S. How do we monitor oxygenation during the management of PPHN? Alveolar, arterial, mixed venous oxygen tension or peripheral saturation? Children 2020;7(10).
9. Hudson I, Houston A, Aitchison T, et al. Reproducibility of measurements of cardiac output in newborn infants by Doppler ultrasound. Arch Dis Child 1990;65(1 Spec No):15–9.
10. Lieberman JA, Weiskopf RB, Kelley SD, et al. Critical oxygen delivery in conscious humans is less than 7.3 ml O2 x kg(-1) x min(-1). Anesthesiology 2000;92(2):407–13.
11. van Woerkens EC, Trouwborst A, van Lanschot JJ. Profound hemodilution: what is the critical level of hemodilution at which oxygen delivery-dependent oxygen consumption starts in an anesthetized human? Anesth Analg 1992;75(5):818–21.
12. Leone BJ, Spahn DR. Anemia, hemodilution, and oxygen delivery. Anesth Analg 1992;75(5):651–3.

13. Polin R, Abman SH, Rowitch DH, et al. Fetal and neonatal physiology, 2-volume set, vol. 2. Philadelphia, PA: Elsevier; 2021.

14. Wimberley PD. Fetal hemoglobin, 2,3-diphosphoglycerate and oxygen transport in the newborn premature infant. Scand J Clin Lab Invest Suppl 1982;160:1–149.

15. Wardle SP, Yoxall CW, Crawley E, et al. Peripheral oxygenation and anemia in preterm babies. Pediatr Res 1998;44(1):125–31.

16. Wardle SP, Yoxall CW, Weindling AM. Determinants of cerebral fractional oxygen extraction using near infrared spectroscopy in preterm neonates. J Cerebr Blood Flow Metab 2000;20(2):272–9.

17. Pritisanac E, Urlesberger B, Schwaberger B, et al. Fetal hemoglobin and tissue oxygenation measured with near-infrared spectroscopy-a systematic qualitative review. Frontiers in pediatrics 2021;9:710465.

18. Stutchfield CJ, Jain A, Odd D, et al. Foetal haemoglobin, blood transfusion, and retinopathy of prematurity in very preterm infants: a pilot prospective cohort study. Eye (Lond) 2017;31(10):1451–5.

19. Katheria AC, Clark E, Yoder B, et al. Umbilical cord milking in nonvigorous infants: a cluster-randomized crossover trial. Am J Obstet Gynecol 2023;228(2):217, e211-e214.

20. Gao Y, Raj JU. Role of veins in regulation of pulmonary circulation. Am J Physiol Lung Cell Mol Physiol 2005;288(2):L213–26.

21. Gao Y, Raj JU. Regulation of the pulmonary circulation in the fetus and newborn. Physiol Rev 2010;90(4):1291–335.

22. Lumb AB, Thomas CR. Nunn's applied respiratory physiology: chapter 6. Pulmonary circulation. 9th edition. Philadelphia, PA: Elsevier Health Sciences; 2020.

23. Rudolph AM, Yuan S. Response of the pulmonary vasculature to hypoxia and H+ ion concentration changes. J Clin Invest 1966;45(3):399–411.

24. Lakshminrusimha S, Swartz DD, Gugino SF, et al. Oxygen concentration and pulmonary hemodynamics in newborn lambs with pulmonary hypertension. Pediatr Res 2009;66(5):539–44.

25. Lakshminrusimha S, Russell JA, Steinhorn RH, et al. Pulmonary hemodynamics in neonatal lambs resuscitated with 21%, 50%, and 100% oxygen. Pediatr Res 2007;62(3):313–8.

26. Lakshminrusimha S, Konduri GG, Steinhorn RH. Considerations in the management of hypoxemic respiratory failure and persistent pulmonary hypertension in term and late preterm neonates. J Perinatol 2016;36(Suppl 2):S12–9.

27. Rawat M, Chandrasekharan P, Gugino SF, et al. Optimal oxygen targets in term lambs with meconium aspiration syndrome and pulmonary hypertension. Am J Respir Cell Mol Biol 2020;63(4):510–8.

28. Askie LM, Darlow BA, Finer N, et al. Association between oxygen saturation targeting and death or disability in extremely preterm infants in the neonatal oxygenation prospective meta-analysis collaboration. JAMA 2018;319(21):2190–201.

29. Lakshminrusimha S, Manja V, Mathew B, et al. Oxygen targeting in preterm infants: a physiological interpretation. J Perinatol 2015;35(1):8–15.

30. Manja V, Saugstad OD, Lakshminrusimha S. Oxygen saturation targets in preterm infants and outcomes at 18-24 Months: a systematic review. Pediatrics 2017;139(1).

31. Laliberte C, Hanna Y, Ben Fadel N, et al. Target oxygen saturation and development of pulmonary hypertension and increased pulmonary vascular resistance in preterm infants. Pediatr Pulmonol 2019;54(1):73–81.

32. Kanaan U, Srivatsa B, Huckaby J, et al. Association of unit-wide oxygen saturation target on incidence of pulmonary hypertension in very low birthweight premature infants. J Perinatol 2018;38(2):148–53.
33. Abman SH, Wolfe RR, Accurso FJ, et al. Pulmonary vascular response to oxygen in infants with severe bronchopulmonary dysplasia. Pediatrics 1985;75(1):80–4.
34. Abman SH. Monitoring cardiovascular function in infants with chronic lung disease of prematurity. Arch Dis Child Fetal Neonatal Ed 2002;87(1):F15–8.
35. Hansmann G, Koestenberger M, Alastalo TP, et al. 2019 Updated consensus statement on the diagnosis and treatment of pediatric pulmonary hypertension: the European Pediatric Pulmonary Vascular Disease Network (EPPVDN), endorsed by AEPC, ESPR and ISHLT. J Heart Lung Transplant 2019;38(9):879–901.
36. Sjoding MW, Dickson RP, Iwashyna TJ, et al. Racial bias in pulse oximetry measurement. N Engl J Med 2020;383(25):2477–8.
37. Vesoulis Z, Tims A, Lodhi H, et al. Racial discrepancy in pulse oximeter accuracy in preterm infants. J Perinatol 2021;42(1):79–85.
38. Andrist E, Nuppnau M, Barbaro RP, et al. Association of race with pulse oximetry accuracy in hospitalized children. JAMA Netw Open 2022;5(3):e224584.
39. Siefkes H, Sunderji S, Vaughn J, et al. Factors to consider to study preductal oxygen saturation targets in neonatal pulmonary hypertension. Children 2022;9(3):396.
40. Carlo WA, Finer NN, Walsh MC, et al. Target ranges of oxygen saturation in extremely preterm infants. N Engl J Med 2010;362(21):1959–69.
41. Vali P, Underwood M, Lakshminrusimha S. Hemoglobin oxygen saturation targets in the neonatal intensive care unit: is there a light at the end of the tunnel? (1). Can J Physiol Pharmacol 2019;97(3):174–82.
42. Kirpalani H, Bell EF, Hintz SR, et al. Higher or lower hemoglobin transfusion thresholds for preterm infants. N Engl J Med 2020;383(27):2639–51.
43. Lakshminrusimha S, Steinhorn RH, Wedgwood S, et al. Pulmonary hemodynamics and vascular reactivity in asphyxiated term lambs resuscitated with 21 and 100% oxygen. J Appl Physiol (1985) 2011;111(5):1441–7.
44. Lakshminrusimha S, Russell JA, Steinhorn RH, et al. Pulmonary arterial contractility in neonatal lambs increases with 100% oxygen resuscitation. Pediatr Res 2006;59(1):137–41.
45. Lakshminrusimha S, Russell JA, Wedgwood S, et al. Superoxide dismutase improves oxygenation and reduces oxidation in neonatal pulmonary hypertension. Am J Respir Crit Care Med 2006;174(12):1370–7.
46. Abman SH, Hansmann G, Archer SL, et al. Pediatric pulmonary hypertension: guidelines from the American Heart Association and American Thoracic Society. Circulation 2015;132(21):2037–99.
47. Manja V, Lakshminrusimha S, Cook DJ. Oxygen saturation target range for extremely preterm infants: a systematic review and meta-analysis. JAMA Pediatr 2015;169(4):332–40.
48. STOP-ROP. Supplemental therapeutic oxygen for prethreshold retinopathy of prematurity (STOP-ROP), a randomized, controlled trial. I: primary outcomes. Pediatrics 2000;105(2):295–310.
49. Rosenberg AA. Regulation of cerebral blood flow after asphyxia in neonatal lambs. Stroke; A Journal of Cerebral Circulation 1988;19(2):239–44.
50. Rosenberg AA. Cerebral blood flow and O2 metabolism after asphyxia in neonatal lambs. Pediatr Res 1986;20(8):778–82.

51. Kapadia VS, Chalak LF, DuPont TL, et al. Perinatal asphyxia with hyperoxemia within the first hour of life is associated with moderate to severe hypoxic-ischemic encephalopathy. J Pediatr 2013;163(4):949–54.

52. Reiss I, Schaible T, van den Hout L, et al. Standardized postnatal management of infants with congenital diaphragmatic hernia in Europe: the CDH EURO Consortium consensus. Neonatology 2010;98(4):354–64.

53. Boloker J, Bateman DA, Wung JT, et al. Congenital diaphragmatic hernia in 120 infants treated consecutively with permissive hypercapnea/spontaneous respiration/elective repair. J Pediatr Surg 2002;37(3):357–66.

54. Gupta A, Rastogi S, Sahni R, et al. Inhaled nitric oxide and gentle ventilation in the treatment of pulmonary hypertension of the newborn–a single-center, 5-year experience. J Perinatol 2002;22(6):435–41.

55. Hansmann G, Sallmon H, Roehr CC, et al. Pulmonary hypertension in bronchopulmonary dysplasia. Pediatr Res 2021;89(3):446–55.

56. Gentle SJ, Abman SH, Ambalavanan N. Oxygen therapy and pulmonary hypertension in preterm infants. Clin Perinatol 2019;46(3):611–9.

57. Shankaran S, Laptook AR, Ehrenkranz RA, et al. Whole-body hypothermia for neonates with hypoxic-ischemic encephalopathy. N Engl J Med 2005;353(15):1574–84.

58. Lakshminrusimha S, Shankaran S, Laptook A, et al. Pulmonary hypertension associated with hypoxic-ischemic encephalopathy-antecedent characteristics and comorbidities. J Pediatr 2018;196:45–51 e43.

59. Afzal B, Chandrasekharan P, Tancredi DJ, et al. Monitoring gas exchange during hypothermia for hypoxic-ischemic encephalopathy. Pediatr Crit Care Med 2019;20(2):166–71.

60. Cunningham S, Rodriguez A, Adams T, et al. Oxygen saturation targets in infants with bronchiolitis (BIDS): a double-blind, randomised, equivalence trial. Lancet 2015;386(9998):1041–8.

61. Chang I, Thomas K, O'Neill Gutierrez L, et al. Protocol for a randomized multiple center trial of conservative versus liberal oxygenation targets in critically ill children (Oxy-PICU): oxygen in pediatric intensive care. Pediatr Crit Care Med 2022;23(9):736–44.

62. Capellier G, Barrot L, Winizewski H. Oxygenation target in acute respiratory distress syndrome. J Intensive Med 2023;3(3):220–7.

63. Lim MJ, Lakshminrusimha S, Hedriana H, et al. Pregnancy and severe ARDS with COVID-19: epidemiology, diagnosis, outcomes and treatment. Semin Fetal Neonatal Med 2023;28(1):101426.

64. Eid J, Stahl D, Costantine MM, et al. Oxygen saturation in pregnant individuals with COVID-19: time for re-appraisal? Am J Obstet Gynecol 2022;226(6):813–6.

65. Vali P, Lakshminrusimha S. The fetus can teach Us: oxygen and the pulmonary vasculature. Children 2017;4(8):67.

66. Vali P, Underwood M, Lakshminrusimha S. Hemoglobin oxygen saturation targets in the neonatal intensive care unit: is there a light at the end of the tunnel? (1). Can J Physiol Pharmacol 2018;1–9.

67. Rudolph AM. Congenital diseases of the heart: clinical-physiological considerations. 3 edition. West Sussex: John Wiley and Sons Ltd; 2009.

68. Peters MJ, Jones GAL, Wiley D, et al. Conservative versus liberal oxygenation targets in critically ill children: the randomised multiple-centre pilot Oxy-PICU trial. Intensive Care Med 2018;44(8):1240–8.

69. Investigators I-R, the A. New Zealand Intensive Care Society Clinical Trials G, et al. Conservative Oxygen Therapy during Mechanical Ventilation in the ICU. N Engl J Med 2020;382(11):989–98.
70. Barrot L, Asfar P, Mauny F, et al. Liberal or conservative oxygen therapy for acute respiratory distress syndrome. N Engl J Med 2020;382(11):999–1008.
71. Girardis M, Busani S, Damiani E, et al. Effect of conservative vs conventional oxygen therapy on mortality among patients in an intensive care unit: the oxygen-ICU randomized clinical trial. JAMA 2016;316(15):1583–9.

Inhaled Nitric Oxide in Neonatal Pulmonary Hypertension

Michael W. Cookson, MD[a,b,*], John P. Kinsella, MD[a,b]

KEYWORDS

- Inhaled nitric oxide (iNO) • Persistent pulmonary hypertension of the newborn (PPHN)
- Hypoxemic respiratory failure (HRF)

KEY POINTS

- Hypoxemic respiratory failure (HRF) associated with pulmonary hypertension (PH) is a common problem in neonatal intensive care units.
- Selective pulmonary vasodilation with inhaled nitric oxide (iNO) is safe and beneficial in near-term and term neonates with persistent PH of the newborn.
- A thorough diagnostic evaluation requires echocardiography, which is critical because iNO can be detrimental when used in infants with severe left ventricular dysfunction and congenital heart disease with ductal-dependent systemic blood flow.
- Poor responsiveness to iNO therapy in the setting of HRF can be observed in the presence of lung airway and parenchymal disease with insufficient distal lung recruitment or poor distribution of gas throughout the lung; PH that is primarily due to left-to-right extrapulmonary shunt; or in the setting of abnormal cardiac performance and impaired systemic hemodynamics.

INTRODUCTION

Three decades since the first pilot studies showed improvement in oxygenation with the use of inhaled nitric oxide (iNO) in term neonates with persistent pulmonary hypertension of the newborn (PPHN), iNO is now commonly used in the neonatal intensive care unit, and its use is being applied to varied pathologic conditions.[1,2] Subsequent large randomized trials led to the Food and Drug Administration approval of iNO in 1999 for the treatment of neonatal acute hypoxemic respiratory failure (HRF) associated with pulmonary hypertension (PH).[3,4] Due to the application of iNO to an

[a] Department of Pediatrics, Section of Neonatology, University of Colorado, Anschutz School of Medicine and Children's Hospital Colorado, Aurora, CO 80045, USA; [b] Department of Pediatrics, Pediatric Heart Lung Center, University of Colorado Anschutz School of Medicine and Children's Hospital Colorado, Aurora, CO, USA
* Corresponding author. MS8402 Room 4304, 13121 E 17th Avenue, Aurora, CO 80045-2535.
E-mail address: Michael.cookson@cuanschutz.edu

Clin Perinatol 51 (2024) 95–111
https://doi.org/10.1016/j.clp.2023.11.001   perinatology.theclinics.com

increasing number of pathologic states, we will provide a historical perspective of iNO from bench-to-bedside, briefly review the clinical state of neonatal PH, and address the use of iNO in both early and late PH.

A HISTORY: NEONATAL PULMONARY HYPERTENSION PHYSIOLOGY AND NITRIC OXIDE

In the early 1960s, the association of respiratory distress syndrome (RDS) and PH with right-to-left ductal shunting was shown in the landmark studies of Rudolph and colleagues and the clinical observations of Stahlman.[5,6] The field of neonatology has since been transformed by our ability to recognize and manage infants with PH. Various other observations led to descriptions of "persistence of the fetal circulation" characterizing the extrapulmonary right-to-left shunting across the patent ductus arteriosus (PDA) and atria in neonatal PH.[7,8] In 1976, Levin and colleagues further characterized the underlying physiology of PPHN in 6 newborns with minimal lung disease, in whom the presence of extrapulmonary right-to-left shunting at the ductus arteriosus (DA) was demonstrated by cardiac catheterization and simultaneous preductal and postductal arterial oxygen tension assessments.[9]

Soon after, PPHN pathophysiology was recognized as a syndrome not only of those infants with RDS but also involving other pathologic conditions including meconium aspiration syndrome (MAS) and congenital diaphragmatic hernia (CDH).[5,10] Two decades after Rudolph's initial observations, he provided a framework, still used today, classifying PPHN into categories originating from (1) decreased cross-sectional vascular area, (2) normal vascular development associated with increased vasoconstriction or blood viscosity, and (3) increased muscularization.[11] Although these categories are helpful, it is important to emphasize considerable overlap between these mechanisms in the clinical settings and that neonates with HRF and PH may have a pulmonary vascular bed altered by one or multiple physiologic categories. For example, babies with MAS can have striking pulmonary vascular remodeling, and changes in vascular tone and reactivity can contribute to high pulmoanry vascular resistance (PVR) in infants with suspected lung hypoplasia, as with CDH, oligohydramnios, or developmental lung diseases.[12,13]

The advent of nitric oxide (NO) as a therapeutic agent began in the 1970s, pioneered by the research groups of Drs Furchgott, Ignarro, and Murad whose work understanding the signaling axis of nitric oxide synthase (NOS)—NO—guanylate cyclase (GC)—guanosine 3'-5'-cyclic monophosphate (cGMP) was awarded the 1998 Nobel Prize in Physiology or Medicine (**Fig. 1**). The role of endothelial cell signaling arose due to a serendipitous observation made in the laboratory of Furchgott. When aortic sections were not isolated carefully, isolated systemic vessels would lose the ability to vasodilate due to apparent endothelial injury. The laboratory identified that acetylcholine-induced vasodilation was dependent on maintaining an intact endothelial lining during isolation. This endothelial-dependent relaxation was due to the production of endothelial-derived relaxation factor (EDRF).[13,14] However, the chemical structure of EDRF remained elusive. Over time, EDRF was characterized as being NO after demonstrating its ability to increase cGMP by directly stimulating soluble GC (sGC).[15,16] Building on these observations, EDRF was identified to be NO by 2 independent laboratories, both using aortic endothelial cell isolations.[15,16] The vasodilator properties of both species were also recognized to be inhibited by hemoproteins.[17] The identification of NO as the key component of EDRF combined with the knowledge that binding to hemoglobin inactivates NO, suggested that the potent vasodilatory properties of NO were limited to the local vasculature bed.

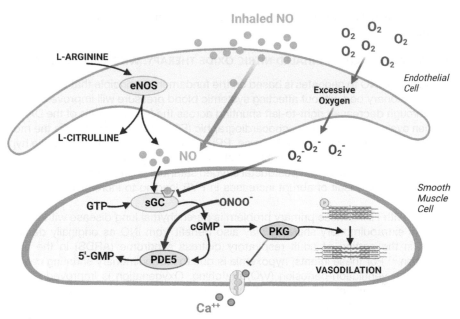

Fig. 1. Endothelial nitric oxide synthase (eNOS) is the key enzyme producing NO within the endothelial lining of the pulmonary vasculature. Endothelial nitric oxide synthase is induced by oxygen, shear stress, and increased pulmonary blood flow among others. Induction of eNOS results in elaboration of NO from L-Arginine. NO endogenous, or exogenous in the form of iNO, diffuses rapidly into the smooth muscle cell. The heme group of sGC binds NO resulting in the conversion of GTP to cGMP. Cyclic GMP stimulates cGMP-dependent protein kinase (PKG)-mediated decreases in intracellular calcium and dephosphorylation of myosin. These actions contribute to smooth muscle relaxation and vasodilation. Phosphodiesterase 5 (PDE5) inactivates cGMP. Excessive oxygen exposure can overwhelm antioxidant handling of the endothelium leading to reactive oxygen species (ROS) (O_2^-). ROS-mediated oxidation of the sGC heme group presents NO-mediated CGMP production. ROS and NO react readily to produce peroxynitrite (ONOO), which enhances PDE5 activity.

EDRF was recognized early to have a critical role in regulating pulmonary vasoreactivity in the perinatal lung. The use of perinatal lamb models taught us that not only did EDRF contribute directly to the fall in PVR during the newborn transition but also that pulmonary arteries undergo maturational changes that alter reactivity to EDRF.[18–20]

Following birth, the breathing of air reduces PVR with an associated increase in pulmonary blood flow essential to the successful transition to extrauterine physiology.[21] Both basal vascular tone and transitional decreases in PVR are dependent on endogenous NO signaling.[19,22] Endothelial nitric oxide synthase (eNOS) is the primary isoform responsible for NO production in the perinatal lung. Lung eNOS expression increases throughout gestation to prime the fetal lung vasculature for postnatal adaptation as the primary organ for gas exchange.[23,24] As with term animals, studies using preterm lambs demonstrated that the fetal pulmonary vascular bed was reactive, and that the transitional decrease in PVR was similarly mediated by endogenous NO.[19,20]

Building on this physiologic experience, gaseous NO, delivered via inhalation (iNO), was demonstrated to acutely and selectively decrease (PVR) in a lamb model of PH and adult humans with PH.[25,26] Neonatal disease models of term PPHN and preterm RDS soon followed, demonstrating that exogenous iNO could selectively dilate the pulmonary vascular bed and improve oxygenation forming the basis of early clinical neonatal trials.[22,27–30]

CLINICAL APPROACH TO INHALED NITRIC OXIDE THERAPY: WHO WILL BENEFIT?

Application of iNO to neonates is based on the fundamental principle that vasodilation of the pulmonary bed without affecting systemic blood pressure will improve oxygenation through decreased right-to-left shunting across the fetal channels of the DA and foramen ovale. Clinical and/or echocardiographic (ECHO) evidence of PH is the most important factor to define before iNO use. PPHN commonly presents with labile hypoxemia and clinical evidence of right-to-left extrapulmonary shunting, demonstrated as a gradient in preductal and postductal oxygen saturations greater than 10%. Labile hypoxemia is the result of abrupt increases in PVR leading to increased right-to-left shunting.

Infants with HRF whose primary problem is parenchymal lung disease without evidence of extrapulmonary shunting may also benefit from iNO as originally demonstrated in the setting of adult respiratory distress syndrome (ARDS) in the adult population.[31] For these infants, hypoxemia is due to intrapulmonary shunting caused by impaired ventilation-perfusion (V/Q) matching. Oxygenation is improved via the "microselective" effect of iNO originating from preferential delivery of iNO to aerated alveoli, inducing local vasodilation, and improving V/Q matching (**Fig. 2**).

The first case reports directed at improving HRF in term neonates with PPHN demonstrated rapid improvements in oxygenation without clinical signs of adverse effects, including systemic hypotension and lung injury.[1,2] Following these initial studies, additional reports of low-dose iNO being adequate to improve and sustain oxygenation were reported and led to a series of randomized trials.[12,32]

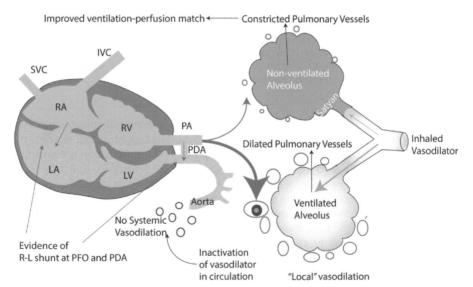

Fig. 2. Selective and microselective effect of iNO. NO after entering the pulmonary circulation is inactivated by hemoglobin (Hb) to form MetHb minimizing systemic vasodilation reducing extrapulmonary right-to-left shunt (selective effect). Inhaled NO also selectively enters ventilated alveoli leading to local vasodilation of adjacent pulmonary vessels (microselective effect) enhancing V/Q matching and reducing intrapulmonary shunt. (Copyright Satyan Lakshminrusimha.)

Multiple randomized controlled trials (RCT) have highlighted the efficacy and safety of iNO for term and near-term (>34 weeks gestational age) infants with HRF. Studies used varied definitions of HRF but most included infants with an oxygenation index greater than 25 (OI: mean airway pressure [cm H_2O] × fraction of inhaled oxygen [Fio_2] × 100 ÷ PaO_2 mm Hg) (**Table 1**). Given the safety profile of iNO, we recommend considering iNO therapy in near-term and term infants identified to have HRF, defined as an OI greater than 25. Although RCTs have not supported decreased extracorporeal membrane oxygenation (ECMO) or death when initiated at a lower OI, it is reasonable to trial iNO with less-severe HRF but only with concurrent ECHO evidence of PH.

DOSE

An appropriate starting dose is 20 ppm in near-term and term infants. The half-life of iNO is 2 to 6 seconds, and response to therapy should be evident within 30 minutes. Using criteria from the various trials, an adequate response to iNO is an increase in PaO_2 greater than 20 mm Hg.[3,33] If there is a lack of response, increasing the dose to 40 or 80 ppm is reasonable but unlikely to significantly increase oxygenation compared with lower doses.[1] These clinical observations were confirmed in neonates with PPHN showing an optimal reduction in pulmonary artery pressures with a dose of 20 ppm as assessed by right heart catheterization.[34] Prolonged exposure to 80 ppm comes with an increased risk of toxicity including methemoglobinemia (MetHb) and increased generation of reactive nitrogen species (ROS).[35]

WEANING

Once an infant has stable hemodynamics with evidence of maintained alveolar gas exchange and pulmonary blood flow, demonstrated by saturations greater than 92%, iNO can be weaned. Adequate oxygenation is demonstrated by decreasing Fio_2 to less than 0.60 while maintaining preductal PaO_2 greater than 60 mm Hg or saturations greater than 92%. Serial ECHOs are helpful to inform the decision to wean based on the resolution of suprasystemic pulmonary artery pressures and improvement in right ventricle (RV) function. Clinically stable infants may not demonstrate clinical signs of rebound PH, and serial ECHOs aid in monitoring for subtle changes during the phase of iNO weaning. We begin gradually weaning the dose at 2 to 4-hour intervals to a goal of 5 ppm. At 5 ppm, the dose is gradually weaned by 1 ppm at similar time intervals. Weaning from 5 ppm to 0 ppm has been associated with hypoxemia.[36] Such abrupt changes in iNO dose can result in "rebound vasoconstriction" causing acute hypoxemia, which is best managed by returning the iNO dose to the prior level and repeating trials at lower doses on subsequent days.

Withdrawal of iNO, even from low doses, may result in rapid hemodynamic decompensation and restarting treatment will normally improve pulmonary blood flow and systemic perfusion. It is not uncommon to observe more severe changes in PVR when weaning from 1 ppm to off than is observed during the weaning phase. Preclinical work supports that the oxidative stress incurred by prolonged oxygen exposure directly impairs sCG activity and increases phosphodiesterase 5 (PDE5) activity, contributing to increase vascular tone in the absence of iNO (see **Fig. 1**).[37,38] Given the risk of reduced endogenous signaling, constant reassessment of the clinical benefit gained from iNO is essential to ensure active weaning and reduce cost.

DURATION

The mean duration of iNO use in clinical trials was 2 to 3 days with most infants weaning off within 1 week of initiation.[3,39,40] Duration may need to be extended for individual

Table 1
Dosing, extracorporeal membrane oxygenation use, and death from multicenter, randomized control trials in near-term and term infants with hypoxemic respiratory failure

Study	Control Group	OI at Initiation of iNO	Number		Initial Dose	ECMO (%)		Mortality (%)	
			Control	iNO		Control	iNO	Control	iNO
NINOS[3] 1997	100% FiO₂	44	121	114	20	55	39[a]	17	14
Roberts et al,[39] 1997	Nitrogen gas	44	28	30	80	71	40[a]	7	7
Davidson et al,[35] 1998		25	41	114[b]	5, 20, 80	34	22	2	8
Clark et al,[80] 2000		39	122	126	20	64	38[a]	8	7
Konduri et al,[33] 2004		19	149	150	20	12	10	9	7

[a] Five studies comparing iNO to standard care with placebo gas have been reported. The most common cause presenting with HRF was MAS. Clinical or ECHO evidence of PH was not a universal inclusion criterion but all studies excluded critical CHD. Variation in ECMO utilization rates over time reflects the benefits of high-frequency ventilation and surfactant. Inhaled NO has consistently decreased ECMO use in infants with severe HRF. Studies by Davidson and Konduri enrolled infants with a lower OI and did not demonstrate a reduction in ECMO use. A decrease in mortality has not consistently been demonstrated. Significant differences defined as $P < .05$ shown with *.

[b] Davidson et al. enrolled 3 study groups to assess dose response at 5, 20, and 80 ppm, with total enrollment across all groups n = 114.

patients in the setting of pulmonary hypoplasia.[41] Prolonged need for iNO therapy without resolution of disease should lead to a more extensive evaluation to determine whether other developmental lung disease or cardiac disease is contributing to persistent elevations in PVR.

TOXICITY
Nitrogen Dioxide

NO is unstable in ambient air, reacting with oxygen to form nitrogen dioxide (NO_2), with the rate of conversion to NO_2 increasing as oxygen concentration increases.[42] Pulmonary toxicities from NO_2 include altered surfactant metabolism, epithelial dysfunction, and inflammation.[43] Despite concerns for NO_2 toxicity, standardization of real-time monitoring has led to minimal NO_2 exposure. Significant elevations in NO_2 levels have been reported only when used at NO doses greater than 40 ppm.[35]

Methemoglobinemia

Exposure of NO to circulating erythrocytes results in the formation of nitrosyl hemoglobin and rapidly becomes oxidized to MetHb. When using standard doses, the production of MetHb more than 2.5% is uncommon in near-term and term neonates.[35] It is not necessary for close monitoring of MetHb levels in these neonates at standard doses when iNO duration remains less than 5 days. Premature neonates are at an increased risk for elevated MetHb levels due to reduced expression of MetHb reductase, and monitoring of MetHb levels every few days is reasonable.[43,44]

Platelet Inhibition

NO-induced platelet dysfunction has been reported both *in vivo* and *in vitro*, raising concerns about the use of iNO in preterm neonates.[45–47] Bleeding time may be acutely increased at typical doses of iNO but is short-lived in neonates without clinical consequence.[18]

CONTRAINDICATIONS

Diligence must be maintained when considering the use of iNO because there are a few pathologies presenting with critical hypoxemia but in whom the addition of iNO will be detrimental (**Fig. 3**).

Methemoglobinemia

NO oxidation of hemoglobin from the ferrous to ferric state results in MetHb in which the oxygen binding capacity of hemoglobin is impaired, leading to a left-shifted hemoglobin oxygen dissociation curve and decreased tissue oxygen delivery. Accumulation of MetHb to greater than 10% can result in methemoglobinemia, characterized by tissue hypoxia; however, this may not be clinically apparent with cyanosis until levels reach greater than 15% to 20%. We recommend weaning iNO when MetHb levels become greater than 3%. Although rare, congenital forms of methemoglobinemia due to genetic deficiencies in cytochrome b5 reductase or cytochrome b5 may present as critical hypoxemia.[49] Oxygen carrying capacity may be further decreased if iNO is used in these neonates.

Severe Left Ventricular Dysfunction

The use of iNO for infants with HRF and evidence of left ventricular (LV) systolic or diastolic dysfunction without added measures to improve cardiac function may worsen hypoxemia (**Fig. 4**). The presence of LV dysfunction decreases antegrade pulmonary venous flow resulting in pulmonary venous hypertension, or "postcapillary" PH.

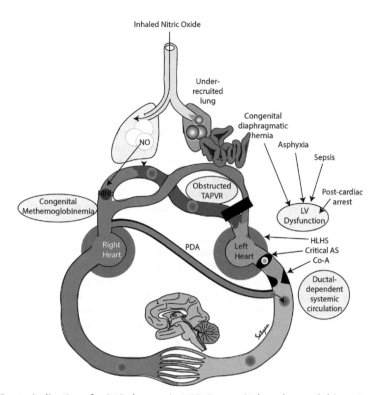

Fig. 3. Contraindications for iNO therapy in HRF. Congenital methemoglobinemia or MetHb reductase deficiency can be exacerbated by iNO therapy worsening hypoxemia. LV dysfunction and pulmonary venous hypertension are worsened by iNO due to pulmonary edema. Ductal-dependent systemic circulation as seen in hypoplastic left heart syndrome (HLHS), critical aortic stenosis (AS), or coarctation of the aorta (Co-A) maintain their systemic circulation through a right-to-left shunt across the patent ductus arteriosus (PDA). Reduced pulmonary arterial pressure by iNO abolishes this shunt and causes systemic hypoperfusion. (Copyright Satyan Lakshminrusimha.)

Pulmonary edema secondary to pulmonary venous hypertension may worsen gas exchange and contribute to increased precapillary PVR. The use of iNO can increase pulmonary artery flow but will not cause sustained improvements in oxygenation due to worsening pulmonary edema and pulmonary venous congestion. Those at risk for LV dysfunction include infants with CDH, hypoxemic-ischemic encephalopathy, sepsis, and in postcardiac arrest populations. ECHO signs suggestive of poor LV function include right-to-left ductal shunting but with left-to-right atrial shunting, mitral valve regurgitation, and left atrial dilation. Physiologic benefit may be better obtained with the use of milrinone, a phosphodiesterase 3 inhibitor, that decreases PVR, decreases LV afterload through systemic vasodilation, and can improve LV myocardial performance.[50–52] In emergent situations, a trial of iNO is warranted while awaiting ECHO evaluation. Minimal improvement in, or worsening, hypoxemia with the initiation of iNO is a sign suggestive of LV dysfunction, warranting discontinuation of iNO.

Congenital Heart Disease

Maintenance of tissue oxygen delivery in cyanotic congenital heart disease (CHD) with ductal-dependent systemic blood flow (eg, HLHS, coarctation) is reliant on right-to-left

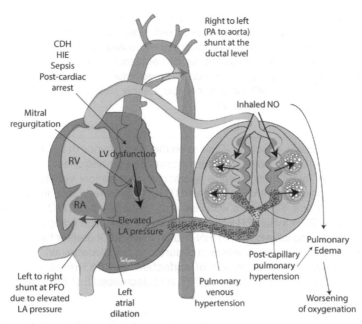

Fig. 4. Pathophysiology of LV dysfunction and pulmonary postcapillary or venous hypertension. ECHO features of LV dysfunction in PPHN include a right-to-left shunt at PDA and a left-to-right shunt at patent foramen ovale (PFO) due to elevated left atrial (LA) pressure. Use of iNO results in worsening of pulmonary edema and hypoxemia. (Copyright Satyan Lakshminrusimha.)

shunting across the DA. Prostaglandin initiated to maintain patency acts as a nonspecific vasodilator.[53] The addition of iNO in the setting of ductal-dependent CHD may significantly reduce or reverse the right-to-left shunt, resulting in decreased systemic blood flow and acute decompensation. Specific diagnoses to evaluate with ECHO before iNO use include hypoplastic left heart syndrome, critical aortic stenosis, and arch abnormalities including interrupted aortic arch or critical coarctation. As discussed earlier, worsening, or minimally changed oxygenation with the initiation of iNO may indicate LV dysfunction but may also be indicative of total anomalous pulmonary venous return (TAPVR) with obstructed pulmonary veins. Compared with LV dysfunction, TAPVR requires urgent evaluation for surgical intervention.

SUPPORTIVE MANAGEMENT OF PULMONARY HYPERTENSION

Despite the efficacy in improving oxygenation, it is clear from past studies that the benefit of iNO depends on first optimizing lung recruitment, systemic hemodynamics, and cardiac performance.[54]

Respiratory Support

Up to 40% of infants will not respond to iNO, with the most common reason for an inadequate response being poor alveolar delivery secondary to an underrecruited lung. Most infants presenting with PH have contributions from underlying lung disease. Specific ventilator strategies depend on the blend of underlying airways and lung parenchymal disease. Optimal lung recruitment to establish gas exchange and improve functional residual capacity is not only essential to treat HRF but may also mitigate the need for pulmonary vasodilator therapy. At low lung volumes, extra-alveolar pulmonary vascular compression will lead to hypoxemia, and similarly, marked hyperinflation contributes to capillary compression and intrapulmonary shunting. Some infants benefit from high-frequency ventilation to increase lung recruitment and maintain FRC while avoiding stretch-induced injury to the lung.[54–56] Following optimal lung recruitment, iNO therapy can be reliably delivered using both conventional and high-frequency ventilators.[40]

Surfactant

Because the therapeutic effect of iNO relies on the maintenance of the alveolar-capillary gas exchange interface, surfactant should be considered when chest x-rays do not support optimal lung recruitment despite aggressive mechanical ventilation. A pre-iNO multicenter randomized controlled trial (MRCT) reported a reduction in ECMO with the use of early surfactant. Surfactant was less likely to decrease ECMO use when the OI was greater than 20 or when PH was not due to lung disease (idiopathic PPHN).[57] A recent MRCT enrolling infants with PPHN and an average OI greater than 35 compared the efficacy of iNO with coadministration of surfactant or placebo (air). Compared with the placebo group, coadministration of surfactant and iNO resulted in decreased treatment failure, improved response to iNO, and decreased ECMO or death.[58]

Oxygen Therapy

During periods of acute PH, when increased right-to-left shunting and decreased left ventricular output may compromise end-organ perfusion, optimization of O_2 delivery to tissues is imperative. As such, O_2 remains the first-line therapy for acute PH. O_2 has potent vasodilator effects and causes selective pulmonary vasodilation through direct activation of calcium-activated K+ channels and enhanced NO production after birth.[59,60] However, even relatively brief periods of hyperoxia may contribute to oxidative stress, impair NO-cGMP signaling, augment inflammation and exacerbate pulmonary vascular injury.[61] In addition to improving pulmonary hemodynamics and V/Q matching, the ability of iNO to lower the need for higher levels of supplemental oxygen may indirectly protect the lung.

Augmentation of Systemic Blood Pressure

Many infants with HRF and PH present with systemic hypotension. Improvement in systemic blood pressure can reduce extrapulmonary right-to-left shunting. The degree of shunting is relative to the pressure differential between systemic and pulmonary vascular beds. Improving systemic blood pressure will reduce the right-to-left pressure gradient improving pulmonary arterial blood flow. Judicious use of vasoactive medications will reduce the untoward physiologic effects because there are variable dose responses in infants and many induce pulmonary vasoconstriction.[62]

INHALED NITRIC OXIDE BEYOND EARLY USE IN NEAR-TERM AND TERM NEONATES
Early Inhaled Nitric Oxide: Premature Neonates with Severe PPHN

The incidence of PPHN has an inverse relationship to the degree of prematurity although it may be common in extremely preterm infants.[63] A recent observational study demonstrated that iNO therapy is equally effective in improving oxygenation in preterm and term neonates.[64] Infants with suspected lung hypoplasia due to prolonged rupture of membranes or oligohydramnios are most likely to benefit.[65] Multiple case series in this population have shown improved oxygenation, leading to recommendations for selective use in preterm infants with confirmed PPHN and suspected pulmonary hypoplasia.[66–68]

In contrast to near-term and term infants, the initial starting dose of iNO in premature infants is 5 ppm.[44,69] Dose escalation to 10 ppm may be required for infants demonstrating a partial response, determined as an increase in Pao_2 10 to 20 mm Hg.[44] Higher dose, 20 ppm, has been studied in premature neonates but it is critical to address that iNO was initiated at 20 ppm after 1 week of life during which the risk for severe IVH is highest and this study did not report on acute changes in oxygenation or evidence of extrapulmonary shunting.[70]

Caution is advised both when initiating and weaning iNO in premature neonates due to rapid hemodynamic changes that contribute to an increased risk of IVH.[44] When used at studied doses of 5 to 10 ppm, RCTs have not demonstrated an increased risk for severe intraventricular hemorrhage (IVH) or bleeding, with some showing a significant reduction in severe IVH.[69,71]

Early Inhaled Nitric Oxide: Prevention of Bronchopulmonary Dysplasia

Preclinical work demonstrated improvements in lung and vascular growth, decreased inflammation, and reduced oxidant stress due to iNO exposure suggesting potential clinical benefit in preventing bronchopulmonary dysplasia (BPD).[72–74] Multiple RCTs have investigated the role of prophylactic iNO to prevent BPD but due to mixed results, iNO is not currently recommended as preventative therapy.[75] However, unlike the near-term and term studies aimed at including infants with pulmonary hypertensive physiology, none of the studies in preterm neonates utilized ECHO screening as criteria for trial entry. The mixed results of trials focused on HRF and not on pulmonary hypertensive physiology, highlight the importance of using serial ECHO studies to guide iNO therapy. Inhaled NO may have a role in decreasing BPD risk when used selectively in preterm neonates when assessed within the broader context of serial hemodynamic assessments.[76]

Late Inhaled Nitric Oxide: Pulmonary Hypertension

A subset of infants with BPD or CDH will develop late PH. Prolonged use of iNO, delivered invasively or noninvasively, to sustain low PVR, may be considered to maintain right ventricular–pulmonary artery coupling.[77] The evolution of late PH in infants with BPD or CDH is variable and complicated by acute PH episodes precipitated by physiologic stress. While improving respiratory support, iNO can be used to treat acute PH episodes but these patients may require other pulmonary vasodilator therapies, such as inhaled prostacyclin, sildenafil, or endothelin-receptor antagonists.

Stabilization During Extracorporeal Membrane Oxygenation Referral

Despite sustained improvements in oxygenation and systemic tissue oxygen delivery with iNO use, some infants may still require ECMO. In some infants who are partial or poor responders to iNO therapy, or in the setting of impaired cardiac performance, maintenance of iNO in transport may decrease hospital length of stay.[78] Delivery of iNO using various conventional and high-frequency oscillatory transport ventilators has been studied and deemed safe for both ground and air transport.[79] Before transfer, it is critical to maintain iNO delivery because discontinuation of iNO before or during transport can be detrimental even if the clinical response has been minimal.[79]

SUMMARY

Tremendous gains in our understanding of the pathologic mechanisms leading to neonatal PH, focused on NO signaling, have led to wide adoption of iNO use in neonatal care. Many studies have demonstrated the clinical benefit of iNO while high-lighting its wide safety margin in near-term and term infants. Careful patient selection based on underlying physiology and ECHO guidance will continue to support ongoing research to delineate neonatal and infant populations likely to benefit from iNO. Premature neonates with severe PH, especially with a history of prolonged rupture of membranes or oligohydramnios can benefit from iNO. Inhaled NO provides clinical stability during transport to ECMO centers and during cannulation.

ACKNOWLEDGMENTS

M.W. Cookson wrote the initial draft, designed, and integrated figures. J.P. Kinsella reviewed and edited the article. S. Lakshminrusimha edited initial drafts and added figures.

Best Practice Box

- Inhaled NO is a potent and selective pulmonary vasodilator with minimal systemic toxicity in both preterm and term infants.
- The benefits of iNO therapy are reliant on comprehensive care of the infant through optimizing cardiopulmonary support.
- Premature infants with suspected pulmonary hypoplasia may benefit from early use of iNO.

FUNDING

Supported in part by the American Academy of Pediatrics, United States (AAP) Marshall Klaus Neonatal-Perinatal Research Award (MWC) and by grants T32HL160508-01 (MWC) from the NHLBI. Contents are the authors' sole responsibility and do not necessarily represent official views of the NIH or AAP. Supported by NIH, United States/NCATS Colorado CTSA Grant Number UL1 TR002535 (JPK). Contents are the authors' sole responsibility and do not necessarily represent official NIH views. M.W. Cookson and J.P. Kinsella are members of the Pediatric Pulmonary Hypertension Network.

DISCLOSURE

M.W. Cookson: None. J.P. Kinsella was awarded an investigator initiated grant by Mallinckrodt to create a registry for PH in premature newborns.

REFERENCES

1. Roberts JD, Polaner DM, Lang P, et al. Inhaled nitric oxide in persistent pulmonary hypertension of the newborn. Lancet 1992;340(8823):818–9.
2. Kinsella JP, Neish SR, Shaffer E, et al. Low-dose inhalation nitric oxide in persistent pulmonary hypertension of the newborn. Lancet 1992;340(8823):819–20.
3. Inhaled nitric oxide in full-term and nearly full-term infants with hypoxic respiratory failure. N Engl J Med 1997;336(9):597–604.
4. Clark RH, Kueser TJ, Walker MW, et al. Low-dose nitric oxide therapy for persistent pulmonary hypertension of the newborn. Clinical Inhaled Nitric Oxide Research Group. N Engl J Med 2000;342(7):469–74.
5. Stahlman M. Treatment of cardiovascular disorders of the newborn. Pediatr Clin North Am 1964;11(2):363–400.

6. Rudolph AM, Drorbaugh JE, Auld PA, et al. Studies on the circulation in the neonatal period. The circulation in the respiratory distress syndrome. Pediatrics 1961;27:551–66.

7. Roberton NR, Hallidie-Smith KA, Davis JA. Severe respiratory distress syndrome mimicking cyanotic heart-disease in term babies. Lancet 1967;2(7526):1108–10.

8. Gersony W, Duc GV, Sinclair JC. "PFC" syndrome (persistance of the fetal circulation). Circulation 1969;40:111.

9. Levin DL, Heymann MA, Kitterman JA, et al. Persistent pulmonary hypertension of the newborn infant. J Pediatr 1976;89(4):626–30.

10. Harrison MR, de Lorimier AA. Congenital diaphragmatic hernia. Surg Clin North Am 1981;61(5):1023–35.

11. Rudolph AM. High pulmonary vascular resistance after birth: I. Pathophysiologic considerations and etiologic classification. Clin Pediatr (Phila) 1980;19(9):585–90.

12. Kinsella JP, Neish SR, Ivy DD, et al. Clinical responses to prolonged treatment of persistent pulmonary hypertension of the newborn with low doses of inhaled nitric oxide. J Pediatr 1993;123(1):103–8.

13. Mous DS, Buscop-Van Kempen MJ, Wijnen RMH, et al. Changes in vasoactive pathways in congenital diaphragmatic hernia associated pulmonary hypertension explain unresponsiveness to pharmacotherapy. Respir Res 2017;18(1). https://doi.org/10.1186/s12931-017-0670-2.

14. Furchgott RF, Zawadzki JV. The obligatory role of endothelial cells in the relaxation of arterial smooth muscle by acetylcholine. Nature 1980;288(5789):373–6.

15. Palmer RMJ, Ferrige AG, Moncada S. Nitric oxide release accounts for the biological activity of endothelium-derived relaxing factor. Nature 1987;327(6122):524–6.

16. Ignarro LJ, Buga GM, Wood KS, et al. Endothelium-derived relaxing factor produced and released from artery and vein is nitric oxide. Proc Natl Acad Sci USA 1987;84(24):9265–9.

17. Furchgott RF, Cherry PD, Zawadzki JV, et al. Endothelial cells as mediators of vasodilation of arteries. J Cardiovasc Pharmacol 1984;6(Suppl 2):S336–43.

18. Cornfield DN, Chatfield BA, McQueston JA, et al. Effects of birth-related stimuli on L-arginine-dependent pulmonary vasodilation in ovine fetus. Am J Physiol 1992;262(5 Pt 2):H1474–81.

19. Abman SH, Chatfield BA, Hall SL, et al. Role of endothelium-derived relaxing factor during transition of pulmonary circulation at birth. Am J Physiol 1990;259(6 Pt 2):H1921–7.

20. Abman SH, Chatfield BA, Rodman DM, et al. Maturational changes in endothelium-derived relaxing factor activity of ovine pulmonary arteries in vitro. Am J Physiol 1991;260(4 Pt 1):L280–5.

21. Fineman JR, Soifer SJ, Heymann MA. The role of pulmonary vascular endothelium in perinatal pulmonary circulatory regulation. Semin Perinatol 1991;15(1):58–62.

22. Kinsella JP, McQueston JA, Rosenberg AA, et al. Hemodynamic effects of exogenous nitric oxide in ovine transitional pulmonary circulation. Am J Physiol 1992;263(3 Pt 2):H875–80.

23. Kinsella JP, Ivy DD, Abman SH. Ontogeny of NO activity and response to inhaled NO in the developing ovine pulmonary circulation. Am J Physiol 1994;267(5 Pt 2):H1955–61.

24. Shaul PW, Afshar S, Gibson LL, et al. Developmental changes in nitric oxide synthase isoform expression and nitric oxide production in fetal baboon lung. Am J Physiol Lung Cell Mol Physiol 2002;283(6):L1192–9.

25. Pepke-Zaba J, Higenbottam TW, Dinh-Xuan AT, et al. Inhaled nitric oxide as a cause of selective pulmonary vasodilatation in pulmonary hypertension. Lancet 1991;338(8776):1173–4.

26. Frostell C, Fratacci MD, Wain JC, et al. Inhaled nitric oxide. A selective pulmonary vasodilator reversing hypoxic pulmonary vasoconstriction. Circulation 1991; 83(6):2038–47.

27. Roberts JD Jr, Chen TY, Kawai N, et al. Inhaled nitric oxide reverses pulmonary vasoconstriction in the hypoxic and acidotic newborn lamb. Circ Res 1993; 72(2):246–54.

28. Villamor E, Le Cras TD, Horan MP, et al. Chronic intrauterine pulmonary hypertension impairs endothelial nitric oxide synthase in the ovine fetus. Am J Physiol 1997;272(5 Pt 1):L1013–20.

29. Zayek M, Cleveland D, Morin FC 3rd. Treatment of persistent pulmonary hypertension in the newborn lamb by inhaled nitric oxide. J Pediatr 1993;122(5 Pt 1): 743–50.

30. Kinsella JP, Parker TA, Galan H, et al. Independent and combined effects of inhaled nitric oxide, liquid perfluorochemical, and high-frequency oscillatory ventilation in premature lambs with respiratory distress syndrome. Chest 1999; 116(1 Suppl):15S–6S.

31. Rossaint R, Falke KJ, Lopez F, et al. Inhaled nitric oxide for the adult respiratory distress syndrome. N Engl J Med 1993;328(6):399–405.

32. Finer NN, Etches PC, Kamstra B, et al. Inhaled nitric oxide in infants referred for extracorporeal membrane oxygenation: dose response. J Pediatr 1994;124(2): 302–8.

33. Konduri GG, Solimano A, Sokol GM, et al. A randomized trial of early versus standard inhaled nitric oxide therapy in term and near-term newborn infants with hypoxic respiratory failure. Pediatrics 2004;113(3 Pt 1):559–64.

34. Tworetzky W, Bristow J, Moore P, et al. Inhaled nitric oxide in neonates with persistent pulmonary hypertension. Lancet 2001;357(9250):118–20.

35. Davidson D, Barefield ES, Kattwinkel J, et al. Inhaled nitric oxide for the early treatment of persistent pulmonary hypertension of the term newborn: a randomized, double-masked, placebo-controlled, dose-response, multicenter study. Pediatrics 1998;101(3):325–34.

36. Sokol GM, Fineberg NS, Wright LL, et al. Changes in arterial oxygen tension when weaning neonates from inhaled nitric oxide. Pediatr Pulmonol 2001;32(1):14–9.

37. Black SM, Heidersbach RS, McMullan DM, et al. Inhaled nitric oxide inhibits NOS activity in lambs: potential mechanism for rebound pulmonary hypertension. Am J Physiol 1999;277(5):H1849–56.

38. Rawat M, Lakshminrusimha S, Vento M. Pulmonary hypertension and oxidative stress: where is the link? Semin Fetal Neonatal Med 2022;27(4):101347.

39. Roberts JD, Fineman JR, Morin FC, et al. Inhaled nitric oxide and persistent pulmonary hypertension of the newborn. the inhaled nitric oxide study group. N Engl J Med 1997;336(9):605–10.

40. Kinsella JP, Truog WE, Walsh WF, et al. Randomized, multicenter trial of inhaled nitric oxide and high-frequency oscillatory ventilation in severe, persistent pulmonary hypertension of the newborn. J Pediatr 1997;131(1 Pt 1):55–62.

41. Goldman AP, Tasker RC, Haworth SG, et al. Four patterns of response to inhaled nitric oxide for persistent pulmonary hypertension of the newborn. Pediatrics 1996;98(4 Pt 1):706–13.
42. Foubert L, Fleming B, Latimer R, et al. Safety guidelines for use of nitric oxide. Lancet 1992;339(8809):1615–6.
43. Frostell CG, Zapol WM. Inhaled nitric oxide, clinical rationale and applications. Adv Pharmacol 1995;34:439–56.
44. Van Meurs KP, Wright LL, Ehrenkranz RA, et al. Inhaled nitric oxide for premature infants with severe respiratory failure. N Engl J Med 2005;353(1):13–22.
45. Van Meurs KP, Rhine WD, Asselin JM, et al. Response of premature infants with severe respiratory failure to inhaled nitric oxide. Preemie NO Collaborative Group. Pediatr Pulmonol 1997;24(5):319–23.
46. Hogman M, Frostell C, Arnberg H, et al. Bleeding time prolongation and NO inhalation. Lancet 1993;341(8861):1664–5.
47. Bassenge E. Antiplatelet effects of endothelium-derived relaxing factor and nitric oxide donors. Eur Heart J 1991;12(Suppl E):12–5.
48. George TN, Johnson KJ, Bates JN, et al. The effect of inhaled nitric oxide therapy on bleeding time and platelet aggregation in neonates. J Pediatr 1998;132(4):731–4.
49. Ward J, Motwani J, Baker N, et al. Congenital methemoglobinemia identified by pulse oximetry screening. Pediatrics 2019;143(3). e20182814.
50. Bischoff AR, Habib S, Mcnamara PJ, et al. Hemodynamic response to milrinone for refractory hypoxemia during therapeutic hypothermia for neonatal hypoxic ischemic encephalopathy. J Perinatol 2021;41(9):2345–54.
51. James AT, Corcoran JD, McNamara PJ, et al. The effect of milrinone on right and left ventricular function when used as a rescue therapy for term infants with pulmonary hypertension. Cardiol Young 2016;26(1):90–9.
52. Kinsella JP, Steinhorn RH, Mullen MP, et al. The left ventricle in congenital diaphragmatic hernia: implications for the management of pulmonary hypertension. J Pediatr 2018;197:17–22.
53. Cookson MW, Abman SH, Kinsella JP, et al. Pulmonary vasodilator strategies in neonates with acute hypoxemic respiratory failure and pulmonary hypertension. Semin Fetal Neonatal Med 2022;27(4):101367.
54. Kinsella JP, Abman SH. Clinical approach to inhaled nitric oxide therapy in the newborn with hypoxemia. J Pediatr 2000;136(6):717–26.
55. Clark RH, Yoder BA, Sell MS. Prospective, randomized comparison of high-frequency oscillation and conventional ventilation in candidates for extracorporeal membrane oxygenation. J Pediatr 1994;124(3):447–54.
56. Kuluz MA, Smith PB, Mears SP, et al. Preliminary observations of the use of high-frequency jet ventilation as rescue therapy in infants with congenital diaphragmatic hernia. J Pediatr Surg 2010;45(4):698–702.
57. Lotze A, Mitchell BR, Bulas DI, et al. Multicenter study of surfactant (beractant) use in the treatment of term infants with severe respiratory failure. Survanta in Term Infants Study Group. J Pediatr 1998;132(1):40–7.
58. González A, Bancalari A, Osorio W, et al. Early use of combined exogenous surfactant and inhaled nitric oxide reduces treatment failure in persistent pulmonary hypertension of the newborn: a randomized controlled trial. J Perinatol 2021; 41(1):32–8.
59. Cornfield DN, Reeve HL, Tolarova S, et al. Oxygen causes fetal pulmonary vasodilation through activation of a calcium-dependent potassium channel. Proc Natl Acad Sci U S A 1996;93(15):8089–94.

60. Cornfield DN. Developmental regulation of oxygen sensing and ion channels in the pulmonary vasculature. Adv Exp Med Biol 2010;661:201–20.

61. Farrow KN, Groh BS, Schumacker PT, et al. Hyperoxia increases phosphodiesterase 5 expression and activity in ovine fetal pulmonary artery smooth muscle cells. Circ Res 2008;102(2):226–33.

62. Giesinger RE, McNamara PJ. Hemodynamic instability in the critically ill neonate: an approach to cardiovascular support based on disease pathophysiology. Semin Perinatol 2016;40(3):174–88.

63. Nakanishi H, Suenaga H, Uchiyama A, et al. Persistent pulmonary hypertension of the newborn in extremely preterm infants: a Japanese cohort study. Arch Dis Child Fetal Neonatal Ed 2018;103(6):F554–61.

64. Nelin L, Kinsella JP, Courtney SE, et al. Use of inhaled nitric oxide in preterm vs term/near-term neonates with pulmonary hypertension: results of the PaTTerN registry study. J Perinatol 2022;42(1):14–8.

65. Peliowski A, Finer NN, Etches PC, et al. Inhaled nitric oxide for premature infants after prolonged rupture of the membranes. J Pediatr 1995;126(3):450–3.

66. Abman SH, Hansmann G, Archer SL, et al. Pediatric pulmonary hypertension. Circulation 2015;132(21):2037–99.

67. Kinsella JP, Steinhorn RH, Krishnan US, et al. Recommendations for the use of inhaled nitric oxide therapy in premature newborns with severe pulmonary hypertension. J Pediatr 2016;170:312–4.

68. Chock VY, Van Meurs KP, Hintz SR, et al. Inhaled nitric oxide for preterm premature rupture of membranes, oligohydramnios, and pulmonary hypoplasia. Am J Perinatol 2009;26(4):317–22.

69. Kinsella JP, Cutter GR, Walsh WF, et al. Early inhaled nitric oxide therapy in premature newborns with respiratory failure. N Engl J Med 2006;355(4):354–64.

70. Ballard RA, Truog WE, Cnaan A, et al. Inhaled nitric oxide in preterm infants undergoing mechanical ventilation. N Engl J Med 2006;355(4):343–53.

71. Kinsella JP, Walsh WF, Bose CL, et al. Inhaled nitric oxide in premature neonates with severe hypoxaemic respiratory failure: a randomised controlled trial. Lancet 1999;354(9184):1061–5.

72. Balasubramaniam V, Maxey AM, Morgan DB, et al. Inhaled NO restores lung structure in eNOS-deficient mice recovering from neonatal hypoxia. Am J Physiol Lung Cell Mol Physiol. Jul 2006;291(1):L119–27.

73. Tourneux P, Markham N, Seedorf G, et al. Inhaled nitric oxide improves lung structure and pulmonary hypertension in a model of bleomycin-induced bronchopulmonary dysplasia in neonatal rats. Am J Physiol Lung Cell Mol Physiol 2009;297(6):L1103–11.

74. Kinsella JP, Parker TA, Galan H, et al. Effects of inhaled nitric oxide on pulmonary edema and lung neutrophil accumulation in severe experimental hyaline membrane disease. Pediatr Res 1997;41(4 Pt 1):457–63.

75. Kumar P, Committee on F, Newborn, American Academy of P. Use of inhaled nitric oxide in preterm infants. Pediatrics 2014;133(1):164–70.

76. Giesinger RE, Rios DR, Chatmethakul T, et al. Impact of early hemodynamic screening on extremely preterm outcomes in a high-performance center. Am J Respir Crit Care Med 2023;208(3):290–300.

77. Kinsella JP, Parker TA, Ivy DD, et al. Noninvasive delivery of inhaled nitric oxide therapy for late pulmonary hypertension in newborn infants with congenital diaphragmatic hernia. J Pediatr 2003;142(4):397–401.

78. Lowe CG, Trautwein JG. Inhaled nitric oxide therapy during the transport of neonates with persistent pulmonary hypertension or severe hypoxic respiratory failure. Eur J Pediatr 2007;166(10):1025–31.
79. Kinsella JP, Griebel J, Schmidt JM, et al. Use of inhaled nitric oxide during interhospital transport of newborns with hypoxemic respiratory failure. Pediatrics 2002;109(1):158–61.
80. Clark RH, Kueser TJ, Walker MW, et al. Low-dose nitric oxide therapy for persistent pulmonary hypertension of the newborn. N Engl J Med 2000;342(7):469–74.

Targeted Therapies for Neonatal Pulmonary Hypertension: Beyond Nitric Oxide

Jeanne Carroll, MD[a], Rohit Rao, MD, MBA[b],
Robin H. Steinhorn, MD[c],*

KEYWORDS

- Pulmonary hypertension • Phosphodiesterase • Prostacyclin • Endothelin
- Pulmonary vasculature

KEY POINTS

- Pulmonary hypertension in the neonate can occur in term or preterm infants and is associated with significant morbidity and mortality.
- Inhaled nitric oxide is the only Food and Drug Administration-approved therapy for neonatal pulmonary hypertension, but treatment failure as determined by need for ECMO therapy occurs in up to 10% of term infants with persistent pulmonary hypertension of the newborn.
- Other available pharmacotherapy for pulmonary hypertension targets three primary pathways: nitric oxide-cyclic guanosine monophosphate, endothelin, and prostacyclin-cyclic adenosine monophosphate.

INTRODUCTION

Pulmonary hypertension (PH) in the neonate is a heterogeneous diagnosis associated with significant morbidity and mortality[1–5] in term and preterm infants. Inhaled nitric oxide (iNO) is the only Food and Drug Administration (FDA)-approved treatment for PH in the neonate. Several additional PH-targeted drug therapies are used in both

a Division of Neonatology, Department of Pediatrics, University of California, San Diego, Rady Children's Hospital-San Diego, 3030 Children's Way, San Diego, CA 92123, USA; b Division of Cardiothoracic Critical Care, Department of Pediatrics, University of California, San Diego, Rady Children's Hospital-San Diego, 3030 Children's Way, San Diego, CA 92123, USA; c Department of Pediatrics, University of California, San Diego, Rady Children's Hospital-San Diego, 3020 Children's Way, San Diego, CA 92123, USA
* Corresponding author.
E-mail address: rsteinhorn@rchsd.org

Clin Perinatol 51 (2024) 113–126
https://doi.org/10.1016/j.clp.2023.11.008
0095-5108/24/© 2023 Elsevier Inc. All rights reserved.

acute and chronic management of PH in the neonate, often based on observational case series or extrapolated experience from adult and pediatric studies.

Pharmacotherapy for PH currently consists of vasodilator drugs and can be divided into groups by the cellular pathways they modulate (**Table 1**). The most relevant pathways are nitric oxide-cyclic guanosine monophosphate (NO-cGMP), endothelin, and prostacyclin-cyclic adenosine monophosphate (prostacyclin-cAMP), which are shown in **Fig. 1**. Immediately after birth, ventilation, oxygenation, and increased pulmonary blood flow trigger endothelial nitric oxide synthase (eNOS) expression and activity, thereby increasing NO production. The effects of NO are primarily mediated through soluble guanylate cyclase (sGC) which converts guanosine triphosphate (GTP) to cGMP, a central mediator responsible for vascular relaxation. Increased cGMP concentrations in turn lead to smooth muscle relaxation.[6] cGMP is broken down by phosphodiesterase 5 (PDE5). PDE5 catalyzes the breakdown and inactivation of cGMP; both sGC and PDE5 reach peak expression and activity in the immediate newborn period to accomplish the pulmonary vascular transition at birth. Disruption to this pathway contributes to acute and chronic PH and can be modified through the use of iNO, PDE5 inhibitors, and sGC stimulators.

Nitric oxide, delivered as an inhaled gas (iNO), has been in clinical use for more than 20 years and has revolutionized the treatment of acute neonatal PH. Although iNO reduces the need for extracorporeal support, it has not been shown to reduce mortality due to the rescue use of extracorporeal membrane oxygenation (ECMO) therapy or length of hospitalization in any clinical trial, and treatment failure occurs in up to 40% of infants. The failure to respond to iNO may indicate inadequate lung recruitment or cardiac dysfunction but may also be due to pulmonary vascular signaling abnormalities downstream of nitric oxide synthesis. In addition to the need for adjunctive therapy for acute neonatal PH, iNO remains impractical for long-term use at home for infants with chronic PH due to conditions such as bronchopulmonary dysplasia (BPD) and congenital diaphragmatic hernia (CDH), and alternatives are needed for this purpose. This review summarizes the current evidence for PH medications beyond iNO that are frequently used and review potential future therapies.

Nitric Oxide-Cyclic Guanosine Monophosphate

Phosphodiesterase-5 inhibitors

Sildenafil, a PDE5 inhibitor that can be administered enterally or intravenously, is a well-established treatment for PH in adults. In a placebo-controlled study, sildenafil was associated with improved 6-minute walk distance and hemodynamics after 12 weeks. These findings were sustained after 3 years in an open-label extension of the trial.[7,8] The STARTS-1 trial studied treatment naïve pediatric patients ages 1 to 17 years with PH randomizing them to placebo or low-, medium-, or high-dose sildenafil for 16 weeks. Peak oxygen consumption, functional class, and hemodynamics were more significantly improved in medium and high-dose patients. The study was extended in STARTS-2 and those on placebo were randomized to low-, medium-, or high-dose sildenafil. This study showed an increase in mortality as sildenafil dose increased, but overall mortality was lower compared with historical data.[9,10] This led to the FDA issuing a warning against the use of sildenafil in pediatric population. However, after accumulation of safety data in adults, the FDA recently concluded that a causal association for the previously observed dose-related effect on mortality risk in pediatric patients was unlikely and approved the use of sildenafil for children ages 1 to 17 years.

There are several small studies on the use of sildenafil in neonates for persistent PH of the newborn (PPHN). In resource-limited settings without access to iNO or ECMO,

Table 1
Pulmonary hypertension pharmacotherapy

Medication	Mechanism of Action	Dose	Side Effects
Nitric Oxide-sGC-cGMP			
Sildenafil	PDE5 inhibitor	PO: 1 mg/kg Q6-8 hr; IV: 0.1-0.25 mg/kg Q6-8 hr or continuous infusion up to 1.6 mg/kg/day	Hypotension, visual disturbance, headache, reflux
Tadalafil	PDE5 inhibitor	PO: 0.5-1 mg/kg Q24 h	Hypotension, headache
Riociguat	sGC stimulator	Limited data. Discontinue PDE5 inhibitors before initiation. PO: Start 0.5 mg daily and titrate up to Q8 hr, then increase dose to max 2 mg Q8 hr	Hypotension, nausea
Endothelin			
Bosentan	ETA and ETB receptor antagonist	PO: 1 mg/kg PO q ˜2 h, increase to 2 mg/kg BID in 2-4 wk if LFTs stable	Liver dysfunction, anemia, hypotension
Macitentan	ETA and ETB receptor antagonist	Limited data. PO: <10 kg: start 1 mg and increase to max 3 mg daily	Anemia, headache, elevated transaminases, hypotension
Ambrisentan	ETA receptor antagonist	Limited data. PO: <20 kg: start ≥5 mg daily	Anemia, headache, edema
Prostacyclin-cAMP			
Epoprostenol	Prostacyclin analog	IV: 1-2 ng/kg/min: increase as tolerated to 50-80 ng/kg/min. Inhaled: 50 ng/kg/min	Hypotension, flushing, diarrhea, airway irritation (inhaled)
Iloprost	Prostacyclin analog	Inhaled: 1-5 mcg Q 2-4 h	Flushing, hypotension, headache, cough
Treprostinil	Prostacyclin analog	IV/SQ: start at 2 ng/kg/min; increase as tolerated to 50-80 ng/kg/min	Hypotension, flushing, vomiting, diarrhea, infusion site pain
Milrinone	PDE3 inhibitor	IV: 0.15 mcg/kg/min - 0.5 mcg/kg/min	Hypotension, arrhythmia, thrombocytopenia
Selexipag	IP receptor agonist	Limited data. PO: <7.5 kg: 25-50 mcg PO Q12 h, increase by 25-50 mcg to goal 200-400 mcg Q 12 h	Jaw pain, nausea, diarrhea, headache

Abbreviations: BID, twice a day; cGMP, cyclic guanosine monophosphate; ET, endothelin; IP, prostacyclin receptor; IV, intravenous; kg, kilogram; LFT, liver function tests; mg, milligram; ng, nanogram; PDE, phosphodiesterase; PO, oral; SC, subcutaneous; sGC, soluble guanylate cyclase.

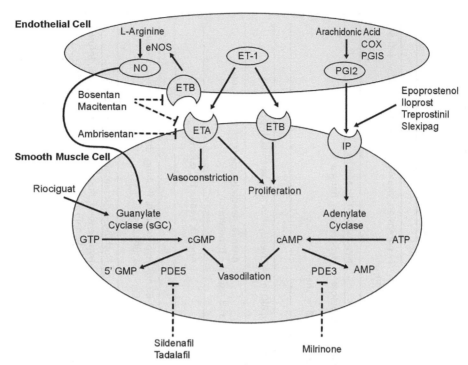

Fig. 1. In the endothelial cell, L-arginine is converted to nitric oxide (NO) by endothelial nitric oxide synthase (eNOS). Nitric oxide then stimulates guanylate cyclase in the smooth muscle cell to increase cyclic guanosine monophosphate (cGMP) which is responsible for vasodilation. cGMP is broken down by phosphodiesterase 5 (PDE5). Endothelin-1 (ET-1) in the endothelial cell acts via endothelin A and B receptors (ETA and ETB). ETA causes vasoconstriction, whereas ETB stimulates eNOS and can increase NO production. Prostacyclin (PGI2) is produced through cyclooxygenase (COX) and prostaglandin I2 synthase (PGIS) activity. It leads to vasodilation via action on the prostacyclin receptor (IP) which stimulates adenylate cyclase which increases cyclic adenosine monophosphate (cAMP). cAMP is responsible for vasodilation and is broken down by phosphodiesterase 3 (PDE3).

the use of sildenafil reduced mortality when compared with placebo (6% vs 40%).[11] When given enterally for acute PPHN, the starting dose is typically 0.5 to 1 mg/kg every 8 hours.[12] An open-label, dose-escalation trial of intravenous (IV) sildenafil alone or in addition to iNO in neonates with PPHN showed the medication was well tolerated with acute improvement in oxygenation. The improvement was most notable in the highest dose cohorts with a loading dose of 0.4 mg/kg over 3 hours followed by maintenance dosing of 1.6 mg/kg/day.[13] However, in a subsequent multicenter randomized-placebo controlled trial of 59 neonates with PPHN, IV sildenafil, given as a loading dose of 0.1 mg/kg followed by maintenance of 0.03 mg/kg/hr (0.72 mg/kg/day, achieving plasma sildenafil concentration approximately half of the prior study), was not superior to placebo in reducing treatment failure or the time on iNO.[14] The lack of benefit in this study may be related to enrollment of patients with an oxygenation index (OI) less than 25, the lower dose of sildenafil (chosen to optimize safety, but lower than the optimal range identified in prior study), or the use of a standardized iNO weaning protocol. The CoDiNOS trial is a large randomized controlled trial comparing the efficacy of sildenafil (loading dose of 0.4 mg/kg over 3 hours followed by maintenance dosing of 1.6 mg/kg/day) versus iNO in infants with CDH less than 7 days of age with acute PH (NL60229.078.17); results remain pending.

The successful use of enteral sildenafil has been reported in infants with chronic PH associated with CDH and BPD. Observational studies have reported hemodynamic and clinical benefit of sildenafil for treatment of PH related to BPD,[15–17] whereas other studies demonstrated echo improvement without robust clinical improvement.[18,19] One large single-center cohort of sildenafil therapy in children included 136 infants with BPD. The median age at initiation was 4 months, and 45% of the infants were able to be weaned off sildenafil due to improvement in PH over time, with a median duration of therapy of 1.75 years.[20] Overall, mortality for this cohort was 26%, with 9/35 deaths due to PH and the rest due to chronic lung disease or other causes.

Despite limited evidence, sildenafil use for BPD-associated PH has increased, and additional safety and efficacy data are needed.[21] In a recent prospective study of pre-term babies (<32 weeks gestation, 3–42 days of age, $n = 9$) at high risk for BPD, a single dose of IV sildenafil (0.25 or 0.125 mg/kg over 90 minutes) was generally well tolerated with one serious adverse event of hypotension.[20] The SIL02 study, a phase 2 multicenter, randomized, placebo-controlled, dose-escalating safety study, is currently enrolling a similar population of high-risk premature infants to determine the safety of up to 34 days of enteral or IV sildenafil (NCT03142568).[22,23] Tadalafil, approved by the FDA for adults with PH, is a longer acting PDE5 inhibitor with once daily dosing but little information is available in the neonatal population.

Soluble guanylate cyclase stimulators

As the vascular benefits of NO are mediated via activation of sGC to increase cGMP, agents that directly target sGC are an attractive approach to overcome NO resistance. Recently, small molecules (stimulators and activators) have been developed that target NO-sGC-cGMP signaling in a number of disease states, including animal models of PPHN.[24,25] sGC stimulators bind to sGC and potentiate NO-mediated cGMP signaling; these agents generally act synergistically with NO and amplify endogenous NO signaling. In contrast to sGC stimulators, sGC activators bind in the heme pocket of the sGC enzyme and directly stimulate sGC by increasing its sensitivity to stimulation by nitric oxide, especially when oxidative stress is present. In addition, poor responses to inhaled NO may be due to impaired sGC due to oxidation; however, sGC activators are able to still stimulate oxidized sGC, thereby improving vasodilation beyond the effect of iNO.

Riociguat is an oral sGC stimulator; it was approved for use in adults with PH in 2013 based on improved hemodynamic markers and 6-minute walk distance.[26] In the pediatric population, safety has been studied in combination with other PH treatments. An open-label phase III trial of 24 patients' age 6 to 17 years demonstrated improved 6-minute walk distance, whereas three patients experienced hypotension.[27] In one small high-risk cohort of infants' ages 1 to 12 months with chronic PH, transitioning from sildenafil to riociguat therapy improved respiratory status, lowered pulmonary arterial pressure, and improved right heart failure without critical hypotension or hypoxia.[28]

Endothelin Pathway

Endothelin-1 (ET-1) is a potent vasoconstrictor produced by endothelial cells. ET-1 expression is increased in lung tissue samples of adults with PH, and arterial concentrations of the peptide are elevated in neonates with PPHN and chronic PH due to severe CDH.[29,30] Factors such as hypoxia and reactive oxygen species stimulate the production of ET-1 while NO and prostacyclin inhibit synthesis. ET-1 acts via two receptors, ET_A and ET_B, both of which can cause smooth muscle cell proliferation. ET_A

additionally causes vasoconstriction, whereas ET_B mediates vasodilation.[31] The ET-1 pathway has been strongly implicated in the development of PH and can be modulated by endothelial receptor antagonists (ERA). In a fetal lamb model of PPHN, ET-1 levels were elevated and selective inhibition of ET_A lead to pulmonary vasodilation.[32] In humans, there are three ERAs available for the treatment of PH: bosentan and macitentan which are nonselective antagonists against ET_A and ET_B and ambrisentan which is a selective inhibitor of ET_A.

In adults, all three ERAs have been shown to improve exercise capacity, hemodynamics, and time to clinical worsening.[33] Bosentan is an oral nonselective ERA and is approved by the FDA for use in children aged 3 years and older. It is the most widely studied ERA in the pediatric and neonatal population. In clinical trials and case series, bosentan has been shown to improve hemodynamics and functional WHO functional class in pediatric patients with PH due to a variety of causes.[34–36] There is conflicting evidence in the setting of PPHN as an adjuvant therapy. A single-center study of 47 iNO-naïve neonates randomized 1:1 to Bosentan or placebo showed improvement in PH and OI in 87.5% of the treatment group versus 20% of the placebo group during the study period.[37] In contrast, the FUTURE-4 multicenter trial found that bosentan as adjunctive therapy for iNO did not improve PPHN outcomes, time on iNO, or time to extubation, possibly in part due to inconsistent intestinal absorption.[38] There were no adverse outcomes in the treatment arm in either study. There is little information on the efficacy of bosentan for chronic PH associated with BPD and CDH. There are even fewer studies on macitentan and ambrisentan in the pediatric population, but early observational studies indicate these medications alone or in combination with other PH therapies may improve PH without serious adverse effects.[39–41]

Bosentan can cause a dose-dependent increase in transaminases which is typically reversible with cessation of the medication in up to 10% of patients and thus requires monthly liver function test (LFT) monitoring. It can also lower the circulating levels of tadalafil and sildenafil in patient on dual therapy.[33] Elevated transaminases seem to be less common in patients younger than 12 year old on bosentan.[42] Ambrisentan and macitentan demonstrate less liver toxicity in adults but more data are needed in children.[33] Additional side effects of ERAs include peripheral edema, headaches, and teratogenicity.

Prostacyclin-Cyclic Adenosine Monophosphate Pathway

Prostacyclin (PGI2) is a metabolite of arachidonic acid, which binds to the prostacyclin receptor (IP) on vascular smooth muscle cells. This stimulates adenylate cyclase which increases cAMP and leads to pulmonary vasodilation. cAMP break down in these cells is mediated by phosphodiesterase 3 (PDE3). Prostacyclin also decreases smooth muscle cell proliferation and platelet aggregation.[43] Prostacyclin levels are decreased and thromboxane, a vasoconstrictor and promoter of platelet aggregation, is increased in adults with primary and secondary PH.[44] There are several drugs aimed at modulating this pathway in the treatment of PH.

Prostacyclin analogs

Epoprostenol, iloprost, and treprostinil are all prostanoids, whereas selexipag is a selective IP agonist. Epoprostenol was one of the earliest PH therapies and has been shown to improve hemodynamics, exercise capacity, and survival in children and adults with PH when used as a continuous IV infusion.[45–47] Long-term therapy improved survival even in those patients who were not acute responders.[45]

The use of IV epoprostenol has been described in observational studies of children with BPD-PH; these infants (median age 234 days) demonstrated tolerance of the medication without serious adverse effects.[48,49] In one retrospective single-center cohort of 36 patients with PPHN refractory to iNO (OI > 25), 15 patients responded to IV epoprostenol and 21 nonresponders died or transitioned to ECMO therapy.[50] Overall, IV PGI2 is rarely used in neonates because of concerns about systemic hypotension and/or ventilation-perfusion mismatch, the need for continuous infusion through a dedicated central line, short half-life of 2 to 5 minutes, and instability at room temperature or neutral pH.

Inhaled epoprostenol delivered continuously has also been shown in small observational studies to improve oxygenation.[51–53] It is commonly used for treatment of acute PH in adults and has been shown to produce transient pulmonary vasodilation and enhanced oxygenation in neonates. In one retrospective single-center cohort study of 43 neonates with PPHN, inhaled epoprostenol administered in addition to iNO improved OI without adverse events.[53] However, there are concerns about airway irritation due to alkalinity of the medication, potential loss of medication into the nebulization circuit, and rebound PH if abruptly discontinued.

Iloprost is an inhaled prostacyclin analog with a half-life of 20 to 30 minutes. In the United States, it is administered via the I-neb adaptive-aerosol delivery (AAD) System. In retrospective case series of neonates with refractory PPHN, inhaled iloprost improved oxygenation in roughly half of the infants with no severe side effects.[54–56] Observational studies of iloprost have also demonstrated benefit in preterm infants with severe respiratory failure and for PH associated with BPD.[57–60]

Treprostinil is available in IV, inhaled, or subcutaneous preparations and is stable at room temperature and neutral pH with a longer half-life of 3 to 6 hours. In both children and adults, subcutaneous administration (which has bioavailability equivalent to IV administration) improved exercise capacity, functional class, and hemodynamics with injection site pain as the most common side effect.[61,62] In a retrospective cohort of 29 patients, inhaled treprostinil given four times per day as an adjuvant to other vasodilator therapy was well tolerated in most children, easy to administer, and significantly improved exercise capacity.[63] There are multiple observational studies describing the use of IV and/or subcutaneous treprostinil in the management of PH associated with CDH. These studies show improvement in hemodynamics without serious adverse effects, suggesting a role in the chronic management of these patients.[64–67] A multicenter, randomized clinical trial studying the safety and efficacy of IV treprostinil as adjunctive therapy for PPHN completed enrollment in late 2022 results remain pending (NCT02261883).

Selexipag is a selective IP agonist that is administered orally. In adults, it is shown to reduce mortality and complications from PH compared with placebo when used alone or in combination with endothelin antagonists or a PDE5 inhibitor.[68] In children, it has been described in observational studies as an option for transition off continuous IV/subcutaneous (SQ) administration of prostacyclin analogs as well as a second- or third-line medication.[69–72] In the largest series, six of ten patients had increased pulmonary vascular resistance index after transition from parenteral prostacyclin to selexipag, indicating importance of closely monitoring after transition and balancing the ease of oral administration with goals of care.[71] Although selexipag use has been reported in infants, there are no studies in neonates.

Phosphodiesterase 3 inhibitor
Milrinone is a PDE3 inhibitor that acts via the prostacyclin-cAMP by decreasing the hydrolysis of cAMP. Increased cAMP in vascular smooth muscle cells and myocardium leads to improved function and decreased vascular resistance. Observational evidence indicates milrinone improves OI and hemodynamics, particularly in those patients who have a poor response to iNO.[73–76] As milrinone can improve both right and left

ventricular function, its greatest utility may be though improving left ventricle (LV) dysfunction and by lowering pulmonary venous pressure. However, the most common complication during initiation of milrinone is systemic hypotension; milrinone should be used with extreme caution in preterm infants due to the risk for systemic hypotension and intraventricular hemorrhage. A randomized placebo controlled trial to investigate milrinone treatment for PPHN was terminated early for low enrollment after 4 years.[77] Milrinone has been proposed as a useful therapy to treat left ventricular dysfunction commonly associated with CDH. Case series have reported variable outcomes after milrinone use for the population[78,79]; a multicenter randomized controlled trial examining the safety and efficacy of milrinone for infants with CDH is currently enrolling patients (NCT02951130).[80]

Other Potential Therapeutic Approaches

L-citrulline, which increases L-arginine, enhances NO production by nitric oxide synthase and could be useful in the treatment or prevention of neonatal PH. Oral L-citrulline improved 6-minute walk distance in adults and reduced PVR in a newborn piglet model of hypoxia-induced PPHN.[81,82] Recent small pharmacokinetic and safety studies in neonates at risk for BPD are paving the way for trials evaluating efficacy.[83]

Reactive oxygen species such as hydrogen peroxide, superoxide, and peroxynitrite cause pulmonary vasoconstriction and play a role in the pathogenesis of PPHN. Increased superoxide levels are detected in the pulmonary arteries of fetal lambs with PPHN. Furthermore, the need for high Fio_2 in neonates with severe respiratory failure and/or PPHN can increase reactive oxygen species (ROS), which decreases eNOS and sGC activity and increases PDE5 activity. This oxidative stress can be minimized by judicious use of inspired oxygen or potentially by the use of targeted antioxidants, such as superoxide dismutase. In a neonatal animal model of PPHN, intratracheal recombinant human superoxide dismutase (rhSOD) restored eNOS expression, improved oxygenation, and induced pulmonary vasodilation.[84,85] In a randomized placebo-controlled trial, premature infants treated at birth with intratracheal rhSOD had less wheezing and fewer hospitalizations at 1 year corrected age, but no human studies have evaluated the efficacy of rhSOD for PH.[86] Oxidative stress also depletes tetrahydrobiopterin (BH4), which causes eNOS "uncoupling" and dysfunction, further amplifying superoxide production and oxidative stress in the pulmonary vasculature. Infants at-risk oxidant stress-mediated PH could theoretically benefit from supplementation with agents such as sapropterin, which is an agent already in use for infants with metabolic disorders. Limited preclinical studies indicate benefit in a piglet model of PPHN.[87]

Data now show that placental changes of maternal vascular under perfusion and fetal growth restriction may be indicators of an antiangiogenic fetal environment that contributes to high risk for BPD and PH in preterm infants.[88,89] In experimental models of antenatal stress that impair lung development, prolonged therapy with recombinant human insulin-like growth factor (IGF-1)/BP3 (binding peptide 3) improved lung structure and function and prevented PH.[90] Phase 2 randomized trials found that infusion of rhIGF-1/rhIGFBP3 through 29 weeks postmenstrual age for prevention of retinopathy of prematurity reduced rates of BPD. However, this was a secondary outcome of the study, and further trials are needed to determine whether this approach reduces BPD-associated PH.

SUMMARY

Although there are multiple FDA-approved medications for adults with PH, iNO remains the only approved treatment in neonates. Bosentan and recently sildenafil are the only FDA-approved agents for the pediatric population. Thus, outside of iNO, PH in the neonate is treated with off-label therapies, often based on data extrapolated from adults or small observational studies. More studies are needed to expand options for the prevention and treatment of PH in the neonate.

Best Practice Box

- Pulmonary vasodilators such as sildenafil and bosentan are not FDA-approved for use during the neonatal period but may be beneficial in (1) pulmonary hypertension with inadequate or ill-sustained response to iNO, (2) to wean iNO and minimize the risk of rebound pulmonary hypertension, (3) need to switch from iNO to an oral agent for chronic therapy, and (4) resource-limited settings with lack of access to iNO.

- In the presence of left ventricular dysfunction and/or pulmonary venous hypertension, iNO may cause pulmonary edema and worsen hypoxemia; adding an agent such as milrinone that lowers systemic vascular resistance may improve PH without worsening pulmonary edema.

- Most intravenous and enterally administered pulmonary vasodilators are associated with the risk of systemic hypotension or worse ventilation-perfusion mismatch in the setting of lung disease, and careful hemodynamic monitoring is needed during their use in neonatal pulmonary hypertension.

DISCLOSURE

None.

REFERENCES

1. Choi EK, Shin SH, Kim EK, et al. Developmental outcomes of preterm infants with bronchopulmonary dysplasia-associated pulmonary hypertension at 18-24 months of corrected age. BMC Pediatr 2019;19(1):26.
2. Altit G, Bhombal S, Feinstein J, et al. Diminished right ventricular function at diagnosis of pulmonary hypertension is associated with mortality in bronchopulmonary dysplasia. Pulm Circ 2019;9(3):1–6.
3. Steurer MA, Jelliffe-Pawlowski LL, Baer RJ, et al. Persistent pulmonary hypertension of the newborn in late preterm and term infants in California. Pediatrics 2017; 139(1):e20161165.
4. Konduri GG, Vohr B, Robertson C, et al. Early inhaled nitric oxide therapy for term and near-term newborn infants with hypoxic respiratory failure: neurodevelopmental follow-up. J Pediatr 2007;150(3):235–40.e1.
5. Khemani E, McElhinney DB, Rhein L, et al. Pulmonary artery hypertension in formerly premature infants with bronchopulmonary dysplasia: clinical features and outcomes in the surfactant era. Pediatrics 2007;120(6):1260–9.
6. Lakshminrusimha S, Steinhorn RH. Pulmonary vascular biology during neonatal transition. Clin Perinatol 1999;26(3):601–19.
7. Rubin LJ, Badesch DB, Fleming TR, et al. Long-term treatment with sildenafil citrate in pulmonary arterial hypertension: the SUPER-2 study. Chest 2011;140(5): 1274–83.
8. Galiè N, Ghofrani HA, Torbicki A, et al. Sildenafil citrate therapy for pulmonary arterial hypertension. N Engl J Med 2005;353(20):2148–57.
9. Barst RJ, Ivy DD, Gaitan G, et al. A randomized, double-blind, placebo-controlled, dose-ranging study of oral sildenafil citrate in treatment-naive children with pulmonary arterial hypertension. Circulation 2012;125(2):324–34.

10. Barst RJ, Beghetti M, Pulido T, et al. STARTS-2: long-term survival with oral silden-afil monotherapy in treatment-naive pediatric pulmonary arterial hypertension. Circulation 2014;129(19):1914–23.

11. Vargas-Origel A, Gómez-Rodríguez G, Aldana-Valenzuela C, et al. The use of sil-denafil in persistent pulmonary hypertension of the newborn. Am J Perinatol 2010;27(3):225–30.

12. Abman SH, Ivy DD, Archer SL, et al. Executive summary of the American heart association and American thoracic society joint guidelines for pediatric pulmo-nary hypertension. Am J Respir Crit Care Med 2016;194(7):898–906.

13. Steinhorn RH, Kinsella JP, Pierce C, et al. Intravenous sildenafil in the treatment of neonates with persistent pulmonary hypertension. J Pediatr 2009;155(6):841–7.e1.

14. Pierce CM, Zhang MH, Jonsson B, et al. Efficacy and safety of IV sildenafil in the treatment of newborn infants with, or at risk of, persistent pulmonary hypertension of the newborn (PPHN): a multicenter, randomized, placebo-controlled trial. J Pediatr 2021;237:154–61.e3.

15. Kadmon G, Schiller O, Dagan T, et al. Pulmonary hypertension specific treatment in infants with bronchopulmonary dysplasia. Pediatr Pulmonol 2017;52(1):77–83.

16. Mourani PM, Sontag MK, Ivy DD, et al. Effects of long-term sildenafil treatment for pulmonary hypertension in infants with chronic lung disease. J Pediatr 2009;154(3):379–84, 384.e1-2.

17. Tan K, Krishnamurthy MB, O'Heney JL, et al. Sildenafil therapy in bronchopulmo-nary dysplasia-associated pulmonary hypertension: a retrospective study of effi-cacy and safety. Eur J Pediatr 2015;174(8):1109–15.

18. Nyp M, Sandritter T, Poppinga N, et al. Sildenafil citrate, bronchopulmonary dysplasia and disordered pulmonary gas exchange: any benefits? J Perinatol 2012;32(1):64–9.

19. Trottier-Boucher MN, Lapointe A, Malo J, et al. Sildenafil for the treatment of pul-monary arterial hypertension in infants with bronchopulmonary dysplasia. Pediatr Cardiol 2015;36(6):1255–60.

20. Cohen JL, Nees SN, Valencia GA, et al. Sildenafil use in children with pulmonary hypertension. J Pediatr 2019;205:29–34.e1.

21. Thompson EJ, Perez K, Hornik CP, et al. Sildenafil exposure in the neonatal inten-sive care unit. Am J Perinatol 2019;36(3):262–7.

22. Lang JE, Hornik CD, Martz K, et al. Safety of sildenafil in premature infants at risk of bronchopulmonary dysplasia: rationale and methods of a phase II randomized trial. Contemp Clin Trials Commun 2022;30:101025.

23. Cochius-den Otter S, Schaible T, Greenough A, et al. The CoDiNOS trial protocol: an international randomised controlled trial of intravenous sildenafil versus inhaled nitric oxide for the treatment of pulmonary hypertension in neonates with congenital diaphragmatic hernia. BMJ Open 2019;9(11):e032122.

24. Buys ES, Zimmer DP, Chickering J, et al. Discovery and development of next gen-eration sGC stimulators with diverse multidimensional pharmacology and broad therapeutic potential. Nitric Oxide 2018;78:72–80.

25. Chester M, Seedorf G, Tourneux P, et al. Cinaciguat, a soluble guanylate cyclase activator, augments cGMP after oxidative stress and causes pulmonary vasodila-tion in neonatal pulmonary hypertension. Am J Physiol Lung Cell Mol Physiol 2011;301(5):L755–64.

26. Ghofrani HA, D'Armini AM, Grimminger F, et al. Riociguat for the treatment of chronic thromboembolic pulmonary hypertension. N Engl J Med 2013;369(4):319–29.

27. García Aguilar H, Gorenflo M, Ivy DD, et al. Riociguat in children with pulmonary arterial hypertension: the PATENT–CHILD study. Pulm Circ 2022;12(3):e12133.
28. Giesinger RE, Stanford AH, Thomas B, et al. Safety and feasibility of riociguat therapy for the treatment of chronic pulmonary arterial hypertension in infancy. J Pediatr 2023;255:224–9.e1.
29. Rosenberg AA, Kennaugh J, Koppenhafer SL, et al. Elevated immunoreactive endothelin-1 levels in newborn infants with persistent pulmonary hypertension. J Pediatr 1993;123(1):109–14.
30. Giaid A, Yanagisawa M, Langleben D, et al. Expression of endothelin-1 in the lungs of patients with pulmonary hypertension. N Engl J Med 1993;328(24): 1732–9.
31. Abman SH. Role of endothelin receptor antagonists in the treatment of pulmonary arterial hypertension. Annu Rev Med 2009;60(1):13–23.
32. Lakshminrusimha S, Mathew B, Leach CL. Pharmacologic strategies in neonatal pulmonary hypertension other than nitric oxide. Semin Perinatol 2016;40(3): 160–73.
33. Humbert M, Kovacs G, Hoeper MM, et al. 2022 ESC/ERS Guidelines for the diagnosis and treatment of pulmonary hypertension. Eur Heart J 2022;43(38): 3618–731.
34. Rosenzweig EB, Ivy DD, Widlitz A, et al. Effects of long-term bosentan in children with pulmonary arterial hypertension. J Am Coll Cardiol 2005;46(4):697–704.
35. Maiya S, Hislop AA, Flynn Y, et al. Response to bosentan in children with pulmonary hypertension. Heart 2006;92(5):664–70.
36. Barst RJ, Ivy D, Dingemanse J, et al. Pharmacokinetics, safety, and efficacy of bosentan in pediatric patients with pulmonary arterial hypertension. Clin Pharmacol Ther 2003;73(4):372–82.
37. Mohamed WA, Ismail M. A randomized, double-blind, placebo-controlled, prospective study of bosentan for the treatment of persistent pulmonary hypertension of the newborn. J Perinatol 2012;32(8):608–13.
38. Steinhorn RH, Fineman J, Kusic-Pajic A, et al. Bosentan as adjunctive therapy for persistent pulmonary hypertension of the newborn: results of the randomized multicenter placebo-controlled exploratory trial. J Pediatr 2016;177:90–6.e3.
39. Albinni S, Heno J, Pavo I, et al. Macitentan in the young—mid-term outcomes of patients with pulmonary hypertensive vascular disease treated in a pediatric tertiary care center. Paediatr Drugs 2023;25(4):467–81.
40. Takatsuki S, Rosenzweig EB, Zuckerman W, et al. Clinical safety, pharmacokinetics, and efficacy of ambrisentan therapy in children with pulmonary arterial hypertension. Pediatr Pulmonol 2013;48(1):27–34.
41. Issapour A, Frank B, Crook S, et al. Safety and tolerability of combination therapy with ambrisentan and tadalafil for the treatment of pulmonary arterial hypertension in children: real-world experience. Pediatr Pulmonol 2022;57(3):724–33.
42. Beghetti M, Hoeper MM, Kiely DG, et al. Safety experience with bosentan in 146 children 2–11 Years old with pulmonary arterial hypertension: results from the European postmarketing surveillance program. Pediatr Res 2008;64(2):200–4.
43. Del Pozo R, Hernandez Gonzalez I, Escribano-Subias P. The prostacyclin pathway in pulmonary arterial hypertension: a clinical review. Expet Rev Respir Med 2017;11(6):491–503.
44. Christman BW, McPherson CD, Newman JH, et al. An imbalance between the excretion of thromboxane and prostacyclin metabolites in pulmonary hypertension. N Engl J Med 1992;327(2):70–5.

45. Barst RJ, Maislin G, Fishman AP. Vasodilator therapy for primary pulmonary hypertension in children. Circulation 1999;99(9):1197–208.
46. Barst RJ, Rubin LJ, McGoon MD, et al. Survival in primary pulmonary hypertension with long-term continuous intravenous prostacyclin. Ann Intern Med 1994; 121(6):409–15.
47. Rosenzweig EB, Kerstein D, Barst RJ. Long-term prostacyclin for pulmonary hypertension with associated congenital heart defects. Circulation 1999;99(14): 1858–65.
48. Nees SN, Rosenzweig EB, Cohen JL, et al. Targeted therapy for pulmonary hypertension in premature infants. Children 2020;7(8):97.
49. Zaidi AN, Dettorre MD, Ceneviva GD, et al. Epoprostenol and home mechanical ventilation for pulmonary hypertension associated with chronic lung disease. Pediatr Pulmonol 2005;40(3):265–9.
50. Ahmad KA, Banales J, Henderson CL, et al. Intravenous epoprostenol improves oxygenation index in patients with persistent pulmonary hypertension of the newborn refractory to nitric oxide. J Perinatol 2018;38(9):1212–9.
51. De Jaegere A, Van Den Anker J. Endotracheal instillation of prostacyclin in preterm infants with persistent pulmonary hypertension. Eur Respir J 1998;12(4): 932–4.
52. Kelly LK, Porta NFM, Goodman DM, et al. Inhaled prostacyclin for term infants with persistent pulmonary hypertension refractory to inhaled nitric oxide. J Pediatr 2002;141(6):830–2.
53. Berger-Caron F, Piedboeuf B, Morissette G, et al. Inhaled epoprostenol for pulmonary hypertension treatment in neonates: a 12-year experience. Am J Perinatol 2019;36(11):1142–9.
54. Ehlen M, Wiebe B. Iloprost in persistent pulmonary hypertension of the newborn. Cardiol Young 2003;13(4):361–3.
55. Verma S, Lumba R, Kazmi SH, et al. Effects of inhaled iloprost for the management of persistent pulmonary hypertension of the newborn. Am J Perinatol 2022;39(13):1441–8.
56. Kahveci H, Yilmaz O, Avsar UZ, et al. Oral sildenafil and inhaled iloprost in the treatment of pulmonary hypertension of the newborn. Pediatr Pulmonol 2014; 49(12):1205–13.
57. Yilmaz O, Kahveci H, Zeybek C, et al. Inhaled iloprost in preterm infants with severe respiratory distress syndrome and pulmonary hypertension. Am J Perinatol 2013;31(04):321–6.
58. Piastra M, De Luca D, De Carolis MP, et al. Nebulized iloprost and noninvasive respiratory support for impending hypoxaemic respiratory failure in formerly preterm infants: a case series. Pediatr Pulmonol 2012;47(8):757–62.
59. Hwang SK, Yung-Chul O, Kim NS, et al. Use of inhaled iloprost in an infant with bronchopulmonary dysplasia and pulmonary artery hypertension. Korean Circ J 2009;39(8):343–5.
60. Gürakan B, Kayıran P, Öztürk N, et al. Therapeutic combination of sildenafil and iloprost in a preterm neonate with pulmonary hypertension. Pediatr Pulmonol 2011;46(6):617–20.
61. Simonneau G, Barst RJ, Galie N, et al. Continuous subcutaneous infusion of treprostinil, a prostacyclin analogue, in patients with pulmonary arterial hypertension. Am J Respir Crit Care Med 2002;165(6):800–4.
62. Levy M, Del Cerro MJ, Nadaud S, et al. Safety, efficacy and Management of subcutaneous treprostinil infusions in the treatment of severe pediatric pulmonary hypertension. Int J Cardiol 2018;264:153–7.

63. Krishnan U, Takatsuki S, Ivy DD, et al. Effectiveness and safety of inhaled treprostinil for the treatment of pulmonary arterial hypertension in children. Am J Cardiol 2012;110(11):1704–9.

64. Olson E, Lusk LA, Fineman JR, et al. Short-term treprostinil use in infants with congenital diaphragmatic hernia following repairs. J Pediatr 2015;167(3):762–4.

65. Carpentier E, Mur S, Aubry E, et al. Safety and tolerability of subcutaneous treprostinil in newborns with congenital diaphragmatic hernia and life-threatening pulmonary hypertension. J Pediatr Surg 2017;52(9):1480–3.

66. Lawrence KM, Hedrick HL, Monk HM, et al. Treprostinil improves persistent pulmonary hypertension associated with congenital diaphragmatic hernia. J Pediatr 2018;200:44–9.

67. De Bie FR, Avitabile CM, Flohr S, et al. Treprostinil in neonates with congenital diaphragmatic hernia-related pulmonary hypertension. J Pediatr 2023;259:113420.

68. Sitbon O, Channick R, Chin KM, et al. Selexipag for the treatment of pulmonary arterial hypertension. N Engl J Med 2015;373(26):2522–33.

69. Youssef D, Richards S, Lague S, et al. A Canadian, retrospective, multicenter experience with selexipag for a heterogeneous group of pediatric pulmonary hypertension patients. Front Pediatr 2023;11:1055158.

70. Rothman A, Cruz G, Evans WN, et al. Hemodynamic and clinical effects of selexipag in children with pulmonary hypertension. Pulm Circ 2020;10(1).

71. Colglazier E, Stevens L, Parker C, et al. Hemodynamic assessment of transitioning from parenteral prostacyclin to selexipag in pediatric pulmonary hypertension. Pulm Circ 2022;12(4):e12159.

72. Koo R, Lo J, Bock MJ. Transition from intravenous treprostinil to enteral selexipag in an infant with pulmonary arterial hypertension. Cardiol Young 2019;29(6):849–51.

73. McNamara PJ, Shivananda SP, Sahni M, et al. Pharmacology of milrinone in neonates with persistent pulmonary hypertension of the newborn and suboptimal response to inhaled nitric oxide*. Pediatr Crit Care Med 2013;14(1):74–84.

74. McNamara PJ, Laique F, Muang-In S, et al. Milrinone improves oxygenation in neonates with severe persistent pulmonary hypertension of the newborn. J Crit Care 2006;21(2):217–22.

75. James AT, Corcoran JD, McNamara PJ, et al. The effect of milrinone on right and left ventricular function when used as a rescue therapy for term infants with pulmonary hypertension. Cardiol Young 2016;26(1):90–9.

76. Dillard J, Pavlek LR, Korada S, et al. Worsened short-term clinical outcomes in a cohort of patients with iNO-unresponsive PPHN: a case for improving iNO responsiveness. J Perinatol 2022;42(1):37–44.

77. EL-Khuffash A, McNamara PJ, Breatnach C, et al. The use of milrinone in neonates with persistent pulmonary hypertension of the newborn - a randomised controlled trial pilot study (MINT 1). J Perinatol 2023;43(2):168–73.

78. Patel N. Use of milrinone to treat cardiac dysfunction in infants with pulmonary hypertension secondary to congenital diaphragmatic hernia: a review of six patients. Neonatology 2012;102(2):130–6.

79. Mears M, Yang M, Yoder BA. Is milrinone effective for infants with mild-to-moderate congenital diaphragmatic hernia? Am J Perinatol 2020;37(03):258–63.

80. Lakshminrusimha S, Keszler M, Kirpalani H, et al. Milrinone in congenital diaphragmatic hernia – a randomized pilot trial: study protocol, review of literature and survey of current practices. Matern Health Neonatol Perinatol 2017;3:27.

81. Sharif Kashani B, Tahmaseb Pour P, Malekmohammad M, et al. Oral l-citrulline malate in patients with idiopathic pulmonary arterial hypertension and Eisenmenger Syndrome: a clinical trial. J Cardiol 2014;64(3):231–5.
82. Fike CD, Dikalova A, Kaplowitz MR, et al. Rescue treatment with L-citrulline inhibits hypoxia-induced pulmonary hypertension in newborn pigs. Am J Respir Cell Mol Biol 2015;53(2):255–64.
83. Fike CD, Aschner JL. Pharmacotherapy for pulmonary hypertension in infants with bronchopulmonary dysplasia: past, present, and future. Pharmaceuticals 2023;16(4):503.
84. Farrow KN, Lakshminrusimha S, Reda WJ, et al. Superoxide dismutase restores eNOS expression and function in resistance pulmonary arteries from neonatal lambs with persistent pulmonary hypertension. Am J Physiol Lung Cell Mol Physiol 2008;295(6):L979–87.
85. Lakshminrusimha S, Russell JA, Wedgwood S, et al. Superoxide dismutase improves oxygenation and reduces oxidation in neonatal pulmonary hypertension. Am J Respir Crit Care Med 2006;174(12):1370–7.
86. Davis JM, Richter SE, Biswas S, et al. Long-term follow-up of premature infants treated with prophylactic, intratracheal recombinant human CuZn superoxide dismutase. J Perinatol 2000;20(4):213–6.
87. Dikalova A, Aschner JL, Kaplowitz MR, et al. Tetrahydrobiopterin oral therapy recouples eNOS and ameliorates chronic hypoxia-induced pulmonary hypertension in newborn pigs. Am J Physiol Lung Cell Mol Physiol 2016;311(4):L743–53.
88. Mestan KK, Check J, Minturn L, et al. Placental pathologic changes of maternal vascular underperfusion in bronchopulmonary dysplasia and pulmonary hypertension. Placenta 2014;35(8):570–4.
89. Check J, Gotteiner N, Liu X, et al. Fetal growth restriction and pulmonary hypertension in premature infants with bronchopulmonary dysplasia. J Perinatol Off J Calif Perinat Assoc 2013;33(7):553–7.
90. Seedorf G, Kim C, Wallace B, et al. rhIGF-1/BP3 preserves lung growth and prevents pulmonary hypertension in experimental bronchopulmonary dysplasia. Am J Respir Crit Care Med 2020;201(9):1120–34.

Asphyxia, Therapeutic Hypothermia, and Pulmonary Hypertension

Regan Geisinger, MD[a,†], Danielle R. Rios, MD, MS[a],
Patrick J. McNamara, MB, BCh, BAO, DCH, MSc, MRCP, MRCPCH[a],
Philip T. Levy, MD[b,*]

KEYWORDS

- Hypoxic ischemic encephalopathy • Therapeutic hypothermia
- Acute pulmonary hypertension • Echocardiography

KEY POINTS

- Neonates with a perinatal hypoxic event and subsequent neonatal encephalopathy are at risk of acute pulmonary hypertension (aPH) in the transitional period.
- The hypoxic insult to cardiopulmonary performance that clinically manifests as aPH may further exacerbate organ damage and contribute to the short-term and long-term neurologic sequelae.
- The phenotypic contributors to aPH following perinatal asphyxia include a combination of parenchymal lung disease (in some cases), hypoxic vasoconstriction of the pulmonary vascular bed, right ventricular dysfunction, and occasionally left heart dysfunction.
- The process of aPH in neonatal encephalopathy is dynamic, evolving with the disease course impacted by the intervention of therapeutic hypothermia during both the cooling and rewarming phases.
- Despite the increased recognition of the risk for aPH, there remains a lack of clarity regarding thresholds for hemodynamic screening, diagnosis, and intervention for aPH in neonatal encephalopathy.

INTRODUCTION

Neonates with a perinatal hypoxic event and subsequent neonatal encephalopathy are at risk of developing acute pulmonary hypertension (aPH) in the early neonatal

[a] Division of Neonatology, Department of Pediatrics, University of Iowa, 200 Hawkins Drive, Iowa City, IA 52242, USA; [b] Division of Newborn Medicine, Department of Pediatrics, Boston Children's Hospital, Harvard Medical School, 300 Longwood Avenue, Hunnewell 436, Boston, MA 02115, USA
[†] In memory, with gratitude.
* Corresponding author.
E-mail address: philip.levy@childrens.harvard.edu

Clin Perinatol 51 (2024) 127–149
https://doi.org/10.1016/j.clp.2023.11.007   perinatology.theclinics.com

period.[1] Clinicians are most often concerned with the hypoxic cerebral injury that results from the lack of adequate blood flow and/or gas exchange immediately before, during, or after delivery, also known as perinatal asphyxia. The injurious processes of perinatal asphyxia may extend to cardiopulmonary performance, which in some patients may clinically manifest as aPH, and further exacerbate organ damage that contributes to the short-term and long-term neurologic sequelae.[2–5] In addition, mortality is higher in infants with combined features of hypoxic ischemic encephalopathy (HIE) and aPH when compared with infants with aPH alone.[6] Accordingly, a high index of suspicion for aPH and its consequences in the immediate postnatal period is important to consider in neonates following a hypoxic ischemic event.

During the past 2 decades, therapeutic hypothermia has become the standard of care for cases where a hypoxic ischemic insult causes moderate or severe encephalopathy.[7] Although perinatal asphyxia may have a negative impact on heart rate, loading conditions, myocardial performance, and vascular interactions, therapeutic hypothermia itself may subsequently modify cardiac performance and pulmonary hemodynamics, exacerbate the aPH, and complicate mechanistic delineation in this high-risk population. Because the biological processes of aPH in neonatal encephalopathy are dynamic and further influenced by both the cooling and rewarming phases of therapeutic hypothermia, the integration of hemodynamic (clinical, biochemical, and echocardiographic) features must be considered to allow for a better assessment of the immediate risk and long-term prognosis. Echocardiography evaluation of cardiac performance and pulmonary vascular hemodynamics may help elucidate cardiopulmonary compromise earlier, enable a more precise approach to therapeutic intervention, monitor treatment response throughout the initial insult and phases of therapeutic hypothermia, and improve overall outcomes.[3,4] This article discusses the impact of perinatal asphyxia on myocardial performance and the pulmonary vascular system, including the causes, risk factors, and hemodynamic assessment of associated aPH. In addition, we discuss the interaction between asphyxia and aPH during each phase of therapeutic hypothermia and highlight important hemodynamic considerations unique to these patients. We provide a physiology-based approach for management of aPH based on recent discoveries and emerging diagnostic methods and therapies.

TERMINOLOGY

Persistent pulmonary hypertension (PPHN) is the terminology typically used for pulmonary hypertension that presents in the immediate postnatal period secondary to abnormal transition of the pulmonary circulation. Although the term "PPHN" may be applicable to patients with hypoxic vasoconstriction of the pulmonary vascular bed and maladaptive pulmonary vasculature leading to failure of the normal postnatal decline in pulmonary vascular resistance (PVR), it misrepresents those cases of pulmonary hypertension that are associated with right[3,4,8] and left heart dysfunction[9,10] in neonates following a perinatal hypoxic event. As such, the phrase "acute pulmonary hypertension" is more suitable in the transitional period because it reflects disturbances of elevated mean pulmonary artery pressure (mPAP) due to a broad range of diseases including right ventricle (RV) or left ventricle (LV) dysfunction, as well as hypoxic pulmonary vasoconstriction, which may result from the perinatal hypoxic insult.[11]

EPIDEMIOLOGY AND RISK FACTORS

HIE affects approximately 1 to 2 per 1000 live births in developed countries and 26 per 1000 in low-resource countries.[12] The incidence of aPH ranges from 13% to 29%

among infants with HIE,[5,6,13–17] which is higher than the incidence of aPH (0.43–6 per thousand live born term infants) in the general population.[18] Acute pulmonary hypertension is more commonly associated with moderate-to-severe HIE.[6] Several reports have investigated the prevalence of aPH since the introduction of therapeutic hypothermia (TH) as standard of care for treatment of moderate/severe HIE.[6,16,19,20] The original trials of TH did not show a higher overall incidence of hypoxemic respiratory failure with presumed pulmonary hypertension.[19] Lakshminrusimha and colleagues[6] reported no difference in the rates of aPH between neonates receiving TH (33.5°C) and those with normothermia in the Neonatal Research Network (National Institute of Child Health and Human Development [NICHD]-NRN) clinical trials. NICHD-NRN optimizing cooling trial showed higher incidence of aPH and extracorporeal membrane oxygenation (ECMO) need with deeper cooling to 32°C.[14] On the contrary, Joanna and colleagues[16] found that aPH was 2.5 times higher in neonates who received TH, and echocardiographic evidence of increased PVR was reported after TH in the observational study by Seghal and colleagues.[20] There is overlap in maternal, fetal, and postnatal risk factors between the phenotypical presentations of neonatal aPH. Maternal and fetal risk factors can affect the development of pulmonary vasculature (eg, maternal diabetes, presence of fetal hypoxemia,[16] maternal age,[5] and outborn status[5]) and how it adapts to extrauterine life (**Table 1**). Additional in utero conditions (eg, placental insufficiency and oligohydramnios) can result in excessive pulmonary vascular muscularization and pulmonary hypoplasia, respectively, which further increase the risk of altered transition and HIE. Perinatal risk factors can lead to injury to the lung parenchyma (eg, respiratory distress syndrome, meconium aspiration,[5,6,16] sepsis,[5] and pulmonary hemorrhage[16]) and affect the molecular pathways responsible for pulmonary vasomotor tone and lead to aPH.[21] Joanna and colleagues[16] found an association between aPH and HIE with several postnatal factors before the initiation of TH, including severe acidosis (presence of hypercarbia on the first postnatal gas) use of medications during delivery room resuscitation, and higher baseline fraction of inspired oxygen (Fio_2; **Fig. 1**). Infants with aPH were more likely to require longer duration of inotropic support[5] and had lower cardiac output,[16] highlighting that the perinatal insult may also cause ventricular dysfunction.[5]

IMPACT OF PERINATAL ASPHYXIA ON PULMONARY VASCULAR VASOREACTIVITY

There are several mechanisms by which perinatal asphyxia and subsequent hypoxia and acidosis prevent the normal relaxation of the pulmonary vascular bed. There is

Table 1
Risk factors for acute pulmonary hypertension in neonates with perinatal asphyxia

Maternal	Fetal	Neonatal
Maternal diabetes	Fetal hypoxemia	Outborn status
Advanced maternal age	Oligohydramnios	Severe acidosis (hypercarbia)
Placental insufficiency		Need for delivery room resuscitation
Maternal drugs (eg, SSRIs) NSAIDs		with pharmacologic agents
Congenital infections		Myocardial dysfunction
		Meconium aspiration syndrome
		Respiratory distress syndrome
		Pulmonary hemorrhage
		Sepsis
		Polycythemia

Abbreviations: NSAIDs, nonsteroidal anti-inflammatory drugs; SSRIs, selective serotonin reuptake inhibitors.

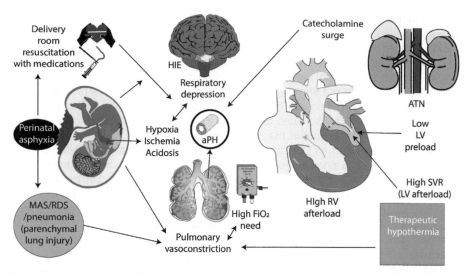

Fig. 1. Pathophysiology of aPH in neonates following perinatal asphyxia. Asphyxia is often associated with parenchymal lung disease such as meconium aspiration syndrome (MAS), respiratory distress syndrome (RDS), or pneumonia or idiopathic aPH contributing to hypoxic pulmonary vasoconstriction. The use of medications (epinephrine) during delivery room resuscitation increases the risk of HIE associated with aPH. ATN, acute tubular necrosis; LV, left ventricle; SVR, systemic vascular resistance. (Image Courtesy of Dr. Satyan Lakshminrusimha.)

an imbalance in favor of production of endothelin 1 with reduced production of nitric oxide that leads to elevated PVR causing deoxygenated blood to be shunted to the systemic vasculature.[22] A "surge of catecholamines" from the adrenal glands produces pulmonary and peripheral vasoconstriction that concentrates blood flow to the brain and further contributes to hypoxemia.[1] Subsequent respiratory depression with late clearance of fluid from the lungs can also increase PVR and reduce the cardiac output to the lungs. As the PVR increases and the aPH worsens, the impairment in oxygenation and pulmonary venous return further compromises the already reduced systemic blood flow from the HIE-induced cardiac injury.[23]

IMPACT OF PERINATAL ASPHYXIA ON MYOCARDIAL PERFORMANCE

Perinatal asphyxia can lead to a specific type of neonatal cardiomyopathy in the anatomically normal heart characterized by ventricular pump failure and dilated heart muscle[9] **(Table 2)**. Heart failure has been documented in 30% to 82% of neonates with severe HIE.[9,24,25] Compared with children and adults, the neonatal myocardium is composed of less-developed contractile mechanisms with disorganized myofibrils, immature calcium handling system, and inadequately compliant collagen **(Fig. 2)**.[9] This places the immature myocardium at increased susceptibility to afterload and extremes of heart rate changes (force–frequency relationship). The etiology of an acquired hypoxic-ischemic myocardial insult is either from the perinatal or coronary insult (stenosis, abnormal origin, or in utero compromise).[26] At the cellular level, hypoxia and acidosis disturbs the physiologic cardiomyocyte metabolism that switches almost completely from glycolytic pathways to oxidation of fatty acids.[27] Redistribution of blood flow with perinatal asphyxia can also lead to decreased perfusion and myocardial ischemia. The myocardial perfusion may be further compromised from the high intramural myocardial pressure secondary to elevated ventricular filling pressures and the low

Table 2
Impact of asphyxia and therapeutic hypothermia on cardiopulmonary status

Hypoxic ischemic insult	Therapeutic Hypothermia	
	Cooling phase	Rewarming phase
Vascular Vasoconstriction of the pulmonary vascular bed	**Vascular** Pulmonary vasoconstriction: ↑ PVR Systemic vasoconstriction: ↑ SVR Decreased cerebral blood flow Redistribution of LVO to brain Cerebral redistribution	**Vascular** Pulmonary vascular vasodilation: ↓ PVR Systemic vasodilation: ↓ SVR Persistent cerebral redistribution
Myocardial RV dysfunction LV dysfunction	**Myocardial** Decreased preload Decreased RV contractility Altered RV–pulmonary vascular coupling Decreased cardiac output **Autonomic** Sinus bradycardia Increased influence of the parasympathetic system **Other** Altered net inotropic response, clearance, and drug metabolism	**Myocardial** Normalization of preload Increased contractility Improved RV – pulmonary vascular coupling Increased LVO/RVO/cardiac output **Autonomic** Increased heart rate **Other** Mobilization (exaggerated) effect of inotropes

Abbreviations: LV, left ventricle; LVO, left ventricle output; PVR, pulmonary vascular resistance; RV, right ventricle; RVO, right ventricle output; SVR, systemic vascular resistance.

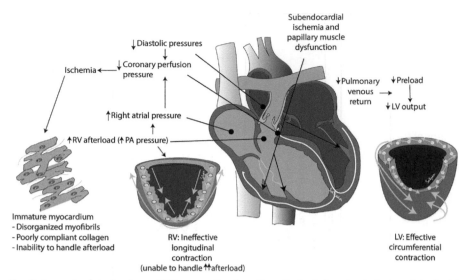

Fig. 2. Impact of asphyxia and TH on cardiac function. Perinatal asphyxia is associated with low diastolic pressure. Acute PH is associated with high right ventricular (RV) and PA pressure in turn leading to increased right atrial pressure. A combination of low diastolic pressure and high right atrial pressure results in low coronary perfusion pressure leading to myocardial ischemia. The RV with longitudinal contraction is less effective in dealing with increased afterload compared with LV with more effective circumferential contraction. Reduced pulmonary venous return due to aPH and deviation of the interventricular septum to the left results in low LV preload. (Image Courtesy of Dr. Satyan Lakshminrusimha.)

systemic diastolic pressure. Morphologically, perinatal asphyxia leads to a dilated cardiomyopathy where the cavity is enlarged with normal or thin wall thickness.[9] The heart can be affected on all levels but there is a preference/tendency for dysfunction at the papillary muscles and subendocardial regions.[26,28] Collectively, these factors predispose the myocardium to diastolic dysfunction and altered compliance with the following impact on the heart: (1) lacking the reserve to cope with reduced preload from low pulmonary venous return, blood loss, and capillary leak and/or (2) not tolerating the abrupt increase in afterload from a combination of hypoxia, sepsis, sedation, adrenal failure, and induced autonomic dysfunction. After the initial perinatal hypoxic insult, myocardial contractility increases and the heart works to enhance blood flow and protect against systemic hypoxia.[29] Myocardial injury will ultimately develop when this "compensation mechanism" fails.[30] Cardiac dysfunction will further worsen following reperfusion injury secondary to reactive oxygen species. Both inflammatory and oxidative stress eventually reduce the contractile responsiveness of the myocardium, causing a significant reduction in cardiac output,[31] hypotension, and further impairment of cerebral blood flow and perfusion of other organs.[29] Differences between RV and LV are outlined in later discussion. In preterm infants with a perinatal asphyxia, the rate of myocardial injury may be higher with known risk factors for diastolic dysfunction and decreased response to altered loading conditions.[32]

PHENOTYPIC ETIOPATHOLOGIES OF ACUTE PULMONARY HYPERTENSION IN HYPOXIC ISCHEMIC ENCEPHALOPATHY

The spectrum of phenotypical presentation for aPH in neonates with HIE is best determined from contributions of PVR, pulmonary blood flow (PBF), and pulmonary capillary wedge pressure (PCWP) on mPAPs by the equation: $mPAP = (PVR \times PBF) + PCWP$.[33] There are 3 potential contributors to aPH that have been observed in neonates with a perinatal hypoxic insult: (1) Hypoxic pulmonary vasoconstriction and elevated PVR[6]; (2) Alterations in right heart performance with altered PBF[3,4]; and (3) Depressed left heart function impacting PCWP.[10] Awareness of the spectrum of these different phenotypes can facilitate appropriate monitoring and management (**Fig. 3**).

Hypoxic Pulmonary Vasoconstriction

In neonates with HIE, the pulmonary vasculature can maladapt after delivery due to either intraparenchymal lung disease processes (eg, meconium aspiration and air leak syndromes) or extraparenchymal disorders (eg, acidosis and sepsis) that affect oxygenation, ventilation, and lung recruitment.[33] The hypoxic vasoconstriction of the pulmonary vasculature leads to elevated PVR. With this phenotype, the pulmonary vasculature is structurally normal but with abnormal vasoreactivity due to mediators promoting vasoconstriction and negating vasodilation, which affect the transitional reduction of RV afterload and the relationship of PVR to systemic vascular resistance (SVR).[34] This phenotype presents with hypoxia and occasionally parenchymal lung disease. For example, meconium aspiration syndrome can interfere with gas exchange, alter lung compliance, and result in raised PVR. In addition, the neonate with HIE may not be able to initiate respirations on their own and is reliant on less-effective positive pressure breaths that can interfere with establishing functional residual capacity. As such, even in the absence of identified lung pathologic condition, proper clearance of fetal lung fluid may be impaired without establishment of pressure gradient for fetal lung fluid to be absorbed (see **Fig. 1**).

Right Heart Disease

Normal RV performance is critical for adequate PBF. The right heart disease that manifests in neonates with HIE may originate from a primary insult to the RV during the initial and reperfusion injury, in addition to its dual response to elevated PVR with hypoxic pulmonary vasoconstriction or ventriculo-ventricular interactions with LV disease.[8] Giesinger and colleagues[3] demonstrated that echocardiographic evidence of RV dysfunction at 24 hours of age in neonates with HIE undergoing TH was an independent

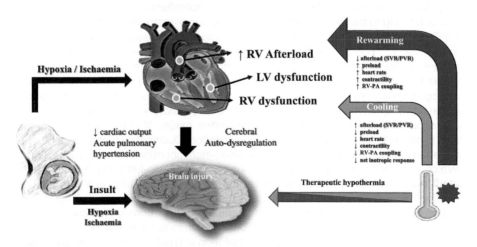

Fig. 3. Phenotypic contributors to aPH following perinatal asphyxia.

predictor of death or abnormal brain MRI in the short term and adverse neurodevelopment into early infancy,[4] even after adjusting for severity of the insult and subsequent disease burden with preserved LV functional parameters and the pseudonormalization of pulmonary hemodynamics.[3] It is plausible that primary RV dysfunction alone has the potential to lead to biventricular enlargement, dilated cardiomyopathy, and further impairment to systemic circulation and end-organ perfusion.[9] The developmental biology of the RV affects how it responds to a primary hypoxic injury during the perinatal transition and aids in classification and management of neonatal aPH.[35] The RV is a thin-walled structure with coarse trabeculations that provide the substrate for the RV to accommodate increases in volume and afterload. Unlike the LV, that has its own unique circumferential fiber pattern to provide the major contributions to stroke volume and enhance cardiac output, the RV relies primarily on a deep longitudinal fiber layer that does not allow for robust responses to changes in afterload (according to the force–frequency relationship) compared with its neighboring LV. The RV experiences greater wall stress for a similar degree of afterload as compared with the LV. In addition, the RV coronary circulation is negatively affected by high right heart pressure and low aortic root pressure seen with impaired pulmonary venous return following perinatal asphyxia. The RV loses its dominance during transition with redistribution of postnatal blood flow, and this leads to increased metabolic demands on the right heart that may not respond favorably to hypoxia and acidosis. As such, the RV becomes dependent on preload with a weakened response to augment cardiac output according to the RV Frank–Starling relationship. Although both the LV and RV may be equally affected by the initial hypoxic insult and reperfusion injury, the cumulative effect may be less well tolerated by the RV due its unique morphology and its immature ability to respond to changes in loading conditions. The RV disease tends to be worse in the first postnatal days and typically resolves during the first week of age.[3,4]

Left Heart Disease

In some neonates with HIE, the LV may also be impacted by the initial perinatal insult.[36] The abnormal LV performance manifests as reduced stroke volume and altered parameters of systolic and diastolic function leading to decreased cardiac output.[1] As mentioned, reactive oxygen species are also present during the reperfusion injury and may reduce contractile responsiveness and lead to further reduction in cardiac output. Severe LV failure with impaired compliance increases left heart preload, according to the Frank–Starling curve, and the overstretched left heart and high PCWP may lead to pulmonary venous congestion and increased pressures in the pulmonary artery.[37] Because of the increased RV afterload, secondary right heart failure may ensue and worsen the aPH. Neonates with HIE and severe LV failure present with hypoxemia, respiratory failure, low cardiac output, and can ultimately progress to cardiogenic shock with failure of compensatory mechanisms. The pulmonary venous congestion and left heart components of this aPH phenotype are usually not responsive to pulmonary vasodilators (eg, inhaled nitric oxide, iNO) because the primary insult is not on the pulmonary arterial (PA) circulation. Diagnostic clues include pulmonary edema on radiograph and persistent left-to-right shunting at the atrial level (indicative of higher left atrial pressure) with simultaneous right-to-left shunting through the patent ductus arteriosus (PDA). In the setting of severe LV failure, infants may have critically low cardiac output; therefore, the systemic circulation is exclusively dependent on right-to-left flow across the PDA and selective pulmonary vasodilators would be harmful. Finally, LV diastolic dysfunction and subsequent increases in PCWP are associated with a higher risk for invasive ventilation and pulmonary disease in infants[38] and are directly correlated with abnormal coupling of the RV to its afterload during the transitional period.[39] The reduced left heart function is often transient, with the most severe cardiovascular abnormalities typically occurring 48 to 72 hours after the initial insult, followed by gradual recovery.[40]

HEMODYNAMICS OF ACUTE PULMONARY HYPERTENSION IN HYPOXIC ISCHEMIC ENCEPHALOPATHY

Perinatal asphyxia–induced aPH results in a "constellation of hemodynamic consequences that manifest as oxygenation failure with cyanosis, severe ventilation perfusion mismatch, low cardiac output in severe cases, and unstable vasoreactivity that leads to instability with handling and agitation."[21] Acute pulmonary hypertension associated with hypoxic pulmonary vasoconstriction (and elevated PVR) and pulmonary venous congestion from left heart dysfunction (elevated PCWP) may both result in a direct increase in RV afterload but require careful delineation because the approach to management is divergent. The challenge for the RV is to remain hemodynamically coupled to the pulmonary circulation in the setting of elevated RV afterload. The RV to pulmonary vasculature coupling is maintained by RV adaptation to increasing pulmonary vascular load by enhancing contractility to maintain PBF.[41] Muscle hypertrophy is a crucial adaptive mechanism that enhances the contractile capabilities of the RV. Prolonged exposure to increased afterload and progressive pressure loading on the RV can lead to maladaptive ventricular remodeling, in which the RV dilates and results in decreased stroke volume followed by an increase in heart rate to maintain cardiac output.[41] This response to high afterload is associated with an increase in RV myocyte stress, dilation, and septal bowing, which further impairs RV function and decreases PBF. In situations where there is an additional primary insult on the RV, the PBF is decreased. RV dysfunction will serve as the catalyst for a cascade of downstream events and "self-perpetuating cycle of declining cardiovascular wellbeing" if untreated.[21] Varying degrees of LV dysfunction can ensue due to the initial perinatal hypoxic insult or "inter-ventricular dependence from LV compaction caused by RV dilation and septal bowing and decreased LV filling from decreased PBF."[33] Ultimately, the neonatal myocardium will not be able to handle complex hemodynamic changes, and the RV uncouples from high afterload, leading to decreased RV performance and overt RV failure.[42]

IMPACT OF THERAPEUTIC HYPOTHERMIA ON ACUTE PULMONARY HYPERTENSION

TH is considered standard of care for neonates suffering from perinatal asphyxia and moderate or severe HIE.[7] The known adverse impact of TH on the cardiopulmonary system is well documented[43,44] with ongoing hemodynamic instability related either to the primary insult, the effects of TH (cooling and/or rewarming), or even the approach to intervention. Although each adverse effect may compromise vital organ perfusion and metabolism and potentially decrease the effectiveness of neuroprotective strategies,[1,45] the risks are outweighed by the benefits to survival and neurodevelopmental outcome.[13] As such, cardiac performance depends on the interaction among preload, afterload, intrinsic myocardial contractility, and heart rate. Therefore, it is important to characterize the hemodynamic changes that can occur during both the cooling and rewarming phases of TH to understand the overall contribution to aPH in this high-risk population (see **Table 2**).

Cooling

The expected physiologic effects during cooling include increased systemic and PVR, reduced cardiac contractility with altered inotropic responses, reduced preload, lower heart rate, and ultimately reduced cardiac output.[43,44]

Increased pulmonary vascular resistance

Hypothermia causes pulmonary vascular constriction and potentially modulates PVR through neuronal mechanisms[46] but this may not be clinically significant in every case.[47] In a lamb model cooled to 30°C, pulmonary artery pressure increased by approximately 50%[48] and in a rodent model, PVR increased 1% per 1°C decrease in body temperature.[48] Increase in blood velocity[49] and catecholamine responses[50] to hypothermia temperatures may also contribute to higher PVR in infants in the cooling phase. Oxygen requirements may increase in patients with aPH due to hypoxic pulmonary vasoconstriction and increased PVR. However, evidences from the original TH studies have not shown a significant increase in aPH.[13] In the only observational human study, Vasquez and Geisinger and colleagues[51] demonstrated that in neonates with HIE, the cooling phase of TH is associated with increased mPAP and worsening pulmonary hemodynamics on echocardiography but RV function was not affected. It is likely that the magnitude by which cooling changes PVR varies by temperature range as observational studies have demonstrated increases in Fio_2 requirement in some but not all neonates with HIE.[43] In addition, experts suggest that initiation of cooling may still modulate the risk of aPH (or exacerbate aPH that is already present) in some patients; therefore, caution is advised in neonates who already display clinical signs of aPH.[4,8,11,36]

Increased systemic vascular resistance

At delivery, the sympathetic system is not yet fully functional because the resting peripheral vascular tone remains high but with decreased beta-adrenergic receptors. Cooling further increases the alpha-adrenergic receptors but blunts the beta-adrenergic effect and affects the intolerance of the myocardial contractility to respond to an increased systemic or PVR (afterload). Ultimately, these processes lead to a reduced net inotropic effect of cardiotropic medications.

Reduced preload

The reduction in preload is multifactorial. The initial perinatal hypoxic insult can increase hydrostatic pressure and lead to increased capillary permeability. The total fluid goal is also restricted when HIE is suspected to minimize metabolic demands and due to coexisting renal dysfunction due to acute tubular necrosis. There is also increased blood sampling during the early cooling phase of TH. A primary insult to RV or a secondary response of the RV to elevated PVR can both lead to reduced stroke capacity, reduced pulmonary venous return, and inferior filling of the LV. Accordingly, stroke volume and cardiac output will be low during the cooling phase based on the Frank–Starling relationship.

Impaired contractility

Cooled neonates have reduced heart function during treatment,[10,52,53] probably to a similar degree as seen in noncooled neonates.[10] Although heart function is reduced during TH, plasma lactate levels that are often high at the start of treatment[10,54] usually improve during cooling,[10] due to reduced metabolic demands at low body temperature. The impairment in contractility results from intolerance to increased afterload, immaturity of the cardiomyocytes, and a blunted beta-adrenergic effect. As such, there is often an altered inotropic response and caution must be used when initiating and titrating certain medications while in the cooling period.[55] For example, neonates with hypoxic respiratory failure and HIE who have undergone TH and are treated with milrinone to augment contractility and reduce pulmonary afterload developed profound reduction of diastolic blood pressure that required escalation of additional cardiotropic support.[55] These effects are postulated to relate to milrinone toxicity secondary to impaired renal clearance.

Lower heart rate

Sinus bradycardia is common during the cooling phase with slow repolarization of the sinoatrial node by reduced intracellular calcium release but does not usually require medical treatment.[13] The decreased effect of the parasympathetic system on the heart during TH also induces moderate bradycardia and leads to decreased stroke volume and reduced metabolic demand on the myocardium.

Altered right ventricle–pulmonary artery coupling

RV function depends on its afterload. With increasing PAP, there is a proportional response in RV systolic function, which is governed by the stress–velocity relationship (ie, RV–PA coupling). The challenge in aPH is for the RV to remain hemodynamically coupled to a compliant pulmonary artery circulation with the degree of RV failure in the first 24 hours directly linked to poor outcomes beyond the neonatal period.[4] Evidence also shows in addition to the initial insult, the cooling phase leads to abnormal RV–PA interactions.[3] This has relevance because when RV–PA coupling is normal, treatment to lower PVR may also enhance RV performance and normalize RV function.

Rewarming

The second phase of TH has its own unique impact on hemodynamics with progressive vasodilation of the systemic and pulmonary vasculature, increases in preload, heart rate, and cardiac output. Although less is known about the hemodynamic impact of rewarming on the brain, observational studies have shown that most intraventricular hemorrhage occurs during the rewarming period and was associated with significant hemodynamic lability.[45] "Rewarming hemodynamics" and how to actively adjust the cardiovascular specific medications throughout the warming period requires further study.[1]

Decreased pulmonary vascular resistance

Rewarming leads to pulmonary vasculature dilation and decreased PVR.[56]

Decreased systemic vascular resistance

Rewarming leads to progressive systemic vasodilation with a decrease in SVR. This is clinically reflected by a lower diastolic component of the blood pressure. As such, the mean blood pressure may actually remain unchanged or decline.[46] Rewarming may be associated with seizures requiring additional antiepileptic medications that may also contribute to hypotension. The lower diastolic blood pressure may affect pharmacologic clearance and metabolism of cardiotropic medications. The mean blood pressure may drop but studies have shown that the redistribution of blood flow to the brain remains constant,[57] with nonsignificant clinical changes in stroke volume and mean blood pressure.[56]

Increased preload

Rewarming results in progressive vasodilation of the systemic and pulmonary vasculature with increased PBF. The total fluids are also slowly increased while some infants are also able to tolerate some enteral nutrition.

Contractility

Rewarming hemodynamics leads to improved cardiac contractility, increased metabolic rate, and cardiac output that are predominately heart rate dependent.[58,59] As such, there may be an "exaggerated" effect of inotropes.

Increased heart rate

Rewarming physiologically raises the heart rate and leads to enhanced stroke volume.[60] Cardiac output actually increases more due to heart rate than stroke volume.[61]

Right ventricle–pulmonary artery coupling

Recent evidence shows infants with more severe HIE show an increase in coupling during the rewarming phase.[3] Interestingly, Geisinger and colleagues[3] also showed that in neonates that underwent TH with normal outcomes, novel echocardiographic measures of coupling were actually preserved. The authors suggest that changes outside of afterload (eg, primary insult on RV performance) may affect RV function in neonates with poor outcomes.[3]

CARDIOPULMONARY ASSESSMENT AND DIAGNOSTIC APPROACH TO ACUTE PULMONARY HYPERTENSION IN HYPOXIC ISCHEMIC ENCEPHALOPATHY

Screening for Acute Pulmonary Hypertension in Hypoxic Ischemic Encephalopathy

There are no consensus guidelines on when to screen for aPH in neonates with HIE, which leads to management variation.[1,62] The diagnosis of aPH in neonates with HIE relies on the assessment of various clinical parameters, biochemical markers, and the use of noninvasive imaging tools. Although the gold standard for diagnosis of PH is cardiac catheterization, its invasive nature makes it a less than ideal modality to screen and monitor aPH in neonates with HIE.[63] Infants with HIE receive a comprehensive laboratory and neurologic evaluation but only some centers routinely perform a complete hemodynamic assessment that includes cardiac biomarkers and echocardiography.[1,62] Unfortunately, the clinical signs of myocardial injury and aPH, as well as electrocardiographic and radiographic findings, are all nonspecific and often insensitive.[64] Specifically, the conventional cardiovascular markers of heart rate and blood pressure are late markers of insufficient cardiac performance. In addition, arterial blood pressure is not reflective of RV function and/or abnormal brain tissue oxygen delivery.[65] Urinary output and plasma lactate are influenced by the primary hypoxic-ischemic insult so they are a less reliable indicator of the adequacy of systemic perfusion. Skin perfusion is modified significantly during TH. Biochemical markers (eg, troponin and creatine kinase-MB) of cardiac injury have been explored in newborns with neonatal encephalopathy and have potential prognostic significance concerning mortality and outcome.[31,64,66–76] However, other than providing insight into contractility, they do not provide real-time information regarding the other major determinants of cardiac performance (eg, loading conditions, heart rate, or morphology). As such, echocardiography remains the primary choice for diagnostic evaluation, follow-up, and analysis of treatment results in neonates with cardiomyopathy associated with perinatal asphyxia. Until recently, echocardiography was only considered in the presence of clinical cardiovascular compromise and/or elevation of biomarkers but recent expert consensus suggests that advanced hemodynamic assessment should be performed early for all infants with HIE treated with TH.[77] Others suggest that a baseline echocardiogram should be obtained at minimum when cardiovascular agents are initiated and/or Fio_2 requirement is greater than 30% but also in moderate to severely impaired infants before or at 24 hours to identify myocardial dysfunction that may not be clinically obvious given the wide variety of competing problems in this high-risk population.[1,23,62]

Echocardiographic Assessment

Echocardiography is used to evaluate myocardial performance and pulmonary hemodynamics and delineate the phenotypes and hemodynamic profile of aPH.[33,78] The characterization of aPH by echocardiography is based on 3 broad categories: (1) evaluation of the severity of PH with indirect assessment of elevated RV afterload and estimation of pulmonary hemodynamics, (2) evaluation of measures of right and left ventricular performance, and (3) appraisal of shunts[78] (**Table 3**). This approach provides

Table 3
Comprehensive evaluation of acute neonatal pulmonary hypertension by echocardiography

Categories	Characteristics
Severity of PH	
Interventricular septal wall configuration[a]	Degree of septal wall flattening in end-systole estimates RVSP in response to changes in RV afterload. Flattening at end-systole suggests >50% systemic RVSP. Posterior systolic bowing into LV suggests suprasystemic RVSP
Eccentricity index (EI)[b]	Ratio of the LV dimensions parallel and perpendicular to the septum in systole and diastole. Elevated PAP if >1.3
Doppler integration of the tricuspid valve (TRJV)	Quantitative estimate of RVSP by the modified Bernoulli equation Quantitative estimate of PVR by the Abbas formula (TRJV:VTI) RVSP estimates PADP
Doppler integration of the pulmonary valve (RVET/PAAT)	Provides reliable non-invasive estimate of mPAP, PVR, and compliance.[c] Normal RVET: PAAT <4
Shunt direction (PDA, ASD, and ventricular septal defect [VSD]: see later discussion)	Size and direction of the flow
Pulmonary/systemic hemodynamics	
Left ventricular output	Normal Range 150–300 mL/min/kg
Right ventricular output	Normal Range 150–300 mL/min/kg
End-organ flow evaluation (MCA, celiac artery Doppler)	Absent or reversed diastolic flow suggestive of high-volume systemic shunts
RV performance[d]	
Morphology	4-chamber view of outflow tracts and linear dimensions of cavity, wall thickness, end-systolic and end-diastolic areas
Fractional area of change (FAC)	Change in cavity dimensions (estimate of RV ejection fraction). Normal RV FAC >35%
Tricuspid annular plane systolic excursion (TAPSE)	Provides an estimate of longitudinal myocardial shortening and RV systolic performance Normal TAPSE >8.5
Tissue Doppler imaging (DI)	Provides quantitative measures of RV systolic (S') and diastolic (E' and A') function
Strain and strain rate	Assessment of RV systolic function (strain), diastolic function (diastolic strain rate), and contractility (systolic strain rate)
RV velocity time integral (VTI)	Estimate of RV stroke volume, reflecting the cumulative inflow of deoxygenated blood and venous return (in the absence of a PDA)
RV-PA coupling (TAPSE/PAAT and Strain/PAAT)	Reliable estimate of invasive coupling hemodynamics
LV Performance	
Morphology	4 chamber view of outflow tracts and linear dimensions of cavity, wall thickness, end-systolic and end-diastolic areas

(continued on next page)

Categories	Characteristics
Table 3 **(continued)**	
Ejection fraction/shortening fraction	Assess LV systolic function Normal EF >55%
Mitral annular plane systolic excursion	Provides an estimate of longitudinal myocardial shortening and LV systolic performance
Tissue DI	Provides quantitative measures of RV systolic (S′) and diastolic (E′ and A′) function.
Strain and strain rate	Assessment of LV systolic function (strain), diastolic function (diastolic strain rate), and contractility (systolic strain rate)
LV VTI	Marker of systemic blood flow
Pulmonary vein Doppler	Assess LV preload
Appraisal of shunt (size and direction of flow)	
PDA	Estimate PASP from systemic pressure, ductal size, characterize restriction patterns
Atrial level shunt (PFO/ASD)	Estimation of RA to LA pressure (direction: right to left shunt indicates right atrial hypertension, left to right shunt indicates higher left atrial pressure)
VSD	Estimate RVSP and PASP from systemic pressure (if applicable)

Abbreviations: FAC, fractional area change; PAAT, pulmonary artery acceleration time; PADP, pulmonary artery diastolic pressure; PASP, pulmonary artery systolic pressure; PFO/ASD, patent foramen ovale/atrial septal defect; RVET, RV ejection time; RVSP, RV systolic pressure; TRJV, tricuspid regurgitant jet velocity.

[a] The degree of septal wall flattening in end-systole provides an estimate of RVSP.

[b] Diastolic LV EI is a reflective marker of RV volume overload and systolic EI reflects RV pressure overload. A pressure-loaded RV in cPH will deviate the septum in systole and reduce the perpendicular dimension resulting with an end-systolic LV EI $\geq$ 1.3.

[c] Visual inspection of the Doppler flow envelope across the RV outflow tract has been shown to be a sensitive predictor of altered pulmonary hemodynamics in neonates with PH. The characteristic midsystolic notch (the "flying W") and its different patterns integrate all the indicators of pulmonary vascular load and RV function and have been used to detect a decline in the RV afterload during the early transitional period in healthy term infants.

[d] RV FAC, TAPSE, tissue DI, and Deformation have all been validated in term and preterm infants with emerging reference patterns in health and disease states.

Adapted with permission from Ruoss JL, Rios DR, Levy PT. Updates on Management for Acute and Chronic Phenotypes of Neonatal Pulmonary Hypertension. Clin Perinatol. 2020;47(3):593-615.

comprehensive information regarding disease severity, responsiveness to therapy, and the relative contributions of pulmonary vascular injury, left heart, and right heart disease in neonates with HIE.[23] All phenotypes may result in exposure of the RV to sustained high afterload that can lead to dilated cardiomyopathy with depressed global function and performance. Recent advances in quantitative echocardiography permit a more comprehensive assessment of myocardial performance in neonatal encephalopathy that could not be previously obtained with conventional imaging.[3,4,9,10,36,40,52,53]

MANAGEMENT OF ACUTE PULMONARY HYPERTENSION IN NEONATES WITH PERINATAL ASPHYXIA

Management of aPH in neonates with perinatal asphyxia requires attention to the phenotypic presentation with an aim to provide sufficient PBF to increase oxygenation and reduce secondary consequences of increased afterload on RV mechanics.[33] The clinical evaluation for aPH begins with a rapid multifaceted approach to identify risk factors, recognize symptoms, and anticipate potential illness. The management consists of 4 principal concepts: (1) supportive cardiorespiratory care (ventilator support, correction of metabolic derangements, sedation and pain management, consideration for surfactant replacement therapy, and treatment of infection), (2) use of pulmonary vasodilators to decrease afterload, (3) cardiotropic support for impaired RV and LV systolic performance, and (4) ECMO if needed[79] (Table 4). It is important to note that the selection of pulmonary vasodilators and cardiotropic medications should be based on the suspected underlying phenotype coupled with the degree of impairment of systemic hemodynamics, ventricular dysfunction, and degree of parenchymal disease (Table 5). Intravenous dobutamine (2.5–10 mcg/kg/min) is the recommended first-line treatment of RV dysfunction. Nonresponders should be transitioned to low-dose epinephrine (0.03–0.05 mg/kg/min) because higher doses of dobutamine are unlikely to benefit and may induce deleterious tachycardia. The selection of

Table 4	
Management of acute pulmonary hypertension in neonates with perinatal asphyxia	
Principle Concepts	**Mechanism**
Supportive cardiorespiratory care	Correction of metabolic derangements that can alter afterload Maintenance of adequate oxygenation Lung recruitment optimization (enhanced ventilation strategies) Cardiovascular support with fluid resuscitation, inotropic agents, or selective systemic vasopressors based on the phenotype[a] Sedation therapies (conservative and pharmacologic) Other[b]
PH targeted therapy (promote pulmonary vasodilation)	NO-cGMP pathway (eg, iNO, sildenafil) Prostacyclin-cAMP pathway (eg, prostacyclin agonist)
Optimization of RV support	Enhanced preload: cautious volume resuscitation Afterload reduction: iNO and PgE1 (if ductus arteriosus is closing or closed to offload RV) Augment RV function: inotropic agents (dobutamine and epinephrine) [c]
Optimization of LV support	Enhanced preload: cautious volume resuscitation Afterload reduction: dobutamine (weak vasodilator) Augment RV function: inotropic agents (dobutamine and epinephrine)
ECMO	VV ECMO: hypoxic respiratory failure without hemodynamic compromise VA ECMO: hypoxic respiratory failure with hemodynamic compromise

[a] Steroid treatment to stabilize blood pressure in inotropic-resistant environments may also be necessary.
[b] Additional therapies to promote pulmonary vasodilation, improve oxygenation, and minimize pulmonary vasoconstriction in specific circumstances include the following: (1) antibiotics (eg, pneumonia and sepsis); (2) red blood cell transfusion for optimization of oxygen delivery; and (3) surfactant replacement therapy (eg, respiratory distress syndrome and meconium aspiration).
[c] Cautious use of milrinone with inotropic support.
Adapted with permission from Ruoss JL, Rios DR, Levy PT. Updates on Management for Acute and Chronic Phenotypes of Neonatal Pulmonary Hypertension. Clin Perinatol. 2020;47(3):593-615.

Table 5
Physiology-based treatment strategies: choice of inotropes in hypoxic ischemic encephalopathy and therapeutic hypothermia

Pathophysiology	Mechanism	Treatment
Hypoxic respiratory failure	aPH ± parenchymal disease	Lung recruitment optimization Surfactant replacement therapy (RDS) Selective pulmonary vasodilators (iNO) Caution with milrinone
Impaired systemic hemodynamics	aPH with hypotension Isolated systolic hypotension Refractory hypotension If TnECHO available Normal function Severe RV dysfunction Severe LV disease/Normal RV function	Dobutamine, epinephrine Hydrocortisone Vasopressin, Norepinephrine Epinephrine, Fluid bolus, PGE Evaluate coronary, myocarditis

Addition of PGE to support the systemic circulation in the setting of severe RV dysfunction, increasing lactate, and evidence of poor end-organ perfusion.

Abbreviations: aPH, acute pulmonary hypertension; iNO, inhaled nitric oxide; LV, left ventricle; PGE, prostaglandins; RDS, respiratory distress syndrome; RV, right ventricle; TnECHO, targetted neonatal echocardiography.

vasopressor support in patients with low diastolic or mean arterial pressure is another important consideration. Intravenous vasopressin or norepinephrine may be appropriate in the setting of preserved LV function with low diastolic blood pressure and aPH. Cautious adjustment of these medications during the rewarming phase should be considered with the known physiologic changes to loading conditions, heart rate, and contractility. Pathophysiology-based approaches will dictate the appropriate therapy. For example, an infant with meconium aspiration and hypoxic pulmonary vasoconstriction may benefit from iNO to decrease the PVR; however, a neonate with isolated moderate-severe LV systolic dysfunction is at risk of deterioration following the initiation of iNO due to the need to maintain a right–left ductal shunt to support systemic blood flow. However, if the LV dysfunction is due to severe RV dysfunction (from a primary insult to the RV or secondary to high PVR), then iNO may still be beneficial. In general, the choice of therapy must be balanced against the goal of optimizing SVR, PVR, and cardiac function. The use of cardiotonic drugs, and the specific agent to use, should be tailored to the individual and based on consideration of the pathophysiologic findings related to end-organ perfusion, loading conditions, and heart function.

Extracorporeal Membrane Oxygenation Utilization

The incidence of ECMO utilization in neonates with HIE and aPH has been reported between 4% and 9%.[14,15] The use of ECMO in these high-risk neonates has been shown to be safe with good survival,[80] although the choice of venovenous (VV) or venoarterial (VA) ECMO may lead to differences in mortality or intracranial hemorrhages.[81] Both VV ECMO and VA ECMO are used for neonatal respiratory failure following perinatal asphyxia but no randomized controlled trial has been done to compare these modalities in this patient population.[82] Interestingly, despite a survey in 2009 that showed that close to 50% of responders from active neonatal centers with ECMO would not offer it as a rescue modality to neonates with moderate-severe HIE,[83] the actual number of neonates with a perinatal insult and aPH that have received ECMO has increased during the past decade.[84] Most outcome data have focused on mortality and/or development of intracranial bleeding but are limited to case reports, small case series, or nested cases in large registries. With the recognition that ECMO may not confer the same risk of intracranial hemorrhage and mortality as one perceived,[84–86] it is no longer contraindicated in neonates with progressive aPH and myocardial dysfunction and should be considered as a rescue therapy. As such, we suggest that when an HIE infant undergoing TH has severe aPH that requires ECMO, the TH should (1) not be discontinued in lieu of avoiding ECMO and (2) continued and managed through the ECMO circuit for the entire period of cooling and rewarming.

SUMMARY

Acute neonatal pulmonary hypertension is a common consequence of perinatal hypoxia that is even more pronounced in neonates with moderate-to-severe HIE. The pathogenesis of the association between perinatal asphyxia and aPH is multifactorial and results from a combination of hypoxic vasoconstriction of the pulmonary vascular bed and primary insults to right or left ventricular performance or other pathophysiologic disorder. The diagnosis of aPH requires clinical awareness of risk factors, recognition of hemodynamic changes, and understanding of the different imaging modalities to provide comprehensive information regarding phenotypes, disease severity, and the influences of pulmonary vascular disease and cardiac dysfunction. Longitudinal assessment can offer valuable physiologic insights into disease progression and response to therapies.

Best Practice Box

What is the current practice?

- Infants with perinatal asphyxia and associated lung disease are closely monitored for hemodynamic instability with consideration for echocardiographic evaluation for diagnosis, follow-up, and analysis of treatment results for acute pulmonary hypertension (aPH), but it is not considered standard of practice at every institution.

Best practices

- Neonates with hypoxic ischemic encephalopathy (HIE) associated aPH may have multiple underlying etiologies that need to be recognized. The approach to management may differ according to the initial insult and during each phase of therapeutic hypothermia (cooling and rewarming).

- Blood pressure is not a reliable predictor of cardiovascular well-being and underlying heart dysfunction.

- Comprehensive assessment of the hemodynamic profiles of aPH include a thorough clinical exam and comprehensive quantitative echocardiography to help guide therapeutic intervention.

- The initial insult, therapeutic hypothermia, and rewarming modulate the major determinants of cardiac performance, afterload, preload, contractility, heart rate, and even morphology. Therefore, careful adjustment of cardiotropic agents and pulmonary vasodilators is recommended in neonates with aPH and myocardial dysfunction.

What changes in current practice are likely to improve outcomes?

- In depth understanding of underlying risk factors and etiopathologies that contribute to the disease phenotype and utilization of non-invasive tools and clinical assessment to guide patient-targeted therapies based on hemodynamic profiles during the cooling and rewarming phases of therapeutic hypothermia.

- Early hemodynamic screening with echocardiography to delineate the contribution of hypoxic pulmonary vasoconstriction from right ventricle (RV) or left ventricle (LV) dysfunction to the clinical manifestation of aPH seen following perinatal asphyxia.
- aPH is often exacerbated by TH leading to increased RV afterload and reduced LV preload.

Is there a clinical algorithm?

- Although there is increased recognition of the impact of aPH in neonates with HIE on short- and long – term neurological outcomes, there is no universal algorithm for screening, diagnosis, or the approach to intervention based on phenotypic presentation.

Major recommendations

- A high index of suspicion for cardiopulmonary dysfunction and aPH is important in the neonate with clinical and biochemical evidence of a hypoxic ischemic insult.
- Neonates with a perinatal hypoxic event at risk for aPH should have screening, and if clinically indicated, serial echocardiograms should be performed to assess severity and response to treatment following the initial hypoxic insult and during both the cooling and rewarming phases of therapeutic hypothermia.
- Therapeutic hypothermia and rewarming modify loading conditions and blood flow and careful adjustment of inotropic agents is recommended with avoidance of those that contribute to increased pulmonary artery pressures as able.
- A combination of pulmonary vasodilators to reduce RV afterload and inotropes supporting ventricular function and vasoactive agents supporting SVR is needed to optimize hemodynamics in aPH during TH. Caution must be exercised while using pulmonary vasodilators in the presence of LV dysfunction.

Summary statement

- It is important to understand the underlying etiopathologies, unique hemodynamic profiles of different endotypes, and novel assessments in order to guide targeted management and improve outcomes in neonates following perinatal hypoxic event and risk for aPH.

DISCLOSURE

The authors have nothing to disclose.

REFERENCES

1. Giesinger RE, Deshpande P, McNamara P, et al. Hypoxic-ischemic encephalopathy and therapeutic hypothermia: the hemodynamic perspective. J Pediatr 2017;180:22–30.e2. Elsevier Inc.
2. Kanik E, Ozer EA, Bakiler AR, et al. Assessment of myocardial dysfunction in neonates with hypoxic-ischemic encephalopathy: is it a significant predictor of mortality? J Matern Fetal Neonatal Med 2009;22(3):239–42.
3. Giesinger RE. Impaired right ventricular function is associated with adverse outcome following hypoxic ischemic encephalopathy. Am J Respir Crit Care Med 2019;200:1294–305.
4. Giesinger RE, El Shahed AI, Castaldo MP, et al. Neurodevelopmental outcome following hypoxic ischaemic encephalopathy and therapeutic hypothermia is related to right ventricular performance at 24-hour postnatal age. Arch Dis Child Fetal Neonatal Ed 2022;107(1):70–5.
5. Yum SK, Seo YM, Kwun Y, et al. Therapeutic hypothermia in infants with hypoxic-ischemic encephalopathy and reversible persistent pulmonary hypertension: short-term hospital outcomes. J Matern Fetal Neonatal Med 2018;31(23):3108–14.

6. Lakshminrusimha S, Shankaran S, Laptook A, et al. Pulmonary hypertension associated with hypoxic-ischemic encephalopathy-antecedent characteristics and comorbidities. J Pediatr 2018;196:45–51.e43.
7. Shankaran S, Pappas A, McDonald SA, et al. Childhood outcomes after hypothermia for neonatal encephalopathy. N Engl J Med 2012;366(22):2085–92.
8. Altit G, Levy PT. Cardiopulmonary impact of hypoxic ischemic encephalopathy in newborn infants. The emerging role of early hemodynamic assessment in determining adverse neurological outcomes. Am J Respir Crit Care Med 2019;200(10): 1206–7.
9. Levy P, Tissot C, Eriksen BH, et al. Application of neonatologist performed echocardiography in the assessment and management of neonatal heart failure unrelated to congenital heart disease. Nature Publishing Group: Springer US; 2018. p. 1–11.
10. Nestaas E, Skranes JH, Stoylen A, et al. The myocardial function during and after whole-body therapeutic hypothermia for hypoxic-ischemic encephalopathy, a cohort study. Early Hum Dev 2014;90(5):247–52.
11. Giesinger RE, More K, Odame J, et al. Controversies in the identification and management of acute pulmonary hypertension in preterm neonates. In. Nature Publishing Group, vol. 82. Nature Publishing Group; 2017. p. 901–14.
12. Lawn JE, Bahl R, Bergstrom S, et al. Setting research priorities to reduce almost one million deaths from birth asphyxia by 2015. PLoS Med 2011;8(1):e1000389.
13. Jacobs SE, Berg M, Hunt R, et al. Cooling for newborns with hypoxic ischaemic encephalopathy. Cochrane Database Syst Rev 2013;1:CD003311.
14. Shankaran S, Laptook AR, Pappas A, et al. Effect of depth and duration of cooling on deaths in the NICU among neonates with hypoxic ischemic encephalopathy: a randomized clinical trial. JAMA 2014;312(24):2629–39.
15. Shankaran S, Pappas A, Laptook AR, et al. Outcomes of safety and effectiveness in a multicenter randomized, controlled trial of whole-body hypothermia for neonatal hypoxic-ischemic encephalopathy. Pediatrics 2008;122(4):e791–8.
16. Joanna RGV, Lopriore E, Te Pas AB, et al. Persistent pulmonary hypertension in neonates with perinatal asphyxia and therapeutic hypothermia: a frequent and perilous combination. J Matern Fetal Neonatal Med 2022;35(25):4969–75.
17. Agarwal P, Shankaran S, Laptook AR, et al. Outcomes of infants with hypoxic ischemic encephalopathy and persistent pulmonary hypertension of the newborn: results from three NICHD studies. J Perinatol 2021;41(3):502–11.
18. Bendapudi P, Rao GG, Greenough A. Diagnosis and management of persistent pulmonary hypertension of the newborn. In: Paediatric respiratory reviews16. 2015. p. 157–61.
19. Thoresen M. Hypothermia after perinatal asphyxia: selection for treatment and cooling protocol. J Pediatr 2011;158(2 Suppl):e45–9.
20. Sehgal A, Linduska N, Huynh C. Cardiac adaptation in asphyxiated infants treated with therapeutic hypothermia. J Neonatal Perinat Med 2019;12(2):117–25.
21. Ruoss JL, Rios DR, Levy PT. Updates on management for acute and chronic phenotypes of neonatal pulmonary hypertension. Clin Perinatol 2020;47(3):593–615.
22. Lapointe A, Barrington KJ. Pulmonary hypertension and the asphyxiated newborn. J Pediatr 2011;158:e19–24.
23. Kluckow M. Functional echocardiography in assessment of the cardiovascular system in asphyxiated neonates. J Pediatr 2011;158:e13–8. Mosby, Inc.
24. Barberi I, Calabro MP, Cordaro S, et al. Myocardial ischaemia in neonates with perinatal asphyxia. Electrocardiographic, echocardiographic and enzymatic correlations. Eur J Pediatr 1999;158(9):742–7.

25. Shah P, Riphagen S, Beyene J, et al. Multiorgan dysfunction in infants with post-asphyxial hypoxic-ischaemic encephalopathy. Arch Dis Child Fetal Neonatal Ed 2004;89:F152–5.
26. Syamsundar P, Vyvasagar D. Perinatal cardiology. In:2015:1-10.
27. Tan CMJ, Lewandowski AJ. The transitional heart: from early embryonic and fetal development to neonatal life. Fetal Diagn Ther 2020;47(5):373–86.
28. Donnelly WH, Bucciarelli RL, Nelson RM. Ischemic papillary muscle necrosis in stressed newborn infants. JPediatr 1980;96(2):295–300.
29. Armstrong K, Franklin O, Sweetman D, et al. Cardiovascular dysfunction in infants with neonatal encephalopathy: table 1. Arch Dis Child 2012;97:372–5.
30. Roberto Antonucci APMDP. Perinatal asphyxia in the term newborn. In:2014:1-14.
31. Rajakumar PS, Vishnu BB, Sridhar MG, et al. Electrocardiographic and echocardiographic changes in perinatal asphyxia. Indian JPediatr 2009;76(3):261–4.
32. Kluckow M. Low systemic blood flow and pathophysiology of the preterm transitional circulation. Early Hum Dev 2005;81:429–37.
33. Jain A, McNamara PJ. Persistent pulmonary hypertension of the newborn: advances in diagnosis and treatment. Semin Fetal Neonatal Med 2015;20(4):262–71.
34. Levy PT, Levin J, Leeman KT, et al. Diagnosis and management of pulmonary hypertension in infants with bronchopulmonary dysplasia. Semin Fetal Neonatal Med 2022;27(4):101351.
35. Goss KN, Everett AD, Mourani PM, et al. Addressing the challenges of phenotyping pediatric pulmonary vascular disease. Pulm Circ 2017;7(1):7–19.
36. Altit G, Bonifacio SL, Guimaraes CV, et al. Altered biventricular function in neonatal hypoxic-ischaemic encephalopathy: a case-control echocardiographic study. Cardiol Young 2022;1–10.
37. Levene M, de Vries L. Hypoxic-ischemic encephalopathy. Fanaroff and Martin's Neonatal-Perinatal Medicine, Disease of the Fetus and Infant 2016;10:1.
38. Bussmann NBC, Levy PT, McCallion N, et al. Early diastolic dysfunction and respiratory morbidity in premature infants: an observational study. J Perinatol 2018;38:1205–11.
39. Bussmann N, El-Khuffash A, Breatnach CR, et al. Left ventricular diastolic function influences right ventricular — pulmonary vascular coupling in premature infants. In. Early Hum Dev, vol. 128. Elsevier; 2018. p. 35–40.
40. Nestaas E, Stoylen A, Brunvand L, et al. Longitudinal strain and strain rate by tissue Doppler are more sensitive indices than fractional shortening for assessing the reduced myocardial function in asphyxiated neonates. Cardiol Young 2011;21(1):1–7.
41. Vonk Noordegraaf A, Westerhof BE, Westerhof N. The relationship between the right ventricle and its load in pulmonary hypertension. J Am Coll Cardiol 2017;69(2):236–43.
42. El-Khuffash A, McNamara PJ. Hemodynamic assessment and monitoring of premature infants. Clin Perinatol 2017;44:377–93.
43. Thoresen M, Whitelaw A. Cardiovascular changes during mild therapeutic hypothermia and rewarming in infants with hypoxic-ischemic encephalopathy. Pediatrics 2000;106(1 Pt 1):92–9.
44. Gebauer CM, Knuepfer M, Robel-Tillig E, et al. Hemodynamics among neonates with hypoxic-ischemic encephalopathy during whole-body hypothermia and passive rewarming. Pediatrics 2006;117:843–50.
45. Al Yazidi G, Boudes E, Tan X, et al. Intraventricular hemorrhage in asphyxiated newborns treated with hypothermia: a look into incidence, timing and risk factors. BMC Pediatr 2015;15:106.

46. Benumof JL, Wahrenbrock EA. Dependency of hypoxic pulmonary vasoconstriction on temperature. J Appl Physiol Respir Environ Exerc Physiol 1977;42(1):56–8.
47. Ovali F. Hemodynamic changes and evaluation during hypoxic-ischemic encephalopathy and therapeutic hypothermia. Early Hum Dev 2022;167:105563.
48. Toubas PL, Hof RP, Heymann MA, et al. Effects of hypothermia and rewarming on the neonatal circulation. Arch Fr Pediatr 1978;35(10 Suppl):84–92.
49. Poulos ND, Mollitt DL. The nature and reversibility of hypothermia-induced alterations of blood viscosity. J Trauma 1991;31(7):996–8, discussion 998-1000.
50. Schubert A. Side effects of mild hypothermia. J Neurosurg Anesthesiol 1995;7(2):139–47.
51. Vasquez A., Buchoff A.R., McNamara P.H., et al., *Impact of therapeutic hypothermia on echocardiography indices of pulmonary hemodynamics, PAS Meeting 2022*, 236, 22.
52. Czernik C, Rhode S, Helfer S, et al. Left ventricular longitudinal strain and strain rate measured by 2-D speckle tracking echocardiography in neonates during whole-body hypothermia. Ultrasound Med Biol 2013;39(8):1343–9.
53. Sehgal A, Wong F, Menahem S. Speckle tracking derived strain in infants with severe perinatal asphyxia: a comparative case control study. Cardiovasc Ultrasound 2013;11:34.
54. Sehgal A, Wong F, Mehta S. Reduced cardiac output and its correlation with coronary blood flow and troponin in asphyxiated infants treated with therapeutic hypothermia. Eur J Pediatr 2012;171(10):1511–7.
55. Bischoff AR, Habib S, McNamara PJ, et al. Hemodynamic response to milrinone for refractory hypoxemia during therapeutic hypothermia for neonatal hypoxic ischemic encephalopathy. J Perinatol 2021;41(9):2345–54.
56. Forman E, Breatnach CR, Ryan S, et al. Noninvasive continuous cardiac output and cerebral perfusion monitoring in term infants with neonatal encephalopathy: assessment of feasibility and reliability. Pediatr Res 2017;82(5):789–95.
57. Hochwald O, Jabr M, Osiovich H, et al. Preferential cephalic redistribution of left ventricular cardiac output during therapeutic hypothermia for perinatal hypoxic-ischemic encephalopathy. J Pediatr 2014;164(5):999–1004.e1001.
58. Zanelli S, Buck M, Fairchild K. Physiologic and pharmacologic considerations for hypothermia therapy in neonates. J Perinatol 2011;31(6):377–86.
59. Yoon JH, Lee EJ, Yum SK, et al. Impacts of therapeutic hypothermia on cardiovascular hemodynamics in newborns with hypoxic-ischemic encephalopathy: a case control study using echocardiography. J Matern Fetal Neonatal Med 2018;31(16):2175–82.
60. Bhagat I, Sarkar S. Multiple organ dysfunction during therapeutic cooling of asphyxiated infants. NeoReviews 2019;20(11):e653–60.
61. Gupta S, Donn SM. Assessment of neonatal perfusion. Semin Fetal Neonatal Med 2020;25(5):101144.
62. Colthorpe A, Latiff A, Subhedar N, et al. Management of cardiovascular dysfunction in neonates with hypoxic ischaemic encephalopathy; a national survey of current practice in the UK. J Perinatol 2022;42(12):1695–6.
63. Levy PT, Patel MD, Groh G, et al. Pulmonary artery acceleration time provides a reliable estimate of invasive pulmonary hemodynamics in children. J Am Soc Echocardiogr 2016;29:1056–65.
64. Matter M, Abdel-Hady H, Attia G, et al. Myocardial performance in asphyxiated full-term infants assessed by Doppler tissue imaging. Pediatr Cardiol 2010;31(5):634–42.

65. Giesinger RE, El-Khuffash AF, McNamara PJ. Arterial pressure is not reflective of right ventricular function in neonates with hypoxic ischemic encephalopathy treated with therapeutic hypothermia. J Perinatol 2023;43(2):162–7.
66. Wei Y, Xu J, Xu T, et al. Left ventricular systolic function of newborns with asphyxia evaluated by tissue Doppler imaging. Pediatr Cardiol 2009;30(6):741–6.
67. Montaldo P, Rosso R, Chello G, et al. Cardiac troponin I concentrations as a marker of neurodevelopmental outcome at 18 months in newborns with perinatal asphyxia. J Perinatol 2014;34:292–5.
68. Costa S, Zecca E, De RG, et al. Is serum troponin T a useful marker of myocardial damage in newborn infants with perinatal asphyxia? Acta Paediatr 2007;96(2): 181–4.
69. Szymankiewicz M, Matuszczak-Wleklak M, Hodgman JE, et al. Usefulness of cardiac troponin T and echocardiography in the diagnosis of hypoxic myocardial injury of full-term neonates. Biol Neonate 2005;88(1):19–23.
70. Turker G, Babaoğlu K, Gokalp AS, et al. Cord blood cardiac troponin I as an early predictor of short-term outcome in perinatal hypoxia. Neonatology 2004;86:131–7.
71. Shastri AT, Samarasekara S, Muniraman H, et al. Cardiac troponin I concentrations in neonates with hypoxic-ischaemic encephalopathy. Acta Paediatr 2011; 101:26–9.
72. Gunes T, Ozturk MA, Koklu SM, et al. Troponin-T levels in perinatally asphyxiated infants during the first 15 days of life. Acta Paediatr 2005;94:1638–43.
73. Agrawal J, Shah GS, Poudel P, et al. Electrocardiographic and enzymatic correlations with outcome in neonates with hypoxic-ischemic encephalopathy. Ital J Pediatr 2012;38:33.
74. Boo N-Y, Hafidz H, Nawawi HM, et al. Comparison of serum cardiac troponin T and creatine kinase MB isoenzyme mass concentrations in asphyxiated term infants during the first 48 h of life. J Paediatr Child Health 2005;41:331–7.
75. Liu X, Chakkarapani E, Stone J, et al. Effect of cardiac compressions and hypothermia treatment on cardiac troponin I in newborns with perinatal asphyxia. Resuscitation 2013;84:1562–7.
76. Neves AL, Henriques-Coelho T, Leite-Moreira A, et al. Cardiac injury biomarkers in paediatric age: are we there yet? Heart Fail Rev 2016;21:771–81.
77. Rios DR, Lapointe A, Schmolzer GM, et al. Hemodynamic optimization for neonates with neonatal encephalopathy caused by a hypoxic ischemic event: physiological and therapeutic considerations. Semin Fetal Neonatal Med 2021;26(4): 101277.
78. Bhattacharya S, Sen S, Levy PT, et al. Comprehensive evaluation of right heart performance and pulmonary hemodynamics in neonatal pulmonary hypertension: evaluation of cardiopulmonary performance in neonatal pulmonary hypertension. Curr Treat Options Cardiovasc Med 2019;21:10.
79. McNamara PJ, Weisz DE, Giesinger RE, et al. Hemodynamics. In: MacDonald MMKS MG, editor. Avery's neonatology: Pathophysiology and management of the newborn. Philadelphia: Wolters Kluwer; 2016. p. 457–86.
80. Agarwal P, Altinok D, Desai J, et al. In-hospital outcomes of neonates with hypoxic-ischemic encephalopathy receiving extracorporeal membrane oxygenation. J Perinatol 2019;39(5):661–5.
81. Agarwal P, Natarajan G, Sullivan K, et al. Venovenous versus venoarterial extracorporeal membrane oxygenation among infants with hypoxic-ischemic encephalopathy: is there a difference in outcome? J Perinatol 2021;41(8):1916–23.
82. Fletcher K, Chapman R, Keene S. An overview of medical ECMO for neonates. Semin Perinatol 2018;42(2):68–79.

83. Chapman RL, Peterec SM, Bizzarro MJ, et al. Patient selection for neonatal extracorporeal membrane oxygenation: beyond severity of illness. J Perinatol 2009; 29(9):606–11.
84. Cuevas Guaman M, Lucke AM, Hagan JL, et al. Bleeding complications and mortality in neonates receiving therapeutic hypothermia and extracorporeal membrane oxygenation. Am J Perinatol 2018;35(3):271–6.
85. Bhandary P, Daniel JM, Skinner SC, et al. Case series of therapeutic hypothermia for neonatal hypoxic-ischemic encephalopathy during extracorporeal life support. Perfusion 2020;35(7):700–6.
86. Massaro A, Rais-Bahrami K, Chang T, et al. Therapeutic hypothermia for neonatal encephalopathy and extracorporeal membrane oxygenation. J Pediatr 2010; 157(3):499–501, 501.e491.

Congenital Diaphragmatic Hernia

Pulmonary Hypertension and Pulmonary Vascular Disease

Shiran S. Moore, MD[a],*, Roberta L. Keller, MD[b,c],
Gabriel Altit, MD[d,e]

KEYWORDS

- Congenital diaphragmatic hernia • Pulmonary hypertension • Ventilation
- Cardiopulmonary interactions • Vasodilators • Inotropes

KEY POINTS

- The management of pulmonary hypertension and altered cardiac function are key in stabilization and long-term prognosis of infants with congenital diaphragmatic hernia.
- Pulmonary vascular disease, cardiopulmonary interactions, and cardiac dysfunction should all be addressed in the evaluation and management.
- The underlying physiology along with frequent reassessment allows for utilization of medical agents and ventilation strategies.

INTRODUCTION

Congenital diaphragmatic hernia (CDH) is characterized by a diaphragmatic defect, associated with abdominal contents herniating into the thorax, with bilateral maldevelopment of pulmonary parenchyma and vasculature.[1,2] Pulmonary hypertension (PH) and altered cardiac function have been associated with an adverse postnatal trajectory and increased mortality.[3–5] This review provides a comprehensive summary of the current understanding of PH in CDH, outlining the underlying pathophysiologic mechanisms, methods for assessing PH severity, optimal management strategies, and prognostic implications.

[a] Neonatology, Dana Dwek Children's Hospital, Tel Aviv Sourasky Medical Center, Weizamann 6, Tel-Aviv, Jaffa 6423906, Israel; [b] Neonatology, UCSF Benioff Children's Hospital, 550 16th Street, #5517, San Francisco, CA 94158, USA; [c] Department of Pediatrics, University of California San Francisco, San Francisco, CA, USA; [d] Neonatology, McGill University Health Centre, Montreal Children's Hospital, 1001 Décarie boulevard, Montreal, H4A Quebec; [e] Department of Pediatrics, McGill University, Montreal, Quebec, Canada
* Corresponding author.
E-mail address: shiransm@tlvmc.gov.il

Clin Perinatol 51 (2024) 151–170
https://doi.org/10.1016/j.clp.2023.10.001
0095-5108/24/© 2023 Elsevier Inc. All rights reserved.
perinatology.theclinics.com

PATHOPHYSIOLOGY

Diaphragmatic precursors develop at approximately 4 weeks of gestation with fusion completed by 12 weeks.[6] While a diaphragmatic defect leads to intra-abdominal contents herniating into the thorax, impeding pulmonary and cardiac growth, this phenomenon does not fully explain bilateral structural pulmonary findings. The current prevailing concept is the "2-hit theory,"[7] which postulates that CDH pathogenesis involves a dual sequence of insults. The first results in developmental arrest of both lungs, while the second primarily affects the ipsilateral lung subsequent to defective diaphragmatic development and compression. The airways, pulmonary vasculature, cardiac structures, and large vessels (pulmonary arteries and aorta) develop alongside in an orchestrated process. Experimental CDH models and postmortem studies demonstrate fewer and smaller caliber bronchioles,[8,9] as well as decreased lung weight, pulmonary arteriole numbers, size, and branching.[10,11] Some animal models demonstrate fetal structural alterations in cardiac dimensions and in the left to right ventricular (LV/RV) balance.[8] Beyond the absolute reduction in vascular surface territory implying a fixed effect in the pulmonary vascular capacitance, the developmental abnormalities include reduced vessel caliber, thickening of muscular media and adventitia, and aberrant functional reactivity.[2,12] These anatomic-histologic changes (variable contributions of abnormal vascular tone and reactivity, in combination with an underdeveloped vascular bed) impede the normal perinatal transition, with decreased pulmonary blood flow (PBF), increased pulmonary vascular resistance (PVR),[13] and persistence of PH (**Fig. 1A**).

Fetal markers of prognosis and mortality are the presence of other major congenital defects (particularly structural cardiac defects), genetic abnormalities, lung size, and liver herniation into the thorax. Specifically, the lung-to-head ratio (LHR) and observed to expected LHR (o/e LHR) have been validated as predictors of postnatal outcomes.[1,14] Prognostication relies predominantly on fetal imaging, with MRI often used in the assessment of lung volume and liver position, which are associated with postnatal survival and morbidity.[15] In severe fetal CDH (LHR or o/e LHR, below 0.6% and 25%, respectively), antenatal intervention can be considered, such as fetal tracheal occlusion (FETO).[1,16,17] Indeed, in severe left CDH, FETO increased survival (40% vs 15%; relative risk [RR] 2.67, confidence interval [CI] 1.22–6.11), despite resulting in preterm delivery.[18]

Fetal echocardiography has provided additional insight into abnormal cardiovascular development in CDH. Preferential streaming of umbilical venous return via the foramen ovale, for instance, is perturbed in CDH,[19] with a greater proportion of blood instead remaining on the right side of the heart. The combination of decreased PBF mediated by increased ductal flow, decreased left heart filling, and LV output, results in the development of a relatively smaller LV.[19–21] Impaired response to maternal hyperoxia is demonstrated in midgestation fetuses with CDH that have neonatal demise, while FETO is associated with improved LV growth and response to hyperoxia.[22–24] Together, these findings suggest that pulmonary vascular disease (PVD) is already present in the fetuses with CDH.

Postnatally, infants with severe CDH present with hypoxemic respiratory failure and shock. The remodeled pulmonary vasculature exhibits the physiology of PVD, with increased sensitivity to vasoconstricting stressors (eg, acidosis, hypoxia) and decreased capacitance with impaired vasorelaxation,[25] thus resulting in increased RV afterload. The failure to transition to normal increase in PBF compromises left atrial (LA) and LV filling and cardiac output, leading to impaired systemic oxygenation and perfusion.[26] This can be further exacerbated by the persistently high RV afterload

A

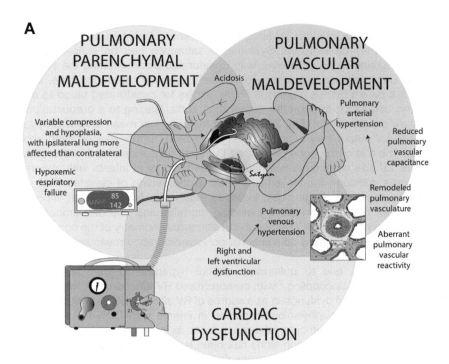

PULMONARY
PARENCHYMAL
MALDEVELOPMENT

Acidosis

PULMONARY
VASCULAR
MALDEVELOPMENT

Pulmonary
arterial
hypertension

Reduced
pulmonary
vascular
capacitance

Variable compression
and hypoplasia,
with ipsilateral lung more
affected than contralateral

Hypoxemic
respiratory
failure

85
142

Remodeled
pulmonary
vasculature

Pulmonary
venous
hypertension

Aberrant
pulmonary
vascular
reactivity

Right and
left ventricular
dysfunction

CARDIAC
DYSFUNCTION

B

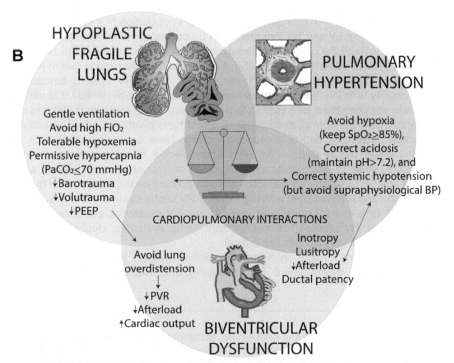

HYPOPLASTIC
FRAGILE
LUNGS

PULMONARY
HYPERTENSION

Gentle ventilation
Avoid high FiO₂
Tolerable hypoxemia
Permissive hypercapnia
(PaCO₂≤70 mmHg)
↓Barotrauma
↓Volutrauma
↓PEEP

Avoid hypoxia
(keep SpO₂≥85%),
Correct acidosis
(maintain pH>7.2), and
Correct systemic hypotension
(but avoid supraphysiological BP)

CARDIOPULMONARY INTERACTIONS

Inotropy
Lusitropy
↓Afterload
Ductal patency

Avoid lung
overdistension
↓
↓PVR
↓Afterload
↑Cardiac output

BIVENTRICULAR
DYSFUNCTION

Fig. 1. Pathophysiology of congenital diaphragmatic hernia (CDH) and recommended targeted clinical management. (*A*) Pathophysiology: variable severity of pulmonary parenchymal

and RV dilation, which impedes LV filling through ventricular interactions, while right atrial pressure may be elevated. Systemic desaturation can be exacerbated by right-to-left shunting at the atrial level, with desaturated blood entering the systemic circulation. The increased pulmonary-to-systemic vascular resistance ratio, in the presence of a patent ductus arteriosus (PDA), allows for desaturated blood to enter the systemic circulation through the descending aorta, leading to a preductal/postductal saturation differential (**Fig. 2**). Systemic hypoxia, low mean arterial pressure, and reduced LV output may impair coronary perfusion, further exacerbating shock physiology. The role of the underdeveloped LV is not fully understood in this clinical scenario, as LV size normalizes postnatally in the majority of infants with abnormal fetal measures, although the LV remains small in the setting of elevated PVR with compromised filling.[21,27] Regardless, impaired ventricular function is an important marker for poor outcomes in CDH, including mortality and use of extracorporeal membrane oxygenation (ECMO), although the abnormal geometry of the compressed LV in the setting of PH makes conventional echocardiography measures of systolic dysfunction less useful.[28]

Elevated afterload due to pulmonary arterial hypertension may lead to RV-pulmonary artery (PA) uncoupling,[2] with compromised RV function.[4] LA hypertension due to LV restriction and dysfunction as a source of RV afterload is another concern.[29] The most common pathophysiology reported in infants with CDH is biventricular dysfunction, implicating ventricular interdependence as a mechanism that contributes to LV dysfunction. LV dysfunction alone has been less commonly described (5% LV alone, 15% RV alone, and 19% biventricular dysfunction).[28] Multiple echocardiographic measurements demonstrate decreased cardiac function in infants with CDH compared to unaffected controls (typically assessed in the first 48 hours),[27,30] while both decreased RV and LV myocardial performance index and cardiac output index have been associated with mortality within the CDH population.[31] Infants transitioning to ECMO had lower LV and RV function, both by conventional echocardiogram measures and by myocardial deformation analysis (strain, a surrogate for contractility).[3,30] Of interest, systolic eccentricity index (EI), a marker of LV deformation due to RV pressure overload, was associated with lower survival, lesser RV systolic function and output (velocity time interval), and more impaired RV global strain while LV strain measures were not correlated with EI.[27] In fact, by strain, only a minority (7/24) had measurements within the normal range, while the rest have biventricular or univentricular dysfunction.[30] Systolic and diastolic dysfunctions have been documented in both ventricles using tissue doppler imaging and speckle tracking echocardiography at<48 hours, while values significantly improved on repeat echocardiogram at 3 to 5 days of age.[27,30] Of note, LV diastolic dysfunction may be underestimated by echocardiography and is associated with high PVR.[32] RV septal strain is more affected than RV free wall or either LV parameter and RV and LV measures correlate with each other.[27,33] Thus, RV afterload is an important factor in cardiac dysfunction in CDH and interventricular interactions are critical.

FETO has become a major antenatal intervention, thought to enhance fetal pulmonary parenchymal development by increasing and maintaining transpulmonary

---

and vascular maldevelopment and dysfunction, accompanied by univentricular or biventricular cardiac dysfunction. (*B*) Management: mechanical ventilation strategy focused on protecting the vulnerable lung while decreasing pulmonary vascular resistance and supporting cardiac function. (Copyright Satyan Lakshminrusimha)

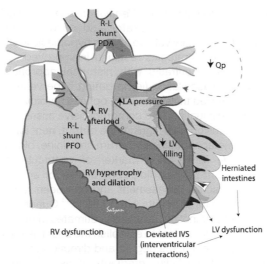

Fig. 2. Cardiac schematic in the setting of pulmonary hypertension due to suprasystemic pulmonary vascular resistance. Right-to-left shunting occurs at level of patent ductus arteriosus (PDA) and atrial septum (patent foramen ovale, PFO) with decreased pulmonary blood flow and pulmonary venous return to the left atrium. Interventricular septum (IVS) is deviated into the left ventricle (LV) due to right heart pressure overload, with both low pulmonary blood flow and deviated IVS contributing to decreased LV filling. Systolic and diastolic cardiac dysfunctions are common. (Copyright Satyan Lakshminrusimha)

distending pressure in utero.[34] As noted, a randomized control trial demonstrated significantly improved survival of FETO over expectant care in severe CDH, although similar benefit was not shown in moderate CDH.[18,35] The physiologic benefits of FETO are not well delineated, although neonatal assessment shows improved lung function, oxygenation, and measures of LV size, compared to newborns with expectant fetal management.[24,36] Improvements in later resolution of PH by echocardiography have also been described in both moderate and severe CDH.[37,38] Experimental models of FETO generally show favorable lung histopathology with respect to lung growth and vascular remodeling,[34] although a recent ovine model of tracheal occlusion recapitulating the contemporary practice of late release of the tracheal balloon prior to delivery did not demonstrate improved perinatal gas exchange despite improved lung function and increased PBF.[39]

MANAGEMENT

Published guidelines[40,41] provide a comprehensive perspective on approaches to postnatal management in CDH, employing a lung-protective, gentle ventilation strategy, including permissive hypercapnia with limitation of ventilator pressure and decreased exposure to hyperoxia using preductal oxygenation for supplemental oxygen titration while allowing for a preductal/postductal oxygen saturation differential (see Fig. 1B). Effective ventilation and airway management are crucial for these infants, emphasizing adequate lung recruitment without causing under-inflation or over-inflation. This balance is essential to prevent significant ventilator-induced lung injuries. Maintaining this equilibrium demands consistent bedside attention, including managing airway secretions, monitoring the ventilator's pressure-volume loops, and carefully adjusting the mean airway pressure based on auscultation, clinical response, and radiographic findings (refer to section on *"Ventilation concepts and cardiopulmonary interactions"*). Strategies to reduce ventilator and oxygen-associated lung injury and inflammation are critical for survival due to lung hypoplasia in CDH, with the implementation of these protective strategies resulting in improved survival over time at several institutions.[42,43] This contrasts with historical approaches aimed toward maximal acute pulmonary vasodilation (ie, targeting hyperventilation, alkalosis and hyperoxia). Without randomized trials regarding optimal cardiovascular management, echocardiography-based evaluation, and comprehensive assessment of adequacy of cardiac output [clinical perfusion, vital signs, urine output, near infrared spectroscopy, blood lactate levels and metabolic acidosis, serum creatinine, blood urea nitrogen and B-type natriuretic peptide (BNP) as a marker of ventricular stress] promote a physiology-guided approach. Echocardiography allows for anatomic and functional cardiac and pulmonary vascular assessment and has been recommended early in the course (<24 hours of life) for all infants with CDH.[40,44] Quantitative echocardiography parameters of RV and LV function, as well as estimates of pulmonary arterial pressure due to elevated PVR are important to establish the baseline condition and monitor changes over time. Assessment of the degree and direction of any shunt at the atrial, ventricular, and ductal levels (including gradients measurement) can further inform regarding PVR to systemic vascular resistance (SVR), as well as relative function and compliance of the ventricles. RV-LV interactions are important to appreciate; a poorly filled LV with low output due to high right heart pressures with displacement of the interventricular septum and low PBF (at times with retrograde ductal flow in the transverse and ascending aorta) results in compromised systemic perfusion and oxygen delivery, even with a non-restrictive PDA. Serial echocardiograms can guide treatment from the initial transition to the chronic management phase in infants with CDH.[2,45,46] Of interest, PH at the initial echocardiogram (<48 hours) does not discriminate between infants that die or receive prolonged respiratory support versus survivors without prolonged respiratory support, while the persistence of PH by echocardiogram is associated with mortality and prolonged need for respiratory support.[47–49]

Ventilation Concepts And Cardiopulmonary Interactions

The Neonatal Resuscitation Program[50] and other published CDH-specific guidelines recommend immediate endotracheal intubation and avoidance of bag-valve or T-piece with mask ventilation at delivery for infants with CDH.[40,41,50] (**Table 1**). Gentle ventilation, using peak pressures ≤25 cm H_2O, and positive end-expiratory pressure (PEEP) no higher than 5 cm H_2O are recommended[40,41] while allowing for permissive hypercapnia, targeting arterial partial pressure of carbon dioxide (Pco_2) ≤70 mm Hg and pH>7.2, although some centers may allow for higher Pco_2 and lower pH, particularly if clinical perfusion and markers of adequate oxygen delivery are reassuring. Gas exchange markers tend to slowly improve if both shorter and longer- term effects of ventilator-associated injury can be minimized. Notably, no tidal volume targets are specified in published guidelines. In the setting of restrictive lung disease due to lung hypoplasia, lower tidal volumes are physiologically appropriate with higher respiratory rates to achieve ventilation targets. However, underdeveloped airways in the context of pulmonary hypoplasia may contribute to higher airway resistance and air-trapping, indicating the need for individualized ventilator strategies. In a small study of milder CDH, Lee and colleagues identified that tidal volume of 5 to 6 mL/kg while on mechanical ventilation was associated with lesser work of breathing than 4 mL/kg.[51] However, this study was not designed to evaluate later outcomes or lung injury, including time to successful extubation. Optimizing mechanical ventilation does not mandate lowering infant work of breathing if the trade-off is prolongation of invasive ventilation.

Table 1
Guidelines for respiratory management and oxygenation and ventilation targets

		Targets	Comments	References
Ventilator settings	CMV Consider HFOV for rescue		VICI trial: less ECMO use, shorter duration of ventilation, and more favorable hemodynamic outcomes with CMV	54,55
	PIP	$\leq$ 25 cm H_2O		40,41
	PEEP	2–5 cm H_2O	PEEP 2 superior to PEEP 5 with respect to lung compliance, oxygenation and pulmonary blood flow	40,41,56
Ventilation		$Paco_2$<70 mm Hg, pH>7.2	Higher $Paco_2$/lower pH may be tolerated during perinatal transition or if perfusion adequate	55
Oxygenation	Monitor preductal (right hand) Allow for preductal/postductal saturation differential	$\geq$85%	$\geq$ 80% during perinatal transition >90%–94% once Fio_2 at "safe" level of 0.4–0.5	40,41

Abbreviations: CMV, conventional mechanical ventilation; ECMO, extracorporeal membrane oxygenation; HFOV, high-frequency oscillatory ventilation; PIP, peak inspiratory pressure; PEEP, positive end expiratory pressure.

Oxygenation targets are usually based on preductal (right hand) measures, with recommended goal oxygen saturations $\geq 85\%$. Some centers target higher saturation goals (>90–94%) if Fio_2 is at a "safer" level, commonly 40% to 50%, as this allows for the pulmonary vasodilatory effects of supplemental oxygen while limiting pulmonary exposure to hyperoxia. Conversely, saturation targets as low as $\geq 80\%$ may be utilized to promote weaning of Fio_2 to limit hyperoxia.[40,41] Of interest, in an experimental ovine model of persistent PH of the newborn (PPHN), prior short exposure to Fio_2 of 1.00 decreased the vasodilator response to inhaled nitric oxide (iNO) in comparison to Fio_2 of 0.21 to 0.50, supporting utilization of lower saturation targets if needed to achieve safer Fio_2 exposure.[52] Guidelines and practice in some centers allow for initial transition over the first several hours, during which lower preductal saturations and higher Pco_2 may be tolerated. In general, oxygenation targets are accepting of a persistent preductal/postductal saturation differential, which would be expected, particularly in more severe CDH, given the prolonged course of resolution of PH.[14] A large preductal/postductal saturation differential (persistently>15–20%) raises concern for a lower mixed venous saturation, which occurs in the setting of decreased oxygen delivery due to increased tissue extraction. In this case, interventions to enhance cardiac output should be considered. Overall, even with adoption of oxygenation and ventilation guidelines, there can be substantial variability in practice and outcomes; among 4 high volume European centers over a 10-year period, survival ranged from 59% to 79%.[53]

The recommended mode of ventilation is conventional mechanical ventilation (CMV). The VICI-trial (High-Frequency Oscillation Versus Conventional Mechanical Ventilation in Newborns with Congenital Diaphragmatic Hernia: A Randomized Clinical Trial), which randomized newborns to CMV versus high-frequency oscillatory ventilation (HFOV), demonstrated increased use of ECMO, longer duration of ventilation, and more hemodynamic compromise with HFOV, with a nonsignificant increase in mortality.[54,55] The trial specified similar oxygenation and ventilation targets as described earlier, with pressure limitation for both CMV and HFOV. Increased hemodynamic compromise in infants randomized to HFOV highlights the importance of cardiopulmonary interactions. Hypoplastic lungs are not generally recruitable in the standard sense, as there is no parenchymal disease, and they are likely readily subject to overdistention, impeding venous return and increasing PVR, which can result in compromised cardiac output. Cardiopulmonary interactions also explain the improved hemodynamics demonstrated with low PEEP in a randomized crossover study of 2 versus 5 cm H_2O PEEP in infants with severe CDH and PH on CMV.[56] Infants had higher lung compliance on 2 cm H_2O PEEP with lower delta pressure and respiratory rate and better ventilation and oxygenation. The PDA had bidirectional flow in both conditions, while echocardiography on low PEEP showed increased PBF and improved left heart filling. Conversely, with appropriate higher ventilator rates in lung hypoplasia, even modest set PEEP may result in overdistention and elevated PVR due to "auto-PEEP."[57] Thus, rapid respiratory rates on the ventilator in the setting of restrictive lung disease are best employed with low-set PEEP (≤ 3 cm H_2O) due to resulting elevated intrinsic PEEP, particularly in underdeveloped airways, as this can lead to gas trapping, potentially increasing PVR. These insights underscore the need for repeated cardiopulmonary assessment.

The VICI trial demonstrates the critical role of ventilator management in supporting newborns with CDH, with respect to mortality and hemodynamic status due to cardiopulmonary interactions. The trial required a prenatal diagnosis of CDH; however, eligibility was not restricted based on fetal assessment of the severity of lung hypoplasia, supporting use of consistent approaches across the spectrum of CDH severity.

Further, data suggest that the severity of fetal lung hypoplasia is associated with the resolution of persistent PH.[14] Thus, attention to the contribution of cardiac dysfunction due to increased afterload, interventricular interactions, and/or innate contractility is an important adjunct to respiratory management in CDH, as it directly impacts oxygen delivery.

Cardiac Output And Function

Decrements in innate contractility of 1 or both ventricles are more common than not, and the necessity of contractility support should be assumed in infants with hemodynamic compromise (**Table 2**). As PH is predominant at the initial echocardiogram and RV afterload is important when considering RV dysfunction, serial assessments will guide management. In the context of significant PH with concern for compromised cardiac output and oxygen delivery, pulmonary vasodilator therapy should be considered. As noted, a decrease in mixed venous saturation (large preductal/postductal saturation differential) should be considered for additional intervention, as it may occur prior to the development of lactic acidosis. Since most infants likely have biventricular dysfunction, agents such as milrinone that provide vasodilatory, inotropic, and lusitropic (cardiac relaxation) support for both ventricles are favored. During perinatal transition, attention should be paid as the small fetal LV may not tolerate aggressive maneuvers to increase PBF, particularly in the setting of more profound acidosis, impairing ventricular function. Allowing for pulmonary transition, decreasing Fio_2 to safer levels as tolerated, and gentle volume loading, followed by pulmonary vasodilator therapy, is prudent. In isolated LV dysfunction, inotropic support and balanced volume loading may improve cardiac output. Given the importance of RV pressure overload to cardiac dysfunction, prostaglandin E1 (PGE) infusion to achieve or maintain ductal patency may allow for the maintenance of cardiac output when PVR is systemic-to-suprasystemic. This approach allows for lower RV afterload, as long as SVR is not manipulated to supraphysiologic levels. There may be a decrease in postductal (lower body) saturation, offset or overcome by increased oxygen delivery due to improvements in cardiac function and output. Data from a single center study support this, with BNP levels decreasing within 24 hours of PGE initiation.[58] It is important

Table 2 Cardiac phenotype and suggested management strategy		
Key Physiology Element	**Strategy**	**Targets**
Normal cardiac function, mild or no PH	Lung protection strategy (for all physiologies)	See **Table 1**
RV dysfunction, significant PH	Pulmonary vasodilators, PGE	Maintain unrestrictive PDA
Biventricular dysfunction	Balance vasodilators, inotropes, and/or PGE. Frequent reassessment	Support contractility, maintain unrestrictive PDA while bilateral or right to left shunt, avoid excessive afterload burden
LV dysfunction	Inotropes to support cardiac output	Support contractility, avoid excessive afterload; avoid iNO in primary LV dysfunction with pulmonary venous hypertension until LV dysfunction is addressed

Abbreviations: LV, left ventricle; PDA, patent ductus arteriosus; PGE, prostaglandin E1; PH, pulmonary hypertension; RV, right ventricle.

to recognize that the physiology is dynamic and ductal patency may be particularly important during transient elevations in PVR with mucous plugging, loss of functional residual capacity during suctioning, and more extended episodes of manipulation such as during CDH repair, even when a preductal/postductal saturation differential is not present at other times.[58,59] Above all, the maintenance of a nonrestrictive PDA allows time for the anticipated decrease in PVR and improvement in cardiac function; interval echocardiograms at 2 to 7 days after PGE initiation show improved LV relaxation, diastolic volume, and myocardial performance index as well as signs of decreased PVR and RV pressure overload with decreased right-to-left ductal flow and displacement of interventricular septum.[30,47,58,59] In addition to lowering RV afterload through communication with the systemic circulation, PGE can function as a pulmonary vasodilator, and importantly, with severe LV dysfunction, allow for circulatory support by the RV. Timing of PGE discontinuation needs to be carefully considered as reversal of ductal shunting with PVR fall may result in excessive PBF and systemic steal, worsening pulmonary mechanics and systemic perfusion. Thus, careful clinical and echocardiographic monitoring are needed, and continuous preductal and postductal saturation monitoring can identify periods when ductal flow shifts.

Pulmonary Vasodilator Therapy

iNO activates guanylate cyclase, leading to the production of cyclic guanosine monophosphate (cGMP) in smooth muscle cells, allowing for selective pulmonary vasodilation and improved ventilation-perfusion matching. However, in a randomized trial, iNO failed to improve oxygenation, avert ECMO, or increase survival in infants with CDH, although management during this period was not focused on gentle ventilation and weaning of Fio_2, and randomization occurred when oxygenation index was in the 40s—conditions which may impact pulmonary vasculature potential for vasodilation.[60] In contrast, contemporary single center retrospective studies have shown that 30% to 40% of infants with CDH have a positive and enduring oxygenation response to iNO.[61,62] Further, iNO responders were less likely to transition to ECMO compared to nonresponders.[61] In consecutive studies from the multicenter CDH Study Group (CDHSG) registry, early iNO initiation (<3 days of age) was associated with increased mortality, although data collection and the statistical approaches in these analyses likely fail to differentiate iNO use as rescue therapy.[63,64] Some have postulated that this may be secondary to pulmonary venous congestion and edema in infants with LV dysfunction, leading to decreased lung function.[45] Left-to-right atrial shunting especially in the setting of right-to-left shunting at the PDA has been proposed as an indirect marker of LV diastolic dysfunction (relative to the RV), leading to cardiopulmonary compromise in the setting of vasodilator therapy. However, Lawrence and colleagues found no differences in pre-iNO echocardiographic LV diastolic measurements in iNO responders versus nonresponders, while abnormal LV systolic function (by shortening fraction, 19% of cohort) was associated with lack of response to iNO.[61] Infants with LV systolic dysfunction were more likely to transition to ECMO support and overall had poorer outcomes, with delayed time to CDH repair and higher mortality, supporting early LV dysfunction as a marker for poor outcome in CDH regardless of iNO therapy. Although Kumar and colleagues found that iNO nonresponders were not more likely to transition to ECMO support, nonresponders had higher mortality.[62] Elevated RV pressure estimates did not decrease in iNO-treated infants by interval echocardiogram on day 3, and despite overall more favorable outcomes in iNO responders, RV pressure estimates increased from pre-iNO echocardiogram, suggesting that iNO may not substantially decrease PVR even among responders, or its effect on PVR may not persist.[62] Guidelines advocate for iNO as a first-line pulmonary vasodilator in those thought to have pulmonary arterial hypertension, with concomitant normal LV function.[40,41] Without clinical improvement, weaning and discontinuation of iNO could be considered.

Other pulmonary vasodilators have been described in the management of infants with refractory PH in the context of CDH. Sildenafil acts in the NO pathway as a selective phosphodiesterase-5 (PDE-5) inhibitor, inhibiting the breakdown of cGMP. Thus, it can potentiate the effect of endogenous or exogenous NO. Small retrospective studies describe variable improvement in oxygenation and cardiac output with sildenafil administration.[65,66] The prostacyclin pathway is another targeted pathway.[40] A CDHSG registry study described increased mortality in infants administered parenteral epoprostenol post-CDH repair, with effects attenuated by adjustment for severity of CDH, suggesting the relationship was due to residual confounding by indication.[67] Treprostinil is a more stable parenteral prostacyclin analogue which can be administered intravenously or subcutaneously. Two single-center retrospective studies described outcomes with initiation of treprostinil at a median of 12 and 19 days of age.[68,69] Over the first month of therapy, branch PA flow, interventricular septal displacement, and measures of RV function improved. Of note, although some improvements were identified within days of treprostinil initiation, these studies describe a time frame over which PH is improving/resolving and BNP is decreasing in infants with CDH without this intervention.[48,70] A recent CDHSG registry study with propensity-matching demonstrated decreased use and duration of ECMO with prostacyclin therapy initiated in the first week of life, although there was no effect on in-hospital mortality.[71]

The final pathway targeted for the treatment of PH is the endothelin pathway. Endothelin-1 is a potent pulmonary vasoconstrictor which is dysregulated in CDH.[47] Bosentan, a receptor antagonist, has been used as therapy for chronic CDH-related PH.[72]

Milrinone

Milrinone is a phosphodiesterase-3 (PDE-3) inhibitor which prevents the breakdown of cyclic adenosine monophosphate (cAMP), leading to pulmonary and systemic vasodilatation and positive inotropic and lusitropic cardiac support. Milrinone effectively dilates PA resistance vessels from an experimental model of PPHN.[73] Further, these vessels exhibit perinatal increases in PDE-3 activity with decreased cAMP levels, an effect rescued by milrinone administration.[74] These effects make milrinone a compelling agent for use in CDH, given elevated PVR and frequent ventricular dysfunction. Two small single-center retrospective studies provide supporting evidence in this respect.[62,75] When initiated in infants on iNO, milrinone was associated with improved oxygenation at 12 to 24 hours, improved diastolic and systolic function, decrease in RV pressure estimate, increase in LV ejection fraction, and maintenance of systemic blood pressures 2 to 3 days after initiation.[75] There is an ongoing randomized phase 2 trial of milrinone in infants with CDH and hypoxic respiratory failure, with target dose of 0.33 to 0.66 mcg/kg/min.[76] Optimal dosing is not established, but in postoperative infants with congenital heart disease, higher dose (0.75 mcg/kg/min) was more effective than low dose (0.25 mcg/kg/min).[77] PDE-3 distribution, abundance, and activity in the neonate may differ from older children, particularly in the setting of hyperoxia; addiotionally, milrinone clearance is decreased and half-life prolonged. In the authors' experience, milrinone initiation at 0.25 mcg/kg/min with titration up to 0.75 to 1 mcg/kg/min is well tolerated with changes every 2 to 6 hours and gentle volume loading at initiation if hypotension occurs.

Postnatal Glucocorticoids

Low cortisol levels (<15 mcg/dL) are common in newborns with CDH (20/34, 59% in a single-center retrospective study).[78] Infants with low cortisol were more likely to have liver herniation, but 88% of infants received steroid supplementation in this cohort, and outcomes and clinical course did not differ by cortisol level. In another single-center study, duration of stress dose steroids was associated with greater mortality in multivariate analysis; steroids did not improve survival with low baseline cortisol levels (<10 mcg/dL), while infants with higher cortisol levels who received steroids had a nonsignificant increase in mortality.[79] Nonetheless, in a lamb PPHN model, hydrocortisone improved oxygenation and ventilation, increased soluble guanylate cyclase, decreased PDE-5 activity, and increased cGMP levels in PA resistance vessels compared to lambs receiving Fio_2 1.0 alone.[80] Hence, in infants with CDH and refractory shock, a judicious course of stress hydrocortisone may be considered as an adjuvant therapy to support hemodynamics. Baseline cortisol level should be obtained prior to steroid administration, recognizing that stress steroids may be harmful when cortisol level is not low.

Inotropes and Vasopressors

Inotropes and vasopressors, while supporting cardiac function and vascular tone, may also be detrimental due to their side-effect profile (**Table 3**). Initiation and titration should be guided by hemodynamics, with close monitoring of clinical perfusion, markers of adequate oxygen delivery, and serial echocardiography. The choice of agents is based on presumed pharmaceutical effects and underlying pathophysiology. Epinephrine, dobutamine, and dopamine act on beta-adrenergic receptors providing some positive inotropic effect. Inotropic support may be best achieved with low doses of intravenous epinephrine or dobutamine, while being mindful of unwanted extreme chronotropy. A fast heart rate may impede filling and diastolic function, as well as increase cardiac oxygen demand. Activation of alpha-receptors (eg, dopamine, epinephrine, or norepinephrine) may result in peripheral systemic vasoconstriction, although lower dose dopamine and epinephrine usually spare this effect. While increased systemic perfusion pressure can improve blood flow to various vascular beds, increases in SVR will increase LV and RV afterload (via the PDA), which may worsen cardiac output and systemic oxygen delivery. When PGE is used in

Table 3 Inotropes and vasoactive agents					
Agent	**HR**	**Contractility**	**SVR/SBP**	**PVR/PBP**	**Suggested Use**
Dobutamine	++	++	=	=	Ventricular dysfunction
Epinephrine	+	+++	+++	++	Ventricular dysfunction with low SBP
Dopamine	+	++	++	+++	Caution when significant PH
Norepinephrine	+	=	+++	+	Low SBP without significant ventricular dysfunction
Vasopressin	=	=	+++	↓/=	Low SBP without significant ventricular dysfunction
Milrinone	=	++	↓↓	↓↓	Severe PH with high/normal SBP

Abbreviations: HR, heart rate; PBP, pulmonary blood pressure; PH, pulmonary hypertension; PVR, pulmonary vascular resistance; SBP, systemic blood pressure; SVR, systemic vascular resistance.

severe PH to unload/protect the RV, systemic vasoconstricting agents should be used with caution, given the high proportion of infants with CDH and hemodynamic compromise who have some degree of RV dysfunction. In this situation, milrinone would be favored for its direct effects on the myocardium and pulmonary vasodilation.

In addition to the systemic circulation, direct effects of vasoconstricting medications on the pulmonary circulation should be considered. Vasopressors, such as norepinephrine and phenylephrine have been considered at low doses to restore the pulmonary-to-systemic pressure ratio and normalize cardiac septal configuration; however, biventricular function, as noted, may be compromised with this strategy and these medications provide limited inotropic support.[2] Vasopressin (adrenergic-independent) has been considered as an agent for the treatment of PPHN, with some advocating that it acts as both a pulmonary vasodilator and a systemic vasoconstrictor; it is not an inotrope. Although there may be developmental regulation in the pulmonary vascular response to vasopressin, experimental data suggest that it acts solely as a systemic vasoconstrictor, without pulmonary vascular effects.[81,82] Further, in a PPHN model, echocardiography demonstrated worsening of functional parameters for both ventricles during vasopressin infusion.[81] In a small single-center study of 11 infants with CDH and catecholamine-resistant hypotension being considered for ECMO support, supraphysiologic systemic blood pressures were achieved with vasopressin infusion, although 5 infants went on ECMO for hypoxemia and/or acidosis, including 3 with severe LV dysfunction.[83] Hyponatremia occurred in infants who received vasopressin infusion for>24 hours. Although there is concern that dopamine can vasoconstrict the pulmonary circulation, a comparative study in asphyxiated newborn piglets of high-dose versus combination moderate-dose dopamine plus low-dose epinephrine showed no benefit of the combination approach, and some high-volume CDH centers continue to use low-to-moderate dose dopamine for circulatory support.[84] Levosimendan, a calcium-sensitizing agent with positive inotropic, lusitropic, and vasodilating effects, was associated with improved oxygenation and stable blood pressure within 24 hours of initiation and improved severity of PH, RV, and LV function after 7 days in an observational cohort.[85] Negative inotropes should be avoided, such as beta-blockers.

Extracorporeal Membrane Oxygenation

ECMO is a rescue strategy for cardiac and/or respiratory failure. Overall mortality is higher in infants that transition to ECMO support, though a recent registry study showed decreased mortality with ECMO in high-risk CDH.[86] Both veno-arterial and veno-venous support can be used, without differences in short-term outcomes at the registry level, although individual institutional experiences may vary.[87]

PROGNOSIS—LATE PULMONARY HYPERTENSION AND CARDIORESPIRATORY PROFILE

The majority of infants with CDH will resolve their PH between 1 to 3 weeks of age, with favorable outcomes despite this delayed perinatal transition.[88] However, infants with evidence of persistent, protracted PH often require prolonged respiratory support and possibly chronic PH therapy.[89] These infants are at higher risk for mortality. Rates of late and chronic PH in this population vary significantly depending on the time of follow-up and PH definition. In a retrospective cohort of 140 infants with CDH, severity of PH at 2 weeks of age predicted mortality, prolonged invasive ventilation beyond 28 days of age, and need for prolonged respiratory support.[48] Rates of chronic PH in CDH survivors in preschool ages vary between 4.5% to 38%.[90] When comparing cardiac catheterization results of CDH infants to infants undergoing PDA closure at 6 to 36 months of age, pulmonary arterial pressure and PVR were significantly higher in those with CDH, and PBF was significantly lower. Only half of these patients had PH signs on echocardiography.[91] This suggests an important role for cardiac catheterization in the long-term follow-up of CDH infants that are dependent on respiratory support.

The effect of fetal intervention on long-term prognosis is not yet described. A recent cohort of children surviving after FETO and a non-FETO comparison group with follow-up to 4 to 6 years demonstrated similar cardiopulmonary and gastrointestinal morbidity across groups.[92]

SUMMARY

PH remains a significant factor dictating management and outcomes in infants with CDH. Respiratory management critically interacts with pulmonary circulation and hemodynamics. Cardiopulmonary status and PH are dynamic, with various types and combinations of cardiac dysfunction contributing to the overall clinical condition, which may fluctuate within the same patient throughout postnatal stabilization. Altered right, left, or biventricular function, with both systolic and diastolic components, arterial disease, and left heart restriction may all contribute. Future studies should evaluate optimal strategies based on the combination of findings, prenatal and postnatal interventions, and the impact on short-term, long-term, and family-driven outcomes.

Best Practice Box

Recommendations for the assessment and management of PH in infants with CDH:

- PH in CDH has a dynamic and shifting clinical phenotype with variable contributions of vascular hypoplasia and arrested growth, abnormal tone and vasoreactivity, and vascular remodeling with possible contribution of pulmonary venous hypertension from left heart dysfunction.

- The authors emphasize the need for frequent reassessment of clinical parameters (perfusion and hemodynamics and changes with interventions), laboratory values (blood gases, lactate, renal function), and imaging (chest radiographs and echocardiography) to guide use of vasoactive and inotropic medications.

- To optimize outcomes of these challenging infants, one should balance gentle ventilation, avoiding hyperoxia with improving cardiopulmonary interactions and treatment tailored to the management of cardiac dysfunction.

- PGE1 infusion to maintain ductal patency can achieve RV afterload reduction, pulmonary vasodilatation, and augmentation of systemic blood flow.

DISCLOSURE

No conflicts of interest to declare.

REFERENCES

1. Chandrasekharan PK, Rawat M, Madappa R, et al. Congenital Diaphragmatic hernia – a review. Maternal Health, Neonatology and Perinatology 2017;3(1). https://doi.org/10.1186/s40748-017-0045-1.

2. Bhombal S, Patel N. Diagnosis & management of pulmonary hypertension in congenital diaphragmatic hernia. Semin Fetal Neonatal Med 2022;27(4):101383.
3. Altit G, Bhombal S, Van Meurs K, et al. Ventricular performance is associated with need for extracorporeal membrane oxygenation in newborns with congenital diaphragmatic hernia. J Pediatr 2017;191:28–34.e1.
4. Aggarwal S, Shanti C, Agarwal P, et al. Echocardiographic measures of ventricular-vascular interactions in congenital diaphragmatic hernia. Early Hum Dev 2022;165:105534.
5. Coughlin MA, Werner NL, Gajarski R, et al. Prenatally diagnosed severe CDH: mortality and morbidity remain high. J Pediatr Surg 2016;51(7):1091–5.
6. Caldeira I, Fernandes-Silva H, Machado-Costa D, et al. Developmental pathways underlying lung development and congenital lung disorders. Cells 2 2021;10(11). https://doi.org/10.3390/cells10112987.
7. Keijzer R, Liu J, Deimling J, et al. Dual-hit hypothesis explains pulmonary hypoplasia in the nitrofen model of congenital diaphragmatic hernia. Am J Pathol 2000;156(4):1299–306.
8. Manso PH, Figueira RL, Prado CM, et al. Early neonatal echocardiographic findings in an experimental rabbit model of congenital diaphragmatic hernia. Braz J Med Biol Res 2015;48(3):234–9.
9. Kitagawa M, Hislop A, Boyden EA, et al. Lung hypoplasia in congenital diaphragmatic hernia. A quantitative study of airway, artery, and alveolar development. Br J Surg 1971;58(5):342–6.
10. Gupta VS, Harting MT. Congenital diaphragmatic hernia-associated pulmonary hypertension. Semin Perinatol 2020;44(1):151167.
11. Acker SN, Seedorf GJ, Abman SH, et al. Pulmonary artery endothelial cell dysfunction and decreased populations of highly proliferative endothelial cells in experimental congenital diaphragmatic hernia. Am J Physiol Lung Cell Mol Physiol 2013;305(12):L943–52.
12. Yamataka T, Puri P. Pulmonary artery structural changes in pulmonary hypertension complicating congenital diaphragmatic hernia. J Pediatr Surg 1997;32(3): 387–90.
13. Cruz-Martinez R, Castañon M, Moreno-Alvarez O, et al. Usefulness of lung-to-head ratio and intrapulmonary arterial Doppler in predicting neonatal morbidity in fetuses with congenital diaphragmatic hernia treated with fetoscopic tracheal occlusion. Ultrasound Obstet Gynecol 2013;41(1):59–65.
14. Lusk LA, Wai KC, Moon-Grady AJ, et al. Fetal ultrasound markers of severity predict resolution of pulmonary hypertension in congenital diaphragmatic hernia. Am J Obstet Gynecol 2015;213(2):216.e1–8.
15. Basta AM, Lusk LA, Keller RL, et al. Fetal stomach position predicts neonatal outcomes in isolated left-sided congenital diaphragmatic hernia. Fetal Diagn Ther 2016;39(4):248–55.
16. Jani J, Nicolaides KH, Keller RL, et al, Antenatal-CDH-Registry Group. Observed to expected lung area to head circumference ratio in the prediction of survival in fetuses with isolated diaphragmatic hernia. Ultrasound Obstet Gynecol 2007; 30(1):67–71.
17. Jani J, Peralta CF, Van Schoubroeck D, et al. Relationship between lung-to-head ratio and lung volume in normal fetuses and fetuses with diaphragmatic hernia. Ultrasound Obstet Gynecol 2006;27(5):545–50.
18. Deprest JA, Nicolaides KH, Benachi A, et al, TOTAL Trial for Severe Hypoplasia Investigators. Randomized trial of fetal surgery for severe left diaphragmatic hernia. N Engl J Med 2021;385(2):107–18.

19. Stressig R, Fimmers R, Eising K, et al. Preferential streaming of the ductus veno-sus and inferior caval vein towards the right heart is associated with left heart un-derdevelopment in human fetuses with left-sided diaphragmatic hernia. Heart. Oct 2010;96(19):1564–8.

20. Byrne FA, Keller RL, Meadows J, et al. Severe left diaphragmatic hernia limits size of fetal left heart more than does right diaphragmatic hernia. Ultrasound Obstet Gynecol 2015;46(6):688–94.

21. Vogel M, McElhinney DB, Marcus E, et al. Significance and outcome of left heart hypoplasia in fetal congenital diaphragmatic hernia. Ultrasound Obstet Gynecol 2010;35(3):310–7.

22. Broth RE, Wood DC, Rasanen J, et al. Prenatal prediction of lethal pulmonary hy-poplasia: the hyperoxygenation test for pulmonary artery reactivity. Am J Obstet Gynecol. Oct 2002;187(4):940–5.

23. Done E, Allegaert K, Lewi P, et al. Maternal hyperoxygenation test in fetuses un-dergoing FETO for severe isolated congenital diaphragmatic hernia. Ultrasound Obstet Gynecol 2011;37(3):264–71.

24. Rocha LA, Byrne FA, Keller RL, et al. Left heart structures in human neonates with congenital diaphragmatic hernia and the effect of fetal endoscopic tracheal oc-clusion. Fetal Diagn Ther 2014;35(1):36–43.

25. Schmidt AF, Rojas-Moscoso JA, Gonçalves FL, et al. Increased contractility and impaired relaxation of the left pulmonary artery in a rabbit model of congenital diaphragmatic hernia. Pediatr Surg Int 2013;29(5):489–94.

26. Kashyap AJ, Crossley KJ, DeKoninck PLJ, et al. Neonatal cardiopulmonary tran-sition in an ovine model of congenital diaphragmatic hernia. Arch Dis Child Fetal Neonatal Ed 2019;104(6):F617–23.

27. Altit G, Bhombal S, Van Meurs K, et al. Diminished cardiac performance and left ventricular dimensions in neonates with congenital diaphragmatic hernia. Pediatr Cardiol 2018;39(5):993–1000.

28. Patel N, Lally PA, Kipfmueller F, et al. Ventricular dysfunction is a critical determi-nant of mortality in congenital diaphragmatic hernia. Am J Respir Crit Care Med 2019;200(12):1522–30.

29. Kinsella JP, Steinhorn RH, Mullen MP, et al, Pediatric Pulmonary Hypertension Network PPHNet. The left ventricle in congenital diaphragmatic hernia: implica-tions for the management of pulmonary hypertension. J Pediatr 2018;197:17–22.

30. Patel N, Massolo AC, Paria A, et al. Early postnatal ventricular dysfunction is associated with disease severity in patients with congenital diaphragmatic her-nia. J Pediatr 2018;203:400–7.e1.

31. Aggarwal S, Stockmann P, Klein MD, et al. Echocardiographic measures of ven-tricular function and pulmonary artery size: prognostic markers of congenital dia-phragmatic hernia? J Perinatol 2011;31(8):561–6.

32. Maia PD, Gien J, Kinsella JP, et al. Hemodynamic characterization of neonates with congenital diaphragmatic hernia-associated pulmonary hypertension by car-diac catheterization. J Pediatr 2023;255:230–5.e2.

33. Massolo AC, Paria A, Hunter L, et al. Ventricular dysfunction, interdependence, and mechanical dispersion in newborn infants with congenital diaphragmatic her-nia. Neonatology 2019;116(1):68–75.

34. Khan PA, Cloutier M, Piedboeuf B. Tracheal occlusion: a review of obstructing fetal lungs to make them grow and mature. Am J Med Genet C Semin Med Genet 2007;145c(2):125–38.

35. Deprest JA, Benachi A, Gratacos E, et al, TOTAL Trial for Moderate Hypoplasia Investigators. Randomized trial of fetal surgery for moderate left diaphragmatic hernia. N Engl J Med 2021;385(2):119–29.
36. Keller RL, Hawgood S, Neuhaus JM, et al. Infant pulmonary function in a randomized trial of fetal tracheal occlusion for severe congenital diaphragmatic hernia. Pediatr Res 2004;56(5):818–25.
37. Donepudi R, Belfort MA, Shamshirsaz AA, et al. Fetal endoscopic tracheal occlusion and pulmonary hypertension in moderate congenital diaphragmatic hernia. J Matern Fetal Neonatal Med 2022;35(25):6967–72.
38. Style CC, Olutoye OO, Belfort MA, et al. Fetal endoscopic tracheal occlusion reduces pulmonary hypertension in severe congenital diaphragmatic hernia. Ultrasound Obstet Gynecol 2019;54(6):752–8.
39. DeKoninck PLJ, Crossley KJ, Kashyap AJ, et al. Effects of tracheal occlusion on the neonatal cardiopulmonary transition in an ovine model of diaphragmatic hernia. Arch Dis Child Fetal Neonatal Ed 2019;104(6):F609–16.
40. Snoek KG, Reiss IK, Greenough A, et al, CDH EURO Consortium. Standardized postnatal management of infants with congenital diaphragmatic hernia in europe: the CDH EURO consortium consensus - 2015 update. Neonatology 2016;110(1):66–74.
41. Puligandla PS, Skarsgard ED, Offringa M, et al. Diagnosis and management of congenital diaphragmatic hernia: a clinical practice guideline. CMAJ 29 2018;190(4):E103–12.
42. Kays DW, Langham MR Jr, Ledbetter DJ, et al. Detrimental effects of standard medical therapy in congenital diaphragmatic hernia. Ann Surg 1999;230(3):340–8, discussion 348-51.
43. Bohn D. Congenital diaphragmatic hernia. Am J Respir Crit Care Med 2002;166(7):911–5.
44. Yang MJ, Fenton S, Russell K, et al. Left-sided congenital diaphragmatic hernia: can we improve survival while decreasing ECMO? J Perinatol 2020;40(6):935–42.
45. Patel N, Massolo AC, Kipfmueller F. Congenital diaphragmatic hernia-associated cardiac dysfunction. Semin Perinatol 2020;44(1):151168.
46. Patel N, Kipfmueller F. Cardiac dysfunction in congenital diaphragmatic hernia: pathophysiology, clinical assessment, and management. Semin Pediatr Surg 2017;26(3):154–8.
47. Keller RL, Tacy TA, Hendricks-Munoz K, et al. Congenital diaphragmatic hernia: endothelin-1, pulmonary hypertension, and disease severity. Am J Respir Crit Care Med 2010;182(4):555–61.
48. Lusk LA, Wai KC, Moon-Grady AJ, et al. Persistence of pulmonary hypertension by echocardiography predicts short-term outcomes in congenital diaphragmatic hernia. J Pediatr 2015;166(2):251–6.e1.
49. Steurer MA, Moon-Grady AJ, Fineman JR, et al. B-type natriuretic peptide: prognostic marker in congenital diaphragmatic hernia. Pediatr Res 2014;76(6):549–54.
50. Textbook of Neonatal Resuscitation. American Academy of Pediatrics.
51. Lee R, Hunt KA, Williams EE, et al. Work of breathing at different tidal volume targets in newborn infants with congenital diaphragmatic hernia. Eur J Pediatr 2022;181(6):2453–8.
52. Lakshminrusimha S, Swartz DD, Gugino SF, et al. Oxygen concentration and pulmonary hemodynamics in newborn lambs with pulmonary hypertension. Pediatr Res 2009;66(5):539–44.

53. Snoek KG, Greenough A, van Rosmalen J, et al. Congenital diaphragmatic hernia: 10-year evaluation of survival, extracorporeal membrane oxygenation, and foetoscopic endotracheal occlusion in four high-volume centres. Neonatology 2018;113(1):63–8.
54. van den Hout L, Tibboel D, Vijfhuize S, et al, CDH-EURO Consortium. The VICI-trial: high frequency oscillation versus conventional mechanical ventilation in newborns with congenital diaphragmatic hernia: an international multicentre randomized controlled trial. BMC Pediatr 2011;11:98.
55. Snoek KG, Capolupo I, van Rosmalen J, et al, CDH EURO Consortium. Conventional mechanical ventilation versus high-frequency oscillatory ventilation for congenital diaphragmatic hernia: a randomized clinical trial (the VICI-trial). Ann Surg 2016;263(5):867–74.
56. Guevorkian D, Mur S, Cavatorta E, et al. Lower distending pressure improves respiratory mechanics in congenital diaphragmatic hernia complicated by persistent pulmonary hypertension. J Pediatr 2018;200:38–43.
57. Boloker J, Bateman DA, Wung JT, et al. Congenital diaphragmatic hernia in 120 infants treated consecutively with permissive hypercapnea/spontaneous respiration/elective repair. J Pediatr Surg 2002;37(3):357–66.
58. Lawrence KM, Berger K, Herkert L, et al. Use of prostaglandin E1 to treat pulmonary hypertension in congenital diaphragmatic hernia. J Pediatr Surg 2019; 54(1):55–9.
59. Inamura N, Kubota A, Ishii R, et al. Efficacy of the circulatory management of an antenatally diagnosed congenital diaphragmatic hernia: outcomes of the proposed strategy. Pediatr Surg Int 2014;30(9):889–94.
60. Inhaled nitric oxide and hypoxic respiratory failure in infants with congenital diaphragmatic hernia. The Neonatal Inhaled Nitric Oxide Study Group (NINOS). Pediatrics 1997;99(6):838–45.
61. Lawrence KM, Monos S, Adams S, et al. Inhaled nitric oxide is associated with improved oxygenation in a subpopulation of infants with congenital diaphragmatic hernia and pulmonary hypertension. J Pediatr 2020;219:167–72.
62. Kumar VHS, Dadiz R, Koumoundouros J, et al. Response to pulmonary vasodilators in infants with congenital diaphragmatic hernia. Pediatr Surg Int 2018;34(7): 735–42.
63. Putnam LR, Tsao K, Morini F, et al, Congenital Diaphragmatic Hernia Study Group. Evaluation of variability in inhaled nitric oxide use and pulmonary hypertension in patients with congenital diaphragmatic hernia. JAMA Pediatr 2016; 170(12):1188–94.
64. Noh CY, Chock VY, Bhombal S, et al, Congenital Diaphragmatic Hernia Study Group. Early nitric oxide is not associated with improved outcomes in congenital diaphragmatic hernia. Pediatr Res 2023. https://doi.org/10.1038/s41390-023-02491-8.
65. Bialkowski A, Moenkemeyer F, Patel N. Intravenous sildenafil in the management of pulmonary hypertension associated with congenital diaphragmatic hernia. Eur J Pediatr Surg 2015;25(2):171–6.
66. Noori S, Friedlich P, Wong P, et al. Cardiovascular effects of sildenafil in neonates and infants with congenital diaphragmatic hernia and pulmonary hypertension. Neonatology 2007;91(2):92–100.
67. Skarda DE, Yoder BA, Anstadt EE, et al. Epoprostenol does not affect mortality in neonates with congenital diaphragmatic hernia. Eur J Pediatr Surg 2015;25(5): 454–9.

68. De Bie FR, Avitabile CM, Flohr S, et al. Treprostinil in neonates with congenital diaphragmatic hernia-related pulmonary hypertension. J Pediatr 2023;12:113420.

69. Carpentier E, Mur S, Aubry E, et al. Safety and tolerability of subcutaneous treprostinil in newborns with congenital diaphragmatic hernia and life-threatening pulmonary hypertension. J Pediatr Surg 2017;52(9):1480–3.

70. Guslits E, Steurer MA, Nawaytou H, et al. Longitudinal B-type natriuretic peptide levels predict outcome in infants with congenital diaphragmatic hernia. J Pediatr 2021;229:191–8.e2.

71. Ramaraj AB, Rice-Townsend SE, Foster CL, et al, Congenital Diaphragmatic Hernia Study Group. Association between early prostacyclin therapy and extracorporeal life support use in patients with congenital diaphragmatic hernia. JAMA Pediatr 2023;177(6):582–9.

72. Lakshminrusimha S, Mathew B, Leach CL. Pharmacologic strategies in neonatal pulmonary hypertension other than nitric oxide. Semin Perinatol 2016;40(3): 160–73.

73. Lakshminrusimha S, Porta NF, Farrow KN, et al. Milrinone enhances relaxation to prostacyclin and iloprost in pulmonary arteries isolated from lambs with persistent pulmonary hypertension of the newborn. Pediatr Crit Care Med 2009;10(1): 106–12.

74. Chen B, Lakshminrusimha S, Czech L, et al. Regulation of phosphodiesterase 3 in the pulmonary arteries during the perinatal period in sheep. Pediatr Res 2009; 66(6):682–7.

75. Patel N. Use of milrinone to treat cardiac dysfunction in infants with pulmonary hypertension secondary to congenital diaphragmatic hernia: a review of six patients. Neonatology 2012;102(2):130–6.

76. Lakshminrusimha S, Keszler M, Kirpalani H, et al. Milrinone in congenital diaphragmatic hernia - a randomized pilot trial: study protocol, review of literature and survey of current practices. Matern Health Neonatol Perinatol 2017;3:27.

77. Hoffman TM, Wernovsky G, Atz AM, et al. Efficacy and safety of milrinone in preventing low cardiac output syndrome in infants and children after corrective surgery for congenital heart disease. Circulation 2003;107(7):996–1002.

78. Kamath BD, Fashaw L, Kinsella JP. Adrenal insufficiency in newborns with congenital diaphragmatic hernia. J Pediatr 2010;156(3):495–7.e1.

79. Robertson JO, Criss CN, Hsieh LB, et al. Steroid use for refractory hypotension in congenital diaphragmatic hernia. Pediatr Surg Int 2017;33(9):981–7.

80. Perez M, Lakshminrusimha S, Wedgwood S, et al. Hydrocortisone normalizes oxygenation and cGMP regulation in lambs with persistent pulmonary hypertension of the newborn. Am J Physiol Lung Cell Mol Physiol 2012;302(6):L595–603.

81. Amer R, Elsayed YN, Graham MR, et al. Effect of vasopressin on a porcine model of persistent pulmonary hypertension of the newborn. Pediatr Pulmonol 2019; 54(3):319–32.

82. Wang M, Shibamoto T, Kuda Y, et al. Systemic vasoconstriction modulates the responses of pulmonary vasculature and airway to vasoconstrictors in anesthetized rats. Exp Lung Res 2015;41(6):324–34.

83. Acker SN, Kinsella JP, Abman SH, et al. Vasopressin improves hemodynamic status in infants with congenital diaphragmatic hernia. J Pediatr 2014;165(1):53–8.e1.

84. Manouchehri N, Bigam DL, Churchill T, et al. A comparison of combination dopamine and epinephrine treatment with high-dose dopamine alone in asphyxiated newborn piglets after resuscitation. Pediatr Res 2013;73(4 Pt 1):435–42.

85. Schroeder L, Gries K, Ebach F, et al. Exploratory assessment of levosimendan in infants with congenital diaphragmatic hernia. Pediatr Crit Care Med 2021;22(7): e382–90.
86. Jancelewicz T, Langham MR Jr, Brindle ME, et al. Survival benefit associated with the use of extracorporeal life support for neonates with congenital diaphragmatic hernia. Ann Surg 2022;275(1):e256–63.
87. Guner YS, Harting MT, Fairbairn K, et al. Outcomes of infants with congenital diaphragmatic hernia treated with venovenous versus venoarterial extracorporeal membrane oxygenation: a propensity score approach. J Pediatr Surg 2018; 53(11):2092–9.
88. Gien J, Kinsella JP. Management of pulmonary hypertension in infants with congenital diaphragmatic hernia. J Perinatol 2016;36(Suppl 2):S28–31.
89. Kinsella JP, Ivy DD, Abman SH. Pulmonary vasodilator therapy in congenital diaphragmatic hernia: acute, late, and chronic pulmonary hypertension. Semin Perinatol 2005;29(2):123–8.
90. Lewis L, Sinha I, Kang SL, et al. Long term outcomes in CDH: cardiopulmonary outcomes and health related quality of life. J Pediatr Surg 2022;57(11):501–9.
91. Zussman ME, Bagby M, Benson DW, et al. Pulmonary vascular resistance in repaired congenital diaphragmatic hernia vs. age-matched controls. Pediatr Res 2012;71(6):697–700.
92. Sferra SR, Nies MK, Miller JL, et al. Morbidity in children after fetoscopic endoluminal tracheal occlusion for severe congenital diaphragmatic hernia: results from a multidisciplinary clinic. J Pediatr Surg 2023;58(1):14–9.

Early Pulmonary Hypertension in Preterm Infants

Srinivasan Mani, MD[a], Hussnain Mirza, MD[b], James Ziegler, MD[c],
Praveen Chandrasekharan, MD, MS[d,e,*]

KEYWORDS

- Pulmonary hypertension • Chronic lung disease • Preterm infants

KEY POINTS

- Pulmonary hypertension (PH) in preterm infants is a heterogeneous disease and is often associated with hypoxic respiratory failure (HRF). It has different phenotypes with diverse pathophysiology requiring precise management appropriate for the underlying phenotype.

- HRF in preterm infants could be secondary to other etiologies such as suboptimal ventilation, atelectasis, hyperinflation, and neonatal infections. Underlying etiology shall be treated first, but specific pulmonary vasodilator therapy can be considered for symptomatic infants if hemodynamic evaluation is consistent with elevated pulmonary vascular resistance (PVR) and PH physiology.

- In some preterm infants, PH is associated with increased pulmonary blood flow with a large left to right ductal shunting or increased pulmonary capillary wedge pressure due to pulmonary venous obstruction or severe cardiac dysfunction. Specific pulmonary vasodilator therapy is contraindicated in these infants.

- Systemic hypotension is common in preterm infants with HRF. Although dopamine is the most commonly used inotrope in infants, it may not be the optimal choice due to the nonselective vasoconstrictive effect that will increase both systemic vascular resistance and PVR. Based on the hemodynamic evaluation by echocardiography, alternative vasopressors and inotropes such as vasopressin, milrinone, norepinephrine, dobutamine, or epinephrine could be considered.

[a] Section of Neonatology, Department of Pediatrics, The University of Toledo/ ProMedica Russell J. Ebeid Children's Hospital, Toledo, OH 43606, USA; [b] Section of Neonatology, Department of Pediatrics, Advent Health for Children/ UCF College of Medicine, Orlando, FL 32408, USA; [c] Division of Cardiovascular Diseases, Department of Pediatrics, Hasbro Children's Hospital/ Brown University, Providence, RI 02903, USA; [d] Division of Neonatology, Department of Pediatrics, Jacobs School of Medicine & Biomedical Sciences, State University of New York at Buffalo, Buffalo, NY 32408, USA; [e] Oishei Children's Hospital, 818 Ellicott Street, Buffalo, NY 14203, USA
* Corresponding author. Oishei Children's Hospital, 818 Ellicott Street, Buffalo, NY 14203.
E-mail address: pkchandr@buffalo.edu

Clin Perinatol 51 (2024) 171–193
https://doi.org/10.1016/j.clp.2023.11.005   perinatology.theclinics.com

INTRODUCTION

Pulmonary hypertension (PH) in preterm infants has unique characteristics because of the interconnections between alveolar and vascular immaturity.[1] The Panama classification of pediatric PH highlighted the interplay of pathologic insults on the growing lung, chromosomal or genetic syndromes, and developmental lung abnormalities in the pathogenesis.[2] The National Heart, Lung, and Blood Institute (NHLBI) workshop in 2012 identified the lack of phenotyping as the significant barrier in research to advance our understanding of pediatric PH.[3] The ensuing research endeavors have advanced our understanding of PH phenotypes in preterm infants. The NHLBI workshop was reconvened in 2017 to enhance insights into pulmonary vascular disease (PVD) through a precision medicine approach and to develop interventions based on novel phenotypes.[4] Recently, different phenotypes of early PH in preterm infants have received increased attention.[5,6]

Echocardiographic evidence of PH without hypoxic respiratory failure (HRF) in preterm infants less than 72 hour of life is considered a physiologic variant,[7] whereas echo evidence of PH after 72 hour of life is termed delayed pulmonary vascular transition (PVT). Persistent PH of the newborns (PPHN), the most common phenotype of PVD in term infants, also occurs in preterm infants.[8] It usually presents before 72 hour of life with HRF. These infants are at high risk of developing myocardial ischemia and cardiac dysfunction due to elevated pulmonary vascular resistance (PVR) and diminished pulmonary blood flow (PBF).

Early PH in preterm infants can be defined as echocardiographic evidence of elevated pulmonary artery pressure (PAP) with or without HRF in the early days of life. Early PH can be differentiated from delayed PVT if a preceding echocardiogram documented a normal PVT. Early PH is associated with bronchopulmonary dysplasia (BPD) or death,[5,9,10] late PH,[11] poor growth, and neurodevelopment.[12]

Per Ohm's law, PAP is based on the PVR, PBF, and pulmonary capillary wedge pressure (PCWP) [PAP= (PVR × PBF) + PCWP]. High PBF due to a significant left to right shunt, for example, PDA, can increase PAP even with normal PVR.[13,14] Higher left atrial pressure due to mitral stenosis or left ventricular (LV) dysfunction may also significantly contribute to PH due to high PCWP.[15] Both of these variants can also present as early PH.

This narrative review aims to summarize the current evidence on pathophysiology, diagnosis and management of early PH, and other close phenotypes (**Box 1**) of PVD in preterm infants, identify knowledge gaps, and suggest future directions for research.

BACKGROUND

The transition of pulmonary and systemic circulatory circuits from functionally parallel to series is a critical event after birth triggered by removal of the placenta and transition of the gas exchange to the lungs. This transition alters the pulmonary circulation from high PVR and low PBF in the fetus to low PVR and increased PBF. This transition that starts at birth is not completed until the factors that aid in the typical fall in PVR act together as programmed.

A study that evaluated changes in the human fetal weight-indexed pulmonary and systemic vascular resistances (SVRs) (RPi and RSi) using Doppler ultrasound found that between gestational age 20 and 30 weeks, there was a 1.5-fold decrease in the RPi.[16] The fall in the PVR observed from the canalicular to the saccular stage of lung development was probably due to the increased density of the lung vasculature associated with lung growth. RPi-to-RSi ratio decreased significantly during the same period but did not change significantly from 30 to 38 weeks. This correlates with an

---

Box 1
Phenotypes of early pulmonary hypertension in preterm infants

I. Physiologic PH
- Echocardiographic evidence of PH at 0 to 72 hour of life without HRF
- No significant pre-post-ductal SpO_2 gradient
- No or minimum risk for adverse clinical outcomes

II. PPHN
- Echocardiographic evidence of PH at 0 to 72 hour of life with HRF
- Pre-post-ductal SpO_2 gradient in the presence of right to left shunting across the PDA
- At risk for cardiac dysfunction, high mortality, late PH, and BPD

III. Delayed PVT
- Echocardiographic evidence of PH at 72 to 96 hour of life without HRF
- No significant pre-post-ductal SpO_2 gradient
- Risk for late PH, BPD, and death

IV. Early PH
- Echocardiographic evidence of PH after 96 hour of life with or without HRF
- Pre-post-ductal SpO_2 gradient in the presence of right-to-left shunting across the PDA
- May be primary disease or secondary to other etiologies like neonatal infections, suboptimal ventilation, or lung recruitment
- Risk for late PH, BPD, and death

V. Flow-Associated PH
- Echocardiographic evidence of PH in association with the excessive PBF due to a significant left-to-right post-tricuspid shunt like ventricular septal defect (VSD) or PDA
- May require respiratory support and higher FiO_2 but do not develop HRF no significant pre-post-ductal SpO_2 gradient
- Risk for late PH, BPD, and death

Abbreviations: HRF, hypoxic respiratory failure; PH, pulmonary hypertension; PPHN, persistent pulmonary hypertension; PVT, pulmonary vascular transition.

---

increase in PVR from 30 weeks to term seen in lamb studies due to increased sensitivity of the pulmonary vasculature to in-utero hypoxemia.[17]

Precisely regulated changes occur in the production of endogenous vasodilator and constrictor mediators at different gestational ages.[18] Endothelin-1 (ET-1) produced by endothelin-converting enzyme-1 (ECE-1) expressing endothelial cells is the predominant vasoconstrictor in the fetus which maintains high basal PVR.[19] Lamb studies have shown that the expression of ECE-1 falls just before birth leading to reduced ET-1-mediated pulmonary vasoconstriction.[20] A human study investigating the expression of ET-1 and its receptors in fetal pulmonary necropsy samples found that ET-1 and the endothelin receptor-A, which induces vasoconstriction, were strongly expressed and stable at various gestational ages and infancy. However, the expression of the endothelin receptor-B, which induces vasodilation, was weak in early gestation, then increased markedly in mid-gestation and remained high for the rest of gestation.[21]

Extraluminal pressure exerted by the lung fluid in the fetus contributes to the increase in PVR by mechanical compression. Lamb studies done to increase the intraluminal pressure by tracheal obstruction (TO) showed a marked reduction in PBF at 7 days of TO. Pressure equalization by draining the lung fluid increased PBF.[22] Studies have shown that phasic changes in the intraluminal pressure caused by accentuated fetal breathing movement decrease the PVR and increase PBF compared with the preceding apneic episodes.[23] So, the egress of the lung fluid and the establishment of rhythmic breathing movements play a role in the drop in PVR after birth.

Inherent nitric oxide from endothelial cells, endothelial nitric oxide synthase (eNOS), and inducible nitric oxide synthase (iNOS) are vital in pulmonary vasodilatation and fall in PVR at birth. The rhythmic distension of the airway epithelium and increase in oxygen tension at birth stimulates the production of iNOS.[24] Fetal lamb studies have shown that mechanical ventilation with 100% oxygen induces pulmonary vasodilation at birth by modulating the non-adenosine triphosphate (ATP)-sensitive potassium channels.[25] In premature animal models, endogenous nitric oxide (eNO) only partially modulates the pulmonary vasodilatation. However, inhaled nitric oxide (iNO) was considered a potent vasodilator that increases the PBF more than 100% oxygen.[26] Thus, multiple factors work in a coordinated fashion to bring about a normal decrease in PVR initiated at birth.

PRETERM BIRTH AND PULMONARY VASCULAR DEVELOPMENT

Sixty percent of preterm births are associated with chorioamnionitis.[27] Studies have demonstrated that chorioamnionitis and funisitis lead to pro-inflammatory activation of the placental endothelium resulting in an altered angiogenic potential in the lungs.[28,29] An immunohistochemical study of the human preterm placentas showed that heat shock protein 70, a marker for cellular stress, is overexpressed in chorioamnionitis, followed by an increased gene transcription of nuclear factor-kB leading to activation of inflammatory cytokines. Further, proangiogenic factors such as vascular endothelial growth factor (VEGF), VEGF R-1, and R-2 were decreased in the placental endothelium.[28] These changes may explain the increased association between chorioamnionitis and early PH in preterm infants.

Postnatal stressors such as mechanical ventilation, hyperoxia, and poor nutrition synergize the prenatal inflammation initiated by intrauterine infection (**Fig. 1**). Preterm lambs exposed to intra-amniotic *Escherichia coli* endotoxin antenatally and mechanically ventilated after delivery showed increased mononuclear infiltrate and elevated IL-6 and IL-8 gene expression in lungs compared with lambs exposed to saline antenatally.[30] Recently, a retrospective clinical study found that in addition to histologic chorioamnionitis, lower birth weight (fetal growth restriction [FGR]) and invasive mechanical ventilation for $\geq$ 14 days are other significant factors associated with PH in the very preterm population.[31]

Preterm premature rupture of membranes (PPROM) in the mid-trimester leading to prolonged oligohydramnios, a risk factor associated with preterm delivery can induce pulmonary hypoplasia. In a study of experimental oligohydramnios in rats, the investigators demonstrated that oligohydramnios induced a decrease in platelet-derived growth factors A and B and elastin synthesis.[32] In a similar laboratory experiment, oligohydramnios caused a decrease in transforming growth factor β1 and collagen synthesis.[33] The defective synthesis of elastin and collagen affecting alveolar development has been proposed as the mechanism for pulmonary hypoplasia.[34] In a mouse model, oligohydramnios affected the differentiation of type 1 lung epithelial cells leading to defective angiogenesis.[35] Inhibition of angiogenesis leads to decreased alveolarization and hypoplastic lungs.[36]

In several clinical studies, oligohydramnios was observed to be a risk factor for both early PH and late PH associated with BPD.[11,37] A recent meta-analysis to identify the risk factors associated with PH in preterm infants diagnosed within 2 weeks of life by clinical and echocardiographic criteria found that oligohydramnios and small for gestational age (SGA) are strong predictors of early PH in preterm infants (see **Fig. 1**).[38]

FGR or SGA is associated with approximately 20% of preterm deliveries. SGA status at birth is associated with early and late PH in preterm infants. In a sheep model of

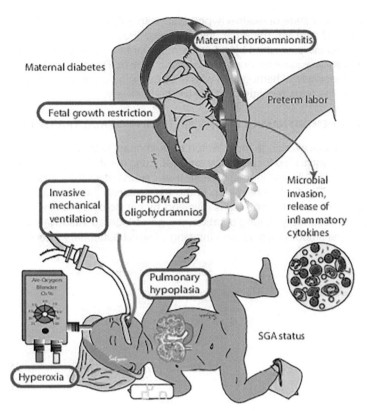

Fig. 1. Risk factors of preterm pulmonary hypertension. The prenatal risk factors include maternal diabetes, maternal chorioamnionitis, oligohydramnios, PPROM, fetal growth restriction, and pulmonary hypoplasia. The postnatal risk factors include small for gestational age, invasive mechanical ventilation, and hyperoxia. (Image Courtesy of Dr. Satyan Lakshminrusimha.)

experimental placental insufficiency, the investigators demonstrated that FGR decreased pulmonary vessel density, affected vascular development, and caused pulmonary artery endothelial cell dysfunction.[39] Observational clinical studies support these findings.[38]

PULMONARY VASCULAR REACTIVITY IN FETAL LIFE

The fetal lungs do not participate in gas exchange. Fetal pulmonary vasoconstriction and the resulting high PVR shunt the blood away from the lungs. High PVR in utero is maintained by several factors such as compression of small pulmonary arteries by fluid-filled alveoli, lack of rhythmic lung distension, relative hypoxemia, presence of thick muscular layer in the small pulmonary arteries in the fetus, and vasoconstrictor mediators like ET-1 and thromboxane counterbalancing the vasodilatory mediators like prostacyclin and eNO oxide to maintain a prominent constrictor tone. PBF is approximately 13% of combined ventricular output at 20 weeks gestation, increases to 25% to 30% at 30 weeks due to pulmonary vascular growth, and decreases again to 21% at 38 weeks due to developing pulmonary vascular reactivity to low fetal PO_2.[16,40]

The fetus is in a state of relative hypoxemia with a PaO_2 of 25 to 28 mm Hg in the aorta compared with the maternal uterine artery (PaO_2 90–100 mm Hg). However, the fetus maintains a constant blood oxygen content to maintain cerebral and tissue oxygen delivery adequate for brain and somatic growth. Reactive pulmonary vasculature and increasing fetal hemoglobin with the advancing pregnancy are essential factors that help the fetus regulate cerebral oxygen delivery.

PULMONARY HEMODYNAMICS DURING PRETERM NEONATAL TRANSITION

Fetal placental gas exchange must switch to pulmonary respiration in the neonate after birth, an essential step for postnatal survival. Lung aeration is the chief trigger leading to decreased PVR and increased PBF that can maintain the LV preload after the cord clamping (**Fig. 2**). The next step in the extra-uterine hemodynamic transition is flow reversal in the ductus arteriosus followed by physiologic closure.

PVR drops secondary to lung aeration, oxygen-triggered vasodilation, rapid involution of medial smooth muscle, and thinning of small pulmonary arteries and loss of

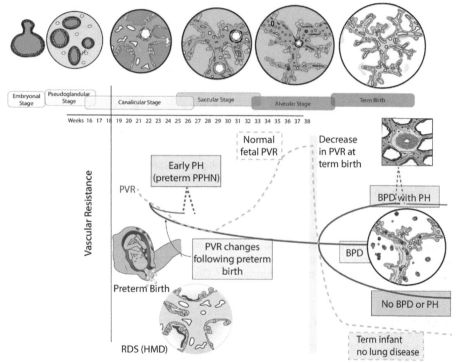

Fig. 2. Prematurity affects the change in the normal course of pulmonary vascular resistance. The illustration shows the various stages of lung development, pulmonary vascular resistance before and after birth, and the effect of bronchopulmonary dysplasia (BPD). Lung aeration after birth triggers a decrease in pulmonary vascular resistance and an increase in pulmonary blood flow that can maintain the left ventricular preload after the cord clamping. Preterm infants with varying degrees of immaturity in lung parenchyma and vasculature, depending on the gestational age at birth, lead to skewed transitions in pulmonary vascular resistance that can present as early pulmonary hypertension and in some cases evolve into late PH with or without BPD. (Image Courtesy of Dr. Satyan Lakshminrusimha.)

fetal lung liquid.[41] Inspired air creates surface tension in the alveoli leading to alveolar recoil, which increases capillary/alveolar wall transmural pressure and subsequently the capillary diameter, leading to a decrease in PVR.[42] The decrease in PVR and the associated increase in PBF are not spatially related to lung aeration,[43] resulting in ventilation/perfusion (V/Q) mismatch in the atelectatic portions of the lung. This is a common scenario during the transition of preterm birth resulting in a more gradual decrease in PVR compared with term infants emphasizing the importance of providing end-expiratory pressure and supplemental oxygen to improve V/Q matching.[44]

In an apneic preterm infant, the expected increase in PBF does not occur. In this scenario, if the umbilical cord is clamped and cut, the LV preload is reduced because of the markedly reduced pulmonary venous return.[42] This predisposes apneic infants to a double hit of hypoxia and ischemia which could possibly be avoided by delayed cord clamping until lung aeration is achieved.[45] However, high-quality clinical evidence supporting such intact cord ventilation practice is lacking and is currently being addressed by several well-designed randomized controlled trials.[46,47]

EARLY PULMONARY VASCULAR DISEASE IN PRETERM INFANTS

Early PVD in preterm infants can present as different phenotypes such as PPHN, delayed PVT, and early PH (see **Box 1**). PPHN is caused by aberration in normal neonatal cardiopulmonary transition resulting in significantly higher PVR, decreased PBF, and evolving cardiac dysfunction. These infants present with HRF that may improve with cardiotropic support and specific pulmonary vasodilator treatment. PPHN, also referred to as acute PH of newborns, can lead to progressive PVD and chronic PH.

Delayed PVT is diagnosed when preterm infants have echocardiographic evidence of elevated PAP without HRF. There is a randomized clinical trial (NCT#03576885) actively enrolling preterm infants to determine if early treatment with iNO can improve the clinical outcomes of extremely preterm infants with delayed PVT. Infants with early PH may have echo evidence of increased PVR that can present with or without HRF. At present, there is no evidence of improved long-term clinical outcomes if these infants are treated with specific pulmonary vasodilators such as iNO, but iNO is commonly used for severe HRF as there are few alternate approaches.

Preterm infants with delayed PVT or early PH may have echo evidence of increased PBF secondary to a significant left to right post-tricuspid shunt like PDA (flow-related PH). These infants may require cardiotropic support to maintain systemic blood pressure, optimized ventilation, and supplemental oxygen.

During hospitalization, preterm infants may develop intermittent or transient PH secondary to underlying etiologies such as sepsis, pneumonia, necrotizing enterocolitis, suboptimal ventilation, or inadequate recruitment of the lungs (atelectasis or hyperinflation). These infants may respond to the pulmonary vasodilators like iNO in the acute phase of illness along with corrective measures to treat underlying etiology.

PREVALENCE OF EARLY PULMONARY HYPERTENSION

The prevalence of early PH in preterm infants is variable, ranging between 8%[10] and 55%[5] based on gestational age or birth weight cutoff chosen for prematurity and timing of echocardiography. A case-control study of infants less than 34 weeks reported a prevalence of 3.3%. A prospective study of preterm infants (n = 277) with birth weight 500 to 1200 g reported a 42% incidence of early PH based on the echocardiographic assessment.[11] A retrospective single-center cohort study from the

Netherlands reported a 26% prevalence of early PH in infants born less than 30 weeks or with birth weight less than 1000 g[48] A recent prospective cohort study from the same center with the same inclusion criteria reported a 55% prevalence of early PH.[5] The vast difference in the reported prevalence of the early PH could be explained by the difference in the timing of the screening echocardiogram. In the absence of any standard guidelines, echocardiographic screening for early PH was performed at different timepoints ranging between 3 days[5] and 6 weeks[9] of life.

RISK FACTORS OF EARLY PULMONARY HYPERTENSION

The prenatal risk factors (see **Fig. 1**) associated with neonatal PH include maternal diabetes,[49] absence of use of maternal antibiotics,[49] higher placental weight,[5] oligohydramnios,[37] PPROM $\geq$ 28 days,[37] and PPROM at less than 26 weeks.[37] The postnatal risk factors associated with neonatal PH are male gender,[37] lower gestational age,[5] SGA,[38] and lower APGAR scores.[5]

"OMICS" IN EARLY PULMONARY HYPERTENSION OF PRETERM

Genetics plays a role in the development of pediatric PH. More than one-third of the cases of pediatric PH are associated with known genes with a significant contribution from de novo variants.[50] Data specific to the neonatal PH are limited. A family-based candidate gene study examined 32 single nucleotide polymorphisms (SNPs) in 12 genes and found that PPHN was associated with genetic variants in corticotropin-releasing hormone receptor 1 and corticotropin-releasing hormone (CRH)-binding protein.[51] A Chinese cohort study including 41 preterm and 74 late preterm and term infants found that three SNPs (rs192759073, rs1047883, and rs2229589) in carbamoyl-phosphate synthetase1 and one SNP (rs1044008) in neurogenic locus notch homolog protein-3 gene were associated with PPHN.[52] A similar study with 112 late preterm and term infants found rs2070699 SNP in the ET-1 gene was associated with PPHN.[53]

HYPOXIC RESPIRATORY FAILURE

Hypoxic respiratory failure (HRF) in neonates is an umbrella term comprising various disease processes leading to hypoxemia and the need for mechanical ventilation. Most studies use a threshold of $\geq$ 60% supplemental oxygen concentration to define HRF.[54] Compared with term infants, preterm babies are at higher risk of death due to HRF.[55] Severe respiratory distress syndrome, congenital pneumonia, sepsis, and PPHN are the most common etiologies for HRF in preterm infants.

Acute lung injury, often a precedent for acute PH in newborns, causes the following pulmonary vascular changes (**Fig. 3**)–endothelial dysfunction, pulmonary vascular occlusion, increased vascular tone, extrinsic vessel occlusion, and vascular remodeling.[56] Endothelial dysfunction is an important precursor for the disease progressing to chronic PH leading to oxidative stress, uncoupling of eNOS, and increased endothelin production (see **Fig. 3**). Acute lung injury propagates endothelial dysfunction through endothelial cell–leukocyte interactions, endothelial cell–platelet–neutrophil interactions, and structural changes between endothelial cells.[57] These pathophysiological interactions lead to intravascular coagulation and inflammation at the microvascular endothelial level. The ensuing chronic inflammation leads to smooth muscle hypertrophy and neomuscularization of previously nonmuscular vessels within the pulmonary vascular bed and adventitial thickening.[58]

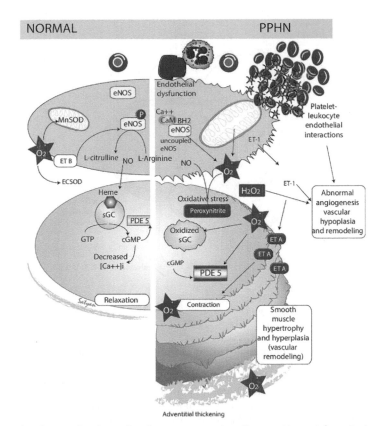

Fig. 3. Molecular mechanism of pulmonary vascular disease. Neonatal acute lung injury leads to pulmonary vascular changes such as endothelial dysfunction, pulmonary vascular occlusion, increased vascular tone, extrinsic vessel occlusion, and vascular remodeling. Endothelial dysfunction leads to oxidative stress, uncoupling of eNOS, and increased endothelin production. Acute lung injury propagates endothelial dysfunction through mechanisms such as endothelial cell–leukocyte interactions and endothelial cell–platelet–neutrophil interactions, leading to intravascular coagulation and inflammation at the microvascular endothelial level. The ensuing chronic inflammation leads to smooth muscle hypertrophy, neovascularization of previously nonmuscular vessels within the pulmonary vascular bed and adventitial thickening. (Image Courtesy of Dr. Satyan Lakshminrusimha.)

CLINICAL FEATURES OF EARLY PULMONARY HYPERTENSION

The clinical features observed in preterm infants with early PH are nonspecific (**Fig. 4**). Preterm infants with early PH may be asymptomatic or present with HRF. They require prolonged ventilator days with a median of approximately 4 weeks.[10] Infants with early PH can present with respiratory distress out of proportion to the severity of the parenchymal lung disease as assessed by the radiological parameters and ventilator requirements.

A difference in the pre- and post-ductal oxygen saturation can be seen by pulse oximetry. Differential oxygen saturation indicates right-to-left shunt across the patent ductus arteriosus (PDA). Sometimes, the oxygen saturation can be low in all four limbs without a pre-/post-ductal difference. This condition can be seen if the extracardiac shunt is insignificant compared with the intracardiac right-to-left shunt across the

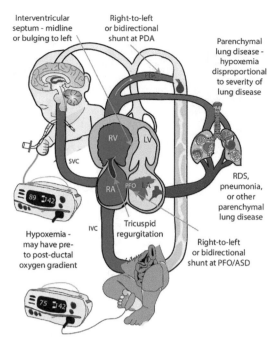

Fig. 4. Clinical and echocardiographic features of pulmonary hypertension. In infants with respiratory distress syndrome, pneumonia, or other parenchymal lung disease, hypoxemia in the presence of a patent ductus arteriosus may present with pre- and post-ductal oxygen gradient. In an infant with PH, an echocardiogram may show tricuspid regurgitation, interventricular septal position (flattening or bulging into the left ventricle), right-to-left, or bidirectional shunt flow across the patent ductus arteriosus (extracardiac) or patent foramen ovale (intracardiac). (Image Courtesy of Dr. Satyan Lakshminrusimha.)

patent foramen ovale (PFO). This variant of early PH has been reported as early PH without ductal shunt.

DIAGNOSTIC EVALUATION
Biomarkers

Natriuretic peptide levels rise due to the atrial strain (atrial natriuretic peptide) or ventricular strain (B-type natriuretic peptide [BNP]). In adults, these markers correspond well with cardiac function and can be used to identify cardiac disease. However, reference ranges for these cardiac biomarkers are not well established in cardiac conditions affecting the extremely preterm infants.[59,60] Some studies show the significance of these biomarkers to determine the cardiac dysfunction[61] or the significance of a PDA.[62] N-terminal pro b-type natriureticpeptide (NT-proBNP) and BNP may have a role in screening and monitoring of infant with late PH associated with BPD,[63] but no correlation was identified between early PH and these biomarkers.[64]

A single-center prospective observational study studied the biological samples of infants born at a gestational age (GA) of 23w0d to 28w6d. The urine samples were analyzed for nitric oxide metabolites and plasma samples for markers of oxidant stress. Plasma amino acid profile was quantified. The study found that the high urine nitric oxide metabolite at day of life (DOL) 3 was associated with an increased risk of PH at 36 weeks. The high plasma citrulline level at DOL 7 was associated with a lower risk of PH.[65]

A multicenter proof of concept study was done in the United States using a discovery, and a validation cohort aimed to quantify and compare levels of potential biomarkers in neonates with BPD, BPD-PH, PH without BPD, and neonates without lung disease at a postmenstrual age (PMA) of 36 weeks. Multiple cytokines, angiopoietin (ANG) 1 and 2, and intracellular chloride channels 1 and 4 proteins were measured using enzyme-linked immunosorbent assay (ELISA) at 36 weeks PMA. The study found higher levels of ANG 2 and lower levels of ANG 1 associated with infants with BPD alone compared with infants with BPD-PH and no lung disease. The study observed decreased monocyte chemoattractant protein-1 and increased interleukin (IL)-1β levels in infants with BPD-PH. Similarly, the BPD-PH group had increased levels of IL-6, IL-8, IL-10, and TNF-α compared with infants with no lung disease.[66] At present, no reliable biomarker of PH in preterm infants is available for clinical application.

Echocardiogram

Echocardiogram is not the gold standard for the precise evaluation of PH. However, for preterm infants, it is the only feasible test especially in the early days of life. However, it is important to understand the limitations of using echocardiograms for evaluation of PH.[67] The objectives of performing an echo in a suspected case of PH are (1) screen for structural malformations, (2) estimate PAP, and (3) assess the cardiac function and estimate cardiac output and blood flow across any shunt like PDA.

After excluding structural heart defects, PAP can be estimated using several echo measures including the tricuspid regurgitation (TR), inter-ventricular septal position, eccentricity index (EI), LV:right ventricular (RV) diameter ratio, RV acceleration or ejection time (RVET), pulmonary artery acceleration time (PAAT), pulmonary artery time interval ratios such as PAAT:RVET, and pressure gradient across a shunt such as VSD or PDA.[68,69] RV function is evaluated by measuring the RV size, RV output, tricuspid annular plane systolic excursions, or speckle tracking. Similarly, LV function and systemic blood flow can be estimated by measuring the LV output. A detailed discussion on all these echo variables is beyond the scope of this article, but we will discuss the most commonly used variables such as TR, septal position, and pressure gradient across a shunt (see **Fig. 4**).

The tricuspid regurgitation (TR) jet measured using a Doppler directly estimates the RV pressure. This is a validated parameter against cardiac catheterization. In the absence of TR jet, pressure gradient across any available post-tricuspid shunt (VSD or PDA) can be used to estimate the PAP. A bidirectional or right-to-left shunt across a PFO/atrial septal defect (ASD) may be due to the PH or secondary to other etiologies like tricuspid stenosis, RV dysfunction, RVOT obstruction, or poor compliance of the right atrium. A qualitative assessment for PH is possible based on the end-systolic septal position at the level of mitral valve chordae in the short axis view (parasternal or subcostal). Septal flattening is considered subsystemic PH, whereas reverse bowing into the LV is considered systemic or supra-systemic PH (see **Fig. 4**). The reliability of septal position can be improved by calculating the EI that is a quantitative index of eccentric LV shape.[70] EI is a reliable and quantitative measure of the septal flattening that may reduce interobserver variability in reporting septal position.[71]

Cardiac Catheterization

Cardiac catheterization with acute pulmonary vasoreactivity testing is the gold standard for evaluation of PH. However, there is no role of cardiac catheterization in the screening or diagnosis of the early PH in extremely preterm infants due to the invasive nature of the test. Cardiac catheterization should be considered in evaluating PH associated with BPD, especially if there is an inadequate response to treatment or other comorbidities are complicating the clinical evaluation.[67] If used, cardiac catheterization would be done under the baby's baseline conditions to assess hemodynamics at rest, during increased cardiac output, following hypoxic exposure, and following vasodilator administration (oxygen and iNO). It would allow gathering baseline data and assessing pulmonary vascular compliance and reactivity. It is important to note that cardiac catheterization is done in an artificial setting, usually with the patient intubated and under general anesthesia and/or high levels of sedation that makes it difficult to fully assess the dynamic pulmonary circulatory changes. Information obtained from cardiac catheterization should be interpreted with these limitations in mind.

MANAGEMENT
General Principles

Preterm infants with FGR, exposure to perinatal infections, and severe respiratory distress syndrome (RDS) are at higher risk for PPHN or acute PH (see **Fig. 1**). A comprehensive evaluation starts with screening for any underlying etiology such as neonatal infections, suboptimal ventilation, or lung recruitment. Optimal clinical management of PH varies based on the underlying etiology, echocardiographic evaluation of hemodynamics, and the phenotype of the PVD. However, there are few general principles in the management of PH including (1) treatment of the underlying diseases such as RDS and neonatal infections, (2) ensuring optimal lung recruitment, (3) optimal ventilation and oxygenation to break the vicious cycle of hypoxemic pulmonary vasoconstriction, and (4) maintain systemic and PBF by supporting the cardiac output. Pulmonary vasodilators and other interventions can be offered based on the underlying pathophysiology of different phenotypes of the PVD.

Ventilation Strategies

Optimizing respiratory support to maintain adequate lung recruitment is very important in managing infants with early PH. Both hyperinflation and atelectasis are associated with increased PVR.[72,73] We must achieve optimal lung inflation to avoid V/Q mismatch and intrapulmonary shunting. This is a physiologic prerequisite for selective pulmonary vasodilators to be efficacious in improving PBF.[69] Coexisting RDS should be treated with an exogenous surfactant. Appropriate respiratory support should be provided to maintain the blood gases in an acceptable range. There is no preference for any specific ventilation mode, but the goal of ventilation should be to keep the lungs optimally inflated (expanded up to 8–9 ribs on chest x-ray), arterial carbon dioxide tension ($PaCO_2$) in the 35 to 50 mm Hg range and pH between 7.3 and 7.4. Correcting respiratory acidosis and maintaining pH in the normal reference range help prevent pulmonary vasoconstriction due to hypercarbia or acidosis. Attention should be paid to the peak inspiratory pressures (PIPs) needed to achieve these goals in conventional ventilation. Infants with reduced lung compliance or lung hypoplasia requiring unusually high PIP should be considered for escalation to high-frequency ventilation that may be synergistic with the action of selective pulmonary vasodilators.

Oxygen and Saturation Targets

An arterial oxygen tension (PaO_2) < 50 mm Hg has been shown to contribute to pulmonary vasoconstriction.[74] Oxygen saturation targets 90% to 97% help to maintain pre-ductal PaO_2 in the 50 to 80 mm Hg range. In this oxygenation range, the benefit of oxygen-induced pulmonary vasodilation is maximal, with minimal risk of injury due to hyperoxia or the oxidative stress. Clinicians should be aware that PaO_2 from the right radial arterial line reflects the pre-ductal oxygenation, whereas the umbilical arterial PaO_2 indicates the post-ductal oxygenation. If the peripheral arterial line on the right upper extremity is not available, titrating supplemental oxygen based on the right upper extremity SpO_2 is a reasonable alternative.

Sedation and Paralysis

On conventional ventilation, minimum sedation may be required to facilitate adequate gas exchange. However, sedation is more likely required for infants on high-frequency ventilation. The use of neuromuscular blockade by vecuronium is not uncommon among the term infants with severe PPHN and HRF.[75] However, there are no data on the safety or efficacy of paralysis in preterm infants with acute PH and HRF and should be avoided with minor exceptions.[76] Close attention to systemic blood pressure is important while providing sedation and neuromuscular blockade.

Systemic Blood Pressure Management

Systemic hypotension in early PH may be secondary to the elevated PVR, increasing the RV afterload, and decreased PBF and, in turn, decreased LV preload. Sepsis, intraventricular hemorrhage, sedation, paralysis, use of high mean airway pressure (MAP), adrenal insufficiency, and hypovolemia or dehydration can contribute to systemic hypotension. RV dysfunction could coexist and contribute to systemic hypotension.[77] Uncorrected hypotensive shock worsens hypoxemia causing further pulmonary vasoconstriction, a vicious cycle leading to high mortality. Detecting RV dysfunction is important to guide us in choosing the inotrope.

Dopamine is the most commonly used inotrope for preterm infants with PH and systemic hypotension.[78] In the dose range of 5 to 10 mcg/kg/min, the inotropic effect of dopamine is predominant due to beta-1 adrenergic receptor stimulation. However, at higher doses (>10 mcg/kg/min), dopamine stimulates alpha-adrenergic receptors non-colectively, resulting in an increased ratio of pulmonary-to-systemic vascular resistance. Increasing SVR has been described as a strategy to decrease the right-to-left shunting across the PDA but is detrimental for the cardiac function. RV afterload is increased due to the increased PVR and decreased right to left ductal shunting. This combination may worsen the myocardial ischemia and RV dysfunction leading to a further decrease in PBF and HRF. Although LV preload decreases secondary to worsening PPHN, increased LV afterload secondary to increase in SVR potentiates the LV dysfunction, further decreasing the cardiac output. This vicious cycle can spiral down fast to reach a point where specific pulmonary vasodilators may not be effective to improve cardiac output. So, the use of dopamine especially in the higher doses should be avoided to treat preterm infants with acute PH.[79,80]

If there is no cardiac dysfunction, cardiac output may be low due to the decreased intrathoracic venous return caused by the use of high MAP. To improve intrathoracic venous return, weaning the MAP or positive end-expiratory pressure (PEEP) can be helpful. Fluid bolus can also improve the diastolic filling and the cardiac output. In infants with systemic hypotension without evidence of RV dysfunction, vasopressin is an excellent first choice but may be associated with oliguria and hyponatremia.[81]

In the presence of RV dysfunction with systemic hypotension, epinephrine is the first choice due to its positive inotropic effects and the ability to increase the SVR without adversely affecting the ratio of pulmonary-to-systemic vascular resistance. Dobutamine and milrinone are pure inotropes without vasopressor effects, are potential choices in the presence of RV dysfunction without systemic hypotension, and can be used as an adjunct along with a vasopressor. Dobutamine has minimal effect on PVR.[82] In the setting of septic shock coexisting with early PH, norepinephrine can be considered.[69]

Inhaled Nitric Oxide

iNO is the first-line pulmonary vasodilator for treating acute PH in term and near-term infants after achieving adequate lung recruitment.[69] However, randomized clinical trials that tested the efficacy of iNO therapy for the prevention of BPD in preterm infants did not enroll patients based on the echocardiographic diagnosis of PH.[83–85] Indiscriminate iNO treatment of preterm infants was not beneficial to decrease the risk of BPD or death. A Cochrane review of 17 RCTs grouped into three categories: early rescue (<3 DOL), early routine use, and late treatment (>5–7 DOL) concluded that early routine use of iNO in preterm infants does not prevent serious brain injury or improve survival without BPD. The meta-analysis found that the late use of iNO to prevent BPD could be effective and further studies were recommended.[86]

The knowledge of early PH in the preterm population and the understanding of various phenotypes were limited during the period of conduct of most of these iNO trials. A single-center retrospective study including preterm infants with HRF treated with iNO (n = 93) found that infants exposed to antenatal steroids and PPROM had improved oxygenation with iNO and better survival without intraventricular hemorrhage (IVH)/periventricular leukomalacia (PVL).[87] A multicenter study of preterm infants (22–28 weeks gestation) with pulmonary hypoplasia found that early treatment with iNO did not improve survival.[84] A meta-analysis found that African American infants had significantly reduced death or BPD with iNO treatment: 49% treated versus 63% control.[88] However, a recent neonatal research network cohort study (n = 1732) reported no racial difference in the mortality or the neurodevelopmental outcomes among the preterm infants treated by iNO.[54]

The American Heart Association, the American Thoracic Society, and the Pediatric Pulmonary Hypertension Network jointly recommend the use of iNO if PH is consistent with the PPHN pathophysiology.[89] At present, it is unclear if iNO treatment for early PH or delayed PVT in extremely preterm infants can improve the clinical outcomes.[90] However, given the safety profile of iNO, if echocardiography confirms PPHN phenotype, it may be prudent to conduct a trial of iNO to assess oxygenation response.[91] Preterm infants with PPROM, oligohydramnios, and suspected pulmonary hypoplasia anecdotally seem to demonstrate improvement in oxygenation.[92]

Use of Systemic Pulmonary Vasodilators

There is a rising trend to use systemic pulmonary vasodilators such as milrinone, sildenafil, or bosentan to treat PH in the newborns.[93] However, limited data are available to determine the efficacy or safety of systemic pulmonary vasodilators in preterm infants specially to treat PPHN or early PH.[94–97] In the settings of atelectasis or heterogenous parenchymal lung disease, systemic pulmonary vasodilators can increase the VQ mismatch by increasing the PBF in the atelectatic or diseased segments of the lung. Milrinone is a nonspecific vasodilator; it can increase PBF by decreasing the PVR but also increases the risk of systemic hypotension and should be used cautiously.[98] Right-to-left shunting can worsen across a significant PDA, if systemic hypotension is relatively higher than the decrease in PVR. The use of the systemic pulmonary vasodilators in this high-risk population is limited until the safety and efficacy can be determined in clinical trials.[95] In resource-limited settings, enteral sildenafil is the mainstay of PPHN management.[99] In settings that lack access to iNO for the treatment of PH, sildenafil provides mortality benefit. A recent open-labeled clinical trial that compared oral and intravenous sildenafil in the treatment of mild to moderate neonatal PH including infants greater than 34 weeks gestation found equal efficacy irrespective of the route of administration. However, the complications such as hypotension and poor cardiac contractility were common with the intravenous administration of silden-afil compared with oral route.[100]

Use of Prostaglandin Infusion

Prostaglandins can decrease the PVR and protect the RV function by ensuring the patency of the ductus arteriosus. However, there is limited evidence to support the prostaglandin infusion to treat preterm infants with PPHN or early PH. Nevertheless, under special circumstances when systemic blood flow is duct-dependent due to se-vere PPHN, and RV dysfunction can be benefitted by keeping the ductus open, judi-cious use of prostaglandin infusion shall be considered.[80]

Steroids

Hydrocortisone is a well-studied steroid in the management of PPHN in term in-fants.[101] Early use of dexamethasone is associated with improved clinical outcomes in term infants with meconium aspiration and PPHN.[102] There is limited evidence to support the general use of dexamethasone to decrease the PVR in preterm infants[103] and its use is associated with hypertrophic cardiomyopathy.

Preterm infants with catecholamine-resistant hypotension are usually treated with hydrocortisone that can improve systemic blood pressure without compromising car-diac function, systemic perfusion, and cerebral or renal blood flow. Hydrocortisone in-creases the catecholamine potency by inhibiting its metabolism and improving microcirculation.[69,104,105] It has been shown to downregulate phosphodiesterase 5 by blocking reactive oxygen species-induced NFκB activity in fetal pulmonary artery smooth muscle cells in a lamb model of PPHN.[106]

Treatment of the Flow-Related Early Pulmonary Hypertension

Diuretic treatment may be helpful to decrease the volume overload for preterm infants with echo evidence of flow associated PH secondary to a large left-to-right shunt across the ductus arteriosus or VSD. Shunt management shall be considered while restricting the total daily fluid intake. Pulmonary vasodilator therapy with iNO is con-traindicated as it can further increase the PBF by decreasing the PVR. However, in some cases of severe hypoxemia in extremely preterm infants, a combination of different phenotypes of PH (flow driven by PDA and resistance driven) may compli-cate management.

OUTCOMES

Early PH in preterm infants is associated with poor survival and a high risk for BPD or death.[48] In a South Korean retrospective study including 247 extremely preterm in-fants, early PH detected with echocardiography at 4 to 7 DOL was an independent risk factor for death before 36 weeks PMA.[37] The mortality rate in this study was 28.4% in the early PH group versus 10.4% in the control group. The risk of BPD-associated PH was 18.9% in the early PH group compared with 5.2% in infants without early PH. In a subgroup of infants with moderate or severe BPD, early PH was an independent predictor of the occurrence of late PH.

These findings were confirmed by a subsequent meta-analysis including preterm infants with early PH (diagnosed in the first 2 weeks of life) was associated with an increased risk of moderate to severe BPD, in-hospital mortality, and late PH.[38] A prospective, observational study of preterm infants with birth weights between 500 and 1250 g ($n = 221$) found that early PH diagnosed by echo at DOL 7 was associated with asthma, reactive airway disease, BPD exacerbation, bronchiolitis, pneumonia, and recurrent hospitalization for a respiratory illness during the first 2 years corrected age.[107] The study also found that the risk of late respiratory morbidities in these infants with early PVD increased eightfold if they had received mechanical ventilation at DOL 7 compared with controls. Chandrasekharan and colleagues have reported high rates of mortality or neurodevelopmental impairment among extremely preterm infants with early hypoxemia irrespective of presence of PH.[54]

KNOWLEDGE GAPS AND FUTURE DIRECTIONS

The technological advances in transcriptomics, metabolomics, and proteomics can be used to classify the pathobiological forms of PH and predict response to vasodilator therapy.[108] Such a multiomics approach can provide research avenues with potential to enhance the understanding of neonatal PH and its phenotypes. The lung transcriptional framework for type I PAH constructed by the PH Breakthrough Initiative network study is a fine example of such an endeavor.[109]

A consensus-based classification of different phenotypes of PH in preterm infants will provide an opportunity to test class-specific treatment strategies (see **Box 1**). A randomized clinical trial is needed to determine the efficacy of iNO for preterm infants with early PH and related phenotypes. Further studies are needed to assess safety and efficacy of systemic steroids and systemic pulmonary vasodilators to treat PH in preterm infants. Research on biomarkers to diagnose and classify early PH will be valuable.

SUMMARY

PH in preterm infants is associated with high mortality and morbidity. Disease has a variable pathophysiology based on the different underlying phenotypes. Timely diagnosis and physiology-based management strategy may improve the clinical outcomes of the extremely preterm infants with PH.

Best Practice Box

- Hemodynamic evaluation and screening for pulmonary hypertension shall be considered for all preterm infants with suboptimal systemic blood pressure or hypoxic respiratory failure within the first week of life.

- It is important to optimize lung recruitment and mechanical ventilation to prevent hypoxia, hypercarbia, and overt V/Q mismatch that can induce the pulmonary hypertension.

- iNO treatment could be considered for preterm infants with HRF due to PPHN pathophysiology especially, if associated with PPROM and oligohydramnios. iNO is contraindicated in flow-related early PH in preterm infants.

- For preterm infants with pulmonary hypertension and systemic hypotension, the choice of vasopressors/inotropes shall be based on hemodynamic evaluation by echocardiogram. Vasopressin and norepinephrine are preferred choices for infants with normal RV function. Epinephrine and dobutamine are recommended for infants with PPHN and RV dysfunction. Dopamine especially at higher dose (>10 mcg/kg/min) should be avoided in preterm infants with PPHN due to the nonselective effects on systemic and pulmonary vascular resistance.

AUTHOR CONTRIBUTIONS

S. Mani conceptualized, wrote the original draft, reviewed, and edited the manuscript. H. Mirza contributed to writing, reviewing, and editing the manuscript. J. Ziegler contributed to manuscript writing, reviewing, and editing. P. Chandrasekharan conceptualized, contributed to writing, reviewed, and edited the manuscript, supervised. All authors approved the final manuscript as submitted and agree to be accountable for all aspects of the work.

DISCLOSURE

Praveen Chandrasekharan was supported by the Eunice Kennedy Shriver National Institute of Child Health and Human Development, United States (NICHD; grant number: R01HD104909). The results of this manuscript are not supported or endorsed by any of the funding institutions.

REFERENCES

1. Abman SH, Hansmann G, Archer SL, et al. Pediatric pulmonary hypertension: guidelines from the American heart association and American thoracic society. Circulation 2015;132(21):2037–99.
2. Cerro MJ, Abman S, Diaz G, et al. A consensus approach to the classification of pediatric pulmonary hypertensive vascular disease: report from the PVRI Pediatric Taskforce, Panama 2011. Pulm Circ 2011;1(2):286–98.
3. Robbins IM, Moore TM, Blaisdell CJ, et al. National heart, lung, and blood institute workshop: improving outcomes for pulmonary vascular disease. Circulation 2012;125(17):2165–70.
4. Newman JH, Rich S, Abman SH, et al. Enhancing insights into pulmonary vascular disease through a precision medicine approach. A joint NHLBI-cardiovascular medical research and education fund workshop report. Am J Respir Crit Care Med 2017;195(12):1661–70.
5. Arjaans S, Fries MWF, Schoots MH, et al. Clinical significance of early pulmonary hypertension in preterm infants. J Pediatr 2022;251:74–81 e3.
6. Mirza H, Mandell EW, Kinsella JP, et al. Pulmonary vascular phenotypes of prematurity: the path to precision medicine. J Pediatr 2023;113444.
7. Mirza H, Garcia JA, Crawford E, et al. Natural history of postnatal cardiopulmonary adaptation in infants born extremely preterm and risk for death or bronchopulmonary dysplasia. J Pediatr 2018;198:187–193 e1.
8. Abman SH. Pulmonary hypertension: the hidden danger for newborns. Neonatology 2021;118(2):211–7.
9. Bhat R, Salas AA, Foster C, et al. Prospective analysis of pulmonary hypertension in extremely low birth weight infants. Pediatrics 2012;129(3):e682–9.
10. Mirza H, Ziegler J, Ford S, et al. Pulmonary hypertension in preterm infants: prevalence and association with bronchopulmonary dysplasia. J Pediatr 2014; 165(5):909–914 e1.
11. Mourani PM, Sontag MK, Younoszai A, et al. Early pulmonary vascular disease in preterm infants at risk for bronchopulmonary dysplasia. Am J Respir Crit Care Med 2015;191(1):87–95.
12. Nakanishi H, Uchiyama A, Kusuda S. Impact of pulmonary hypertension on neurodevelopmental outcome in preterm infants with bronchopulmonary dysplasia: a cohort study. J Perinatol 2016;36(10):890–6.
13. Philip R, Lamba V, Talati A, et al. Pulmonary hypertension with prolonged patency of the ductus arteriosus in preterm infants. Children 2020;7(9).
14. Philip R, Nathaniel Johnson J, Naik R, et al. Effect of patent ductus arteriosus on pulmonary vascular disease. Congenit Heart Dis 2019;14(1):37–41.
15. Mourani PM, Ivy DD, Rosenberg AA, et al. Left ventricular diastolic dysfunction in bronchopulmonary dysplasia. J Pediatr 2008;152(2):291–3.

16. Rasanen J, Wood DC, Weiner S, et al. Role of the pulmonary circulation in the distribution of human fetal cardiac output during the second half of pregnancy. Circulation 1996;94(5):1068–73.

17. Morin FC 3rd, Egan EA. Pulmonary hemodynamics in fetal lambs during development at normal and increased oxygen tension. J Appl Physiol 1992;73(1): 213–8.

18. Lakshminrusimha S, Steinhorn RH. Pulmonary vascular biology during neonatal transition. Clin Perinatol 1999;26(3):601–19.

19. Paradis A, Zhang L. Role of endothelin in uteroplacental circulation and fetal vascular function. Curr Vasc Pharmacol 2013;11(5):594–605.

20. Ivy D, Tanzawa K, Abman SH. Ontogeny of endothelin-converting enzyme gene expression and protein content in the ovine fetal lung. Biol Neonate 2002;81(2): 139–44.

21. Levy M, Maurey C, Chailley-Heu B, et al. Developmental changes in endothelial vasoactive and angiogenic growth factors in the human perinatal lung. Pediatr Res 2005;57(2):248–53.

22. Polglase GR, Wallace MJ, Morgan DL, et al. Increases in lung expansion alter pulmonary hemodynamics in fetal sheep. J Appl Physiol 2006;101(1):273–82.

23. Polglase GR, Wallace MJ, Grant DA, et al. Influence of fetal breathing movements on pulmonary hemodynamics in fetal sheep. Pediatr Res 2004;56(6): 932–8.

24. Rairigh RL, Parker TA, Ivy DD, et al. Role of inducible nitric oxide synthase in the pulmonary vascular response to birth-related stimuli in the ovine fetus. Circ Res 2001;88(7):721–6.

25. Tristani-Firouzi M, Martin EB, Tolarova S, et al. Ventilation-induced pulmonary vasodilation at birth is modulated by potassium channel activity. Am J Physiol 1996;271(6 Pt 2):H2353–9.

26. Kinsella JP, Ivy DD, Abman SH. Ontogeny of NO activity and response to inhaled NO in the developing ovine pulmonary circulation. Am J Physiol 1994; 267(5 Pt 2):H1955–61.

27. Goldenberg RL, Hauth JC, Andrews WW. Intrauterine infection and preterm delivery. N Engl J Med 2000;342(20):1500–7.

28. Kramer BW, Kaemmerer U, Kapp M, et al. Decreased expression of angiogenic factors in placentas with chorioamnionitis after preterm birth. Pediatr Res 2005; 58(3):607–12.

29. Parsons A, Netsanet A, Seedorf G, et al. Understanding the role of placental pathophysiology in the development of bronchopulmonary dysplasia. Am J Physiol Lung Cell Mol Physiol 2022;323(6):L651–8.

30. Ikegami M, Jobe AH. Postnatal lung inflammation increased by ventilation of preterm lambs exposed antenatally to Escherichia coli endotoxin. Pediatr Res 2002;52(3):356–62.

31. Yum SK, Kim MS, Kwun Y, et al. Impact of histologic chorioamnionitis on pulmonary hypertension and respiratory outcomes in preterm infants. Pulm Circ 2018; 8(2). https://doi.org/10.1177/2045894018760166. 2045894018760166.

32. Chen CM, Wang LF, Chou HC, et al. Oligohydramnios decreases platelet-derived growth factor expression in fetal rat lungs. Neonatology 2007;92(3):187–93.

33. Chen CM, Chou HC, Wang LF, et al. Experimental oligohydramnios decreases collagen in hypoplastic fetal rat lungs. Exp Biol Med (Maywood) 2008; 233(11):1334–40.

34. Wu CS, Chen CM, Chou HC. Pulmonary hypoplasia induced by oligohydramnios: findings from animal models and a population-based study. Pediatr Neonatol 2017;58(1):3–7.
35. Najrana T, Ramos LM, Abu Eid R, et al. Oligohydramnios compromises lung cells size and interferes with epithelial-endothelial development. Pediatr Pulmonol 2017;52(6):746–56.
36. Jakkula M, Le Cras TD, Gebb S, et al. Inhibition of angiogenesis decreases alveolarization in the developing rat lung. Am J Physiol Lung Cell Mol Physiol 2000;279(3):L600–7.
37. Kim HH, Sung SI, Yang MS, et al. Early pulmonary hypertension is a risk factor for bronchopulmonary dysplasia-associated late pulmonary hypertension in extremely preterm infants. Sci Rep 2021;11(1):11206.
38. Kim YJ, Shin SH, Park HW, et al. Risk factors of early pulmonary hypertension and its clinical outcomes in preterm infants: a systematic review and meta-analysis. Sci Rep 2022;12(1):14186.
39. Rozance PJ, Seedorf GJ, Brown A, et al. Intrauterine growth restriction decreases pulmonary alveolar and vessel growth and causes pulmonary artery endothelial cell dysfunction in vitro in fetal sheep. Am J Physiol Lung Cell Mol Physiol 2011;301(6):L860–71.
40. Vali P, Lakshminrusimha S. The fetus can teach us: oxygen and the pulmonary vasculature. Children 2017;4(8).
41. Gao Y, Raj JU. Regulation of the pulmonary circulation in the fetus and newborn. Physiol Rev 2010;90(4):1291–335.
42. Hooper SB, te Pas AB, Lang J, et al. Cardiovascular transition at birth: a physiological sequence. Pediatr Res 2015;77(5):608–14.
43. Lang JA, Pearson JT, te Pas AB, et al. Ventilation/perfusion mismatch during lung aeration at birth. J Appl Physiol 2014;117(5):535–43.
44. Hooper SB, Siew ML, Kitchen MJ, et al. Establishing functional residual capacity in the non-breathing infant. Semin Fetal Neonatal Med 2013;18(6):336–43.
45. Bhatt S, Alison BJ, Wallace EM, et al. Delaying cord clamping until ventilation onset improves cardiovascular function at birth in preterm lambs. J Physiol 2013;591(8):2113–26.
46. Lakshminrusimha S, Van Meurs K. Better timing for cord clamping is after onset of lung aeration. Pediatr Res 2015;77(5):615–7.
47. Lakshminrusimha S, Saugstad OD, Vento M. Lung aeration during deferred cord clamping-No additional benefits in infants born preterm? J Pediatr 2023;255:11–5.e6.
48. Arjaans S, Zwart EAH, Roofthooft M, et al. Pulmonary hypertension in extremely preterm infants: a call to standardize echocardiographic screening and follow-up policy. Eur J Pediatr 2021;180(6):1855–65.
49. Sheth S, Goto L, Bhandari V, et al. Factors associated with development of early and late pulmonary hypertension in preterm infants with bronchopulmonary dysplasia. J Perinatol 2020;40(1):138–48.
50. Welch CL, Chung WK. Genetics and genomics of pediatric pulmonary arterial hypertension. Genes 2020;11(10):1213.
51. Byers HM, Dagle JM, Klein JM, et al. Variations in CRHR1 are associated with persistent pulmonary hypertension of the newborn. Pediatr Res 2012;71(2):162–7.
52. Liu X, Mei M, Chen X, et al. Identification of genetic factors underlying persistent pulmonary hypertension of newborns in a cohort of Chinese neonates. Respir Res 2019;20(1):174.

53. Mei M, Cheng G, Sun B, et al. EDN1 gene variant is associated with neonatal persistent pulmonary hypertension. Sci Rep 2016;6(1):29877.

54. Chandrasekharan P, Lakshminrusimha S, Chowdhury D, et al. Early hypoxic respiratory failure in extreme prematurity: mortality and neurodevelopmental outcomes. Pediatrics 2020;146(4).

55. Pandya S, Baser O, Wan G, et al. The burden of hypoxic respiratory failure in preterm and term/near-term infants in the United States 2011-2015. Journal of Health Economics and Outcomes Research 2019;6:130–41.

56. Price LC, McAuley DF, Marino PS, et al. Pathophysiology of pulmonary hypertension in acute lung injury. Am J Physiol Lung Cell Mol Physiol 2012;302(9): L803–15.

57. Dehghani T, Panitch A. Endothelial cells, neutrophils and platelets: getting to the bottom of an inflammatory triangle. Open Biology 2020;10(10):200161.

58. Meyrick B, Brigham KL. Repeated Escherichia coli endotoxin-induced pulmonary inflammation causes chronic pulmonary hypertension in sheep. Structural and functional changes. Lab Invest 1986;55(2):164–76.

59. Vijlbrief DC, Benders MJ, Kemperman H, et al. Use of cardiac biomarkers in neonatology. Pediatr Res 2012;72(4):337–43.

60. Weisz DE, McNamara PJ, El-Khuffash A. Cardiac biomarkers and haemodynamically significant patent ductus arteriosus in preterm infants. Early Hum Dev 2017;105:41–7.

61. Moriichi A, Cho K, Mizushima M, et al. B-type natriuretic peptide levels at birth predict cardiac dysfunction in neonates. Pediatr Int 2012;54(1):89–93.

62. Konig K, Guy KJ, Drew SM, et al. B-type and N-terminal pro-B-type natriuretic peptides are equally useful in assessing patent ductus arteriosus in very preterm infants. Acta Paediatr 2015;104(4):e139–42.

63. Xiong T, Kulkarni M, Gokulakrishnan G, et al. Natriuretic peptides in bronchopulmonary dysplasia: a systematic review. J Perinatol 2020;40(4):607–15.

64. Konig K, Guy KJ, Walsh G, et al. Association of BNP, NTproBNP, and early postnatal pulmonary hypertension in very preterm infants. Pediatr Pulmonol 2016; 51(8):820–4.

65. O'Connor MG, Suthar D, Vera K, et al. Pulmonary hypertension in the premature infant population: analysis of echocardiographic findings and biomarkers. Pediatr Pulmonol 2018;53(3):302–9.

66. Sahni M, Yeboah B, Das P, et al. Novel biomarkers of bronchopulmonary dysplasia and bronchopulmonary dysplasia-associated pulmonary hypertension. J Perinatol 2020;40(11):1634–43.

67. Levy PT, Jain A, Nawaytou H, et al. Risk assessment and monitoring of chronic pulmonary hypertension in premature infants. J Pediatr 2020;217:199–209 e4.

68. Levy PT, Patel MD, Choudhry S, et al. Evidence of echocardiographic markers of pulmonary vascular disease in asymptomatic infants born preterm at one year of age. J Pediatr 2018;197:48–56 e2.

69. Jain A, Giesinger RE, Dakshinamurti S, et al. Care of the critically ill neonate with hypoxemic respiratory failure and acute pulmonary hypertension: framework for practice based on consensus opinion of neonatal hemodynamics working group. J Perinatol 2022;42(1):3–13.

70. Ryan T, Petrovic O, Dillon JC, et al. An echocardiographic index for separation of right ventricular volume and pressure overload. J Am Coll Cardiol 1985;5(4): 918–27.

71. Abraham S, Weismann CG. Left ventricular end-systolic eccentricity index for assessment of pulmonary hypertension in infants. Echocardiography 2016; 33(6):910–5.
72. Creamer KM, McCloud LL, Fisher LE, et al. Ventilation above closing volume reduces pulmonary vascular resistance hysteresis. Am J Respir Crit Care Med 1998;158(4):1114–9.
73. Jardin F, Vieillard-Baron A. Right ventricular function and positive pressure ventilation in clinical practice: from hemodynamic subsets to respirator settings. Intensive Care Med 2003;29(9):1426–34.
74. Lakshminrusimha S, Swartz DD, Gugino SF, et al. Oxygen concentration and pulmonary hemodynamics in newborn lambs with pulmonary hypertension. Pediatr Res 2009;66(5):539–44.
75. Johnson PN, Miller J, Gormley AK. Continuous-infusion neuromuscular blocking agents in critically ill neonates and children. Pharmacotherapy 2011;31(6): 609–20.
76. Sahni M, Richardson CJ, Jain SK. Sustained neuromuscular blockade after vecuronium use in a premature infant. AJP Rep 2015;5(2):e121–3.
77. Storme L, Aubry E, Rakza T, et al. Pathophysiology of persistent pulmonary hypertension of the newborn: impact of the perinatal environment. Archives of Cardiovascular Diseases 2013;106(3):169–77.
78. Burns ML, Stensvold HJ, Risnes K, et al. Inotropic therapy in newborns, A population-based National registry study. Pediatr Crit Care Med 2016;17(10): 948–56.
79. Siefkes HM, Lakshminrusimha S. Management of systemic hypotension in term infants with persistent pulmonary hypertension of the newborn: an illustrated review. Arch Dis Child Fetal Neonatal Ed 2021;106(4):446–55.
80. McNamara PJ, Giesinger RE, Lakshminrusimha S. Dopamine and neonatal pulmonary hypertension-pressing need for a better pressor? J Pediatr 2022;246: 242–50.
81. Mohamed A, Nasef N, Shah V, et al. Vasopressin as a rescue therapy for refractory pulmonary hypertension in neonates: case series. Pediatr Crit Care Med 2014;15(2):148–54.
82. Ruffolo RR Jr. The pharmacology of dobutamine. Am J Med Sci 1987;294(4): 244–8.
83. Kinsella JP, Cutter GR, Walsh WF, et al. Early inhaled nitric oxide therapy in premature newborns with respiratory failure. N Engl J Med 2006;355(4):354–64.
84. Ellsworth KR, Ellsworth MA, Weaver AL, et al. Association of early inhaled nitric oxide with the survival of preterm neonates with pulmonary hypoplasia. JAMA Pediatr 2018;172(7):e180761.
85. Abman SH. Bronchopulmonary dysplasia: "a vascular hypothesis". Am J Respir Crit Care Med 2001;164(10 Pt 1):1755–6.
86. Barrington KJ, Finer N, Pennaforte T. Inhaled nitric oxide for respiratory failure in preterm infants. Cochrane Database Syst Rev 2017;1(1):Cd000509.
87. Chandrasekharan P, Kozielski R, Kumar VH, et al. Early use of inhaled nitric oxide in preterm infants: is there a rationale for selective approach? Am J Perinatol 2017;34(5):428–40.
88. Askie LM, Davies LC, Schreiber MD, et al. Race effects of inhaled nitric oxide in preterm infants: an individual participant data meta-analysis. J Pediatr 2018; 193:34–9.e2.
89. Ballard RA, Truog WE, Cnaan A, et al. Inhaled nitric oxide in preterm infants undergoing mechanical ventilation. N Engl J Med 2006;355(4):343–53.

90. Lakshminrusimha S, Kinsella JP, Krishnan US, et al. Just say No to iNO in preterms-really? J Pediatr 2020;218:243–52.
91. Baczynski M, Jasani B, De Castro C, et al. Association between immediate oxygenation response and survival in preterm infants receiving rescue inhaled nitric oxide therapy for hypoxemia from pulmonary hypertension: a systematic review and meta-analysis. Early Hum Dev 2023;184:105841.
92. Mullaly R, McCallion N, El-Khuffash A. Inhaled nitric oxide in preterm neonates with preterm prelabour rupture of membranes, a systematic review. Acta Paediatr 2023;112(3):358–71.
93. Lakshminrusimha S, Mathew B, Leach CL. Pharmacologic strategies in neonatal pulmonary hypertension other than nitric oxide. Semin Perinatol 2016;40(3):160–73.
94. El-Khuffash A, McNamara PJ, Breatnach C, et al. The use of milrinone in neonates with persistent pulmonary hypertension of the newborn - a randomised controlled trial pilot study (MINT 1). J Perinatol 2023;43(2):168–73.
95. Samiee-Zafarghandy S, Raman SR, van den Anker JN, et al. Safety of milrinone use in neonatal intensive care units. Early Hum Dev 2015;91(1):31–5.
96. Lang JE, Hornik CD, Martz K, et al. Safety of sildenafil in premature infants at risk of bronchopulmonary dysplasia: rationale and methods of a phase II randomized trial. Contemp Clin Trials Commun 2022;30:101025.
97. Rhee SJ, Shin SH, Oh J, et al. Population pharmacokinetic analysis of sildenafil in term and preterm infants with pulmonary arterial hypertension. Sci Rep 2022;12(1):7393.
98. McNamara PJ, Laique F, Muang-In S, et al. Milrinone improves oxygenation in neonates with severe persistent pulmonary hypertension of the newborn. J Crit Care 2006;21(2):217–22.
99. Kelly LE, Ohlsson A, Shah PS. Sildenafil for pulmonary hypertension in neonates. Cochrane Database Syst Rev 2017;8(8):Cd005494.
100. Chetan C, Suryawanshi P, Patnaik S, et al. Oral versus intravenous sildenafil for pulmonary hypertension in neonates: a randomized trial. BMC Pediatr 2022;22(1):311.
101. Alsaleem M, Malik A, Lakshminrusimha S, et al. Hydrocortisone improves oxygenation index and systolic blood pressure in term infants with persistent pulmonary hypertension. Clin Med Insights Pediatr 2019;13. 1179556519888918.
102. da Costa DE, Nair AK, Pai MG, et al. Steroids in full term infants with respiratory failure and pulmonary hypertension due to meconium aspiration syndrome. Eur J Pediatr 2001;160(3):150–3.
103. Sehgal A, Nold MF, Roberts CT, et al. Cardiorespiratory adaptation to low-dose dexamethasone for lung disease in extremely preterm infants: a prospective echocardiographic study. J Physiol 2022;600(19):4361–73.
104. Noori S, Friedlich P, Wong P, et al. Hemodynamic changes after low-dosage hydrocortisone administration in vasopressor-treated preterm and term neonates. Pediatrics 2006;118(4):1456–66.
105. Büchele GL, Silva E, Ospina-Tascón GA, et al. Effects of hydrocortisone on microcirculatory alterations in patients with septic shock. Crit Care Med 2009;37(4):1341–7.
106. Perez M, Wedgwood S, Lakshminrusimha S, et al. Hydrocortisone normalizes phosphodiesterase-5 activity in pulmonary artery smooth muscle cells from lambs with persistent pulmonary hypertension of the newborn. Pulm Circ 2014;4(1):71–81.

107. Mourani PM, Mandell EW, Meier M, et al. Early pulmonary vascular disease in preterm infants is associated with late respiratory outcomes in childhood. Am J Respir Crit Care Med 2019;199(8):1020–7.
108. Hemnes AR. Using omics to understand and treat pulmonary vascular disease. Front Med 2018;5:157.
109. Stearman RS, Bui QM, Speyer G, et al. Systems analysis of the human pulmonary arterial hypertension lung transcriptome. Am J Respir Cell Mol Biol 2019; 60(6):637–49.

Pulmonary Hypertension in Established Bronchopulmonary Dysplasia
Physiologic Approaches to Clinical Care

Steven H. Abman, MD[a],*, Satyan Lakshminrusimha, MD[b]

KEYWORDS

- Oxygen • Hypoxia • Cardiopulmonary interaction
- Hypoxic pulmonary vasoconstriction

KEY POINTS

- Strong laboratory and clinical data suggest that antenatal factors, such as preeclampsia, chorioamnionitis, oligohydramnios, and placental dysfunction leading to fetal growth restriction, increase susceptibility for bronchopulmonary dysplasia (BPD)-associated pulmonary hypertension (PH) after premature birth.
- Early echocardiogram findings of pulmonary vascular disease during the first postnatal week are strongly associated with short-term and long-term complications of prematurity, including high risk for developing BPD, late PH, and a more severe respiratory course with worse long-term outcomes.
- Mechanisms contributing to PH in infants with BPD include high pulmonary vascular tone and vasoreactivity in response to acute or intermittent hypoxia, abnormal lung vascular growth, and vascular structural remodeling.
- In addition to pulmonary vascular disease, abnormalities in lung mechanics and gas exchange, right and left ventricular dysfunction, and shunts across the ductus arteriosus and atrial septum contribute substantially to the development and progression of PH in infants with BPD.
- Echocardiogram metrics and serial assessments of NT-proBNP provide useful tools to diagnose and monitor clinical course during the management of BPD-associated PH, as well as monitoring for such complicating conditions as left ventricular diastolic dysfunction, shunt lesions, and pulmonary vein stenosis.
- Therapeutic strategies should include careful assessment and management of underlying airways and lung disease, cardiac performance, and systemic hemodynamics, prior to initiation of PH-targeted drug therapies.

[a] Department of Pediatrics, The Pediatric Heart Lung Center, University of Colorado Anschutz Medical Campus, Mail Stop B395, 13123 East 16th Avenue, Aurora, CO 80045, USA;
[b] Department of Pediatrics, University of California, UC Davis Children's Hospital, 2516 Stockton Boulevard, Sacramento, CA 95817, USA
* Corresponding author.
E-mail address: Steven.Abman@cuanschutz.edu

Clin Perinatol 51 (2024) 195–216
https://doi.org/10.1016/j.clp.2023.12.002
0095-5108/24/© 2023 Elsevier Inc. All rights reserved.

INTRODUCTION

Major advances in perinatal and *neonatal intensive care* unit (NICU) care have dramatically improved survival of extremely premature infants in the modern post-surfactant era. Despite striking improvements in diagnostics, therapeutics, and bedside care, however, preterm newborns remain at high risk for significant mortality and morbidities, which include the development of bronchopulmonary dysplasia (BPD), the chronic lung disease of prematurity.[1–4] BPD is perhaps the most common sequelae of premature birth, with the incidence remaining at nearly 45% for infants born prior to 29 weeks gestational age, and this rate has not improved over the past decades.[4–7] Importantly, there has been a growing proportion of infants developing more severe forms of BPD, which is most likely due to the increase in survival of extremely premature newborns at 22 to 24 weeks gestation, who are particularly associated with high risk for BPD due to greater fragility of the developing lung at such an early period of lung development.[7]

There has also been a growing recognition of the clinical importance of pulmonary vascular disease (PVD) and the impact of pulmonary hypertension (PH) on the clinical course and outcomes of preterm infants with BPD.[8–11] Even in their original description of BPD in 1967, Northway and colleagues state that "...(of infants with late deaths) all patients had striking cardiomegaly and right ventricular hypertrophy (and that) the pathogenesis of cor pulmonale is puzzling..."[1] PH has long been associated with poor survival in preterm infants with BPD even beyond the severity of underlying lung disease. A diagnosis of PH that persists beyond the first few months of life was linked with mortality rates as high as 40% to 50%, in 1980,[11] which is identical to rates that have been reported in very recent studies as well.[11–17] Importantly, prospective cohort studies show the presence of echocardiographic evidence of PH in 14% to 25% of preterm infants at 36 weeks' post menstrual age (PMA), with especially high rates of PH identified in infants with severe BPD (range: 29%–58%).[11,13,14,16] Finally, as highlighted in a report from the registry of the multicenter Pediatric Pulmonary Hypertension Network, BPD-PH has been recognized as a major public health issue as one of the most common causes of pediatric PH, accounting for nearly 25% of cases in the Registry.[18]

Thus, despite major advances in perinatal and NICU care that have led to improved survival and changes in the nature of BPD over the decades, the diagnosis of PH and its management continue to be a major challenge in infants with established BPD. With evolving or established BPD, PH is often clinically manifested by persistent respiratory distress, the sustained need for high levels of respiratory support, recurrent cyanotic episodes, and other signs. In some infants, the presence of PH with milder lung disease at the time of NICU discharge is associated with high risk for progressive PH, late respiratory problems, the need for hospital readmissions, exercise intolerance, and other morbidities. Although recent recommendations from American Heart Association (AHA) and American Thoracic Society (ATS) guidelines,[19] the Pediatric Pulmonary Hypertension Network[20] and others have outlined current consensus strategies for the monitoring, evaluation, and care of BPD-associated PH, there remains clear acknowledgment that the lack of physiologic, pharmacologic, and randomized clinical trial data limit our current care, and that there is a striking need for further research to better enhance short-term and long-term outcomes. This review provides a brief overview of current understanding of BPD-associated PH, with particular focus on disease pathogenesis and the important role of defining underlying physiologic phenotypes that include cardiac, lung, and lung vascular interactions, which lead to targeted strategies that optimize clinical care.

PATHOGENESIS OF PULMONARY VASCULAR DISEASE IN BRONCHOPULMONARY DYSPLASIA

In addition to central and small airways disease, BPD is characterized by an arrest of vascular and alveolar growth, which contributes to increased susceptibility for the development of PH. However, mechanisms underlying the pathogenesis of PH in BPD are likely multifactorial, and reflect the impact of the interplay between antenatal and postnatal injuries on lung vascular growth, pulmonary arterial remodeling, and vasoreactivity, and contribute to the "vasculopathy" of BPD, which includes the development of early and late PH (**Fig. 1**).

Laboratory and clinical studies demonstrate that early disruption of angiogenesis during the critical period of active lung vascular development during late gestation and after premature birth impairs growth of the distal airspace, leading to high risk for PH as well as BPD (the "vascular hypothesis" of BPD) (**Figs. 2** and **3**).[21–25] Previous studies demonstrate that early disruption of lung vascular growth due to hemodynamic stress *in utero* or by treatment with anti-angiogenesis agents during the early postnatal period cause PH and also impair alveolarization.[21,26,27] For example, partial occlusion of the ductus arteriosus in late gestation fetal sheep reduces vessel density and induces pulmonary artery smooth muscle thickening but also reduces septation and alveolar growth.[28] These changes are associated with severe PH at birth with poor vasodilator responsiveness to mechanical ventilation and oxygen therapy.[28–30]

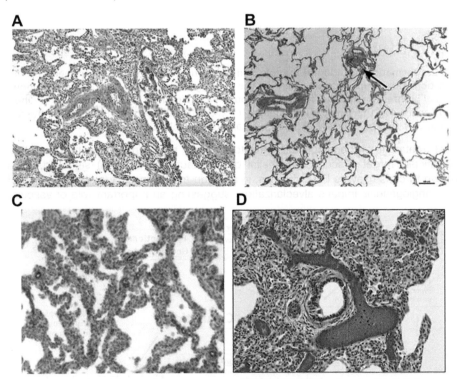

Fig. 1. Diverse histopathologic features of the lung circulation in BPD-associated PH. Pulmonary vascular pathology includes thickening of the vascular media with adventitial thickening (*A*), reduced vascular density with decreased alveolar surface area (*B*), dysmorphic growth of distal lung microvasculature. *Arrow* indicates small pulmonary artery (*C*), and prominent intrapulmonary bronchopulmonary anastomotic vessels (*D*).

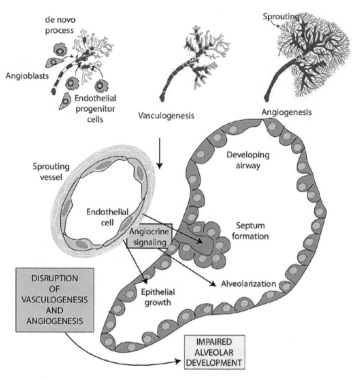

Fig. 2. Schematic illustration of the role of disruption of endothelial and epithelial cell interactions during lung development in the pathogenesis of BPD. The top panel shows normal progression of vessel formation through vasculogenesis and angiogenesis. The bottom panel shows the "angiocrine" signaling between endothelium from a developing vessel and airway. (Image Courtesy of Dr. Satyan Lakshminrusimha.)

Brief treatment with angiogenesis inhibitors shortly after birth, including drugs that specifically target vascular endothelial growth factor-A (VEGF-A) signaling, were shown to cause severe PH.[21,27] Thus, in addition to causing PH, early disruption of lung angiogenesis impairs alveolarization, suggesting an important role of vascular

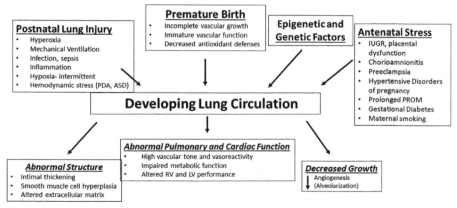

Fig. 3. Multifactorial mechanisms contributing to the pathogenesis of pulmonary vascular disease in BPD.

growth and "angiocrine" signaling for normal development of the distal airspace.[26,31] (see **Fig. 2; Fig. 4**).

Clinically, these laboratory-based findings were reflected from human autopsy findings which demonstrate decreased lung VEGF expression and striking evidence of lung simplification and a dysmorphic vasculature from preterm infants dying with BPD, providing clinical evidence supporting the important role for angiogenesis in the pathobiology of BPD.[24] Laboratory studies further show that endothelial-derived products promote alveolar epithelial growth and septation, highlighting the important role of "angiocrine signaling" during normal lung development, and support the hypothesis that early therapeutic strategies that preserve lung endothelial survival and function in at risk infants may decrease the incidence or severity of BPD and BPD-PH.

Such factors as the severity of prematurity, low birthweight, the diagnosis of small for gestational age, oligohydramnios, and other markers reflecting antenatal stress have been strongly associated with high risk for BPD-associated PH.[32–42] Abnormal placental vascular structure with evidence of placental hypoperfusion is strongly associated with neonatal outcomes of intrauterine growth restriction (IUGR) and increased risk for the development of BPD and BPD- PH.[33–37] Animal models of antenatal stress that mimic chorioamnionitis (inflammation), preeclampsia, and severe IUGR have been shown as sufficient to impair vascular growth and induce long-standing postnatal PH independent of exposure to well-established postnatal stresses, including hyperoxia and ventilator-induced lung injury.[43–45] Clinical studies have further shown that antenatal factors identified at birth,[42,46] cord blood biomarkers of impaired angiogenesis,[47,48] and early echocardiography findings of PH in the days after birth are strongly linked to high risk of BPD, PH, prolonged NICU days, and even late respiratory outcomes during early childhood.[49–56] Thus, antenatal determinants not only cause acute PH and hypoxemic respiratory disease that often contributes to the need for prolonged invasive ventilation and a severe NICU course, but also injury *in utero* can cause sustained disruption of lung and vascular structure throughout infancy, reflecting the sustained impact of fetal programming on the late clinical course. Antenatal stresses, including chorioamnionitis and preeclampsia, in preterm neonates contribute to BPD risk.[38,39] Multiple molecular mechanisms linking antenatal stress to BPD pathogenesis have been identified as potential therapeutic targets for disease

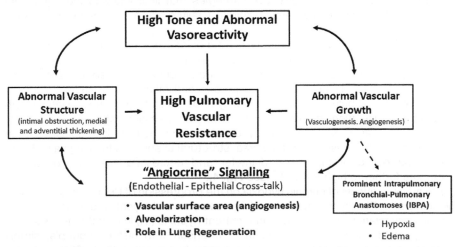

Fig. 4. Physiologic mechanisms contributing to pulmonary vascular disease and the development of PH in BPD.

prevention, including the potential role for augmentation of hypoxia-inducible factor (HIF), insulin-like growth-1 factor (IGF-1), and VEGF signaling pathways.[57–60] Overall, these findings suggest that angiogenesis is necessary for alveolarization during normal lung development, and that injury to the developing pulmonary circulation during a critical period of lung growth can contribute to reduced lung surface area.

Clinically, echocardiography-confirmed signs of early PH and delayed vascular transition are strongly associated with a higher risk for the subsequent development of BPD, late PH, and increased mortality.[49–57,61,62] A prospective study demonstrated that early echocardiographic evidence of increased pulmonary artery pressure even without evidence of severe PH, RV dysfunction, or severe hypoxemia at day 7 is associated with high risk for the subsequent development of BPD and its severity, the presence of PH at 36 weeks' PMA, and late respiratory outcomes during early childhood.[16,49] The combination of the need for invasive ventilation and PH by echocardiogram at postnatal day 7 is especially strongly associated with late morbidities.[49] Thus, early PVD as demonstrated by echocardiographic signs of PH at day 7 of life may provide a useful "biomarker" for identifying preterm infants at high risk for developing severe BPD, late PH, and chronic respiratory disease during early childhood.

In a landmark study, Dr Arjaans and colleagues further examined the idea of whether early PH in preterm infants born at less than 30 weeks gestion during the first week of life is associated with high risk for BPD and other outcomes.[53] This team performed echocardiograms to examine the incidence and nature of early PH, and to then characterize subsequent outcomes. The diagnosis of early PH was made according to standard echocardiographic metrics during the first 3–10 days of postnatal life. Early PH, which was diagnosed in 55% of subjects, was further characterized by 3 phenotypes: 1) Persistent pulmonary hypertension of the newborn (PPHN), as defined by the presence of high pulmonary vascular resistance (PVR) with right-to-left extrapulmonary shunting; 2) PH due high flow as reflected by large left-to-right ductal shunts; and 3) PH without PPHN physiology or high flow. They report that early PH within each of these physiologic groups was associated with severe BPD and/or death before 36 weeks' postmenstrual age, and that the PPHN group had the worst outcomes. Whether specific therapies to match these distinct physiologies in preterm infants with early PH can reduce BPD or BPD-PH remains unknown, but their findings lead to the speculation that selective strategies that limit injury to the pulmonary vasculature during acute hypoxemic respiratory failure may attenuate the subsequent development of BPD or BPD-PH.

Postnatal lung injury due to inflammation and oxidative stress due to hyperoxia and ventilator-induced lung injury further impairs growth, structure, and function of the developing lung circulation after premature birth.[63] Endothelial cells are particularly susceptible to oxidant injury caused by hyperoxia and inflammation, leading to cellular dysfunction. Small pulmonary arteries rapidly undergo striking changes, with smooth muscle cell proliferation, maturation of immature pericytes into mature smooth muscle cells, and increased vascular matrix production from activated fibroblasts.[64,65] In addition to reduced vascular surface area, structural changes in the lung vasculature due to narrowing of the vessel diameter and decreased vascular compliance contribute further to high PVR.[66,67] (see **Fig. 4**).

The adverse effects of chronic hypoxia on the progression of PH in diverse settings, including BPD-PH, are well-established; however, several recent studies now suggest a strong association of even mild or intermittent hypoxia (IH) in its pathogenesis early in the postnatal course after birth. In comparison with historic controls, simply increasing oxygen saturation targets to a slightly higher range (90%–95% vs 88%–92%) during the first weeks of life was associated with a striking reduction in PH in preterm infants.[68] Recent studies have further shown that IH beginning in the first week after birth was associated with an increased risk of developing severe BPD in a large and multi-center cohort of extremely preterm infants.[69] Longer duration of intermittent hypoxemic events was associated both with a diagnosis of BPD-PH and with death among infants with BPD-PH. Gentle and co-workers confirmed these findings in a retrospective case-control single-center study,[70] further suggesting that minimizing the frequency of even brief episodes of hypoxia early in the clinical course may reduce the risk for BPD-PH and improve long-term respiratory outcomes among extremely preterm infants.

Similarly, hemodynamic stress is very well-established as a major cause of PH, especially in the setting of congenital heart disease, but whether high flow through the patent ductus arteriosus (PDA) increases the risk for BPD or BPD-PH in extremely low gestational age newborns has been uncertain. Recent studies suggest that early PH due to high left to right shunt across the PDA is strongly associated with subsequent BPD.[53] A retrospective case-control study showed that in the setting of extremely preterm infants on respiratory support on postnatal day 28, both the presence and a longer duration of a PDA was associated with the development of BPD-PH at NICU discharge.[71] This association of prolonged exposure to a hemodynamically significant PDA being linked with a greater risk for BPD-PH was demonstrated in data from a meta-analysis by using a Bayesian approach to data analysis.[72] These studies suggest that early closure of the PDA, especially in the setting of a reduced pulmonary vascular bed, may be a targetable strategy for attenuating BPD-PH in at-risk infants.

In addition to the potential adverse pulmonary vascular impact due to high flow through the PDA, Vyas-Read and colleagues have shown that increased left-to-right flow through a persistent atrial septal defect (ASD) was more common in preterm infants who developed BPD-PH than matched subjects without an ASD.[73] Observational studies suggest that ASD closures in preterm infants with severe BPD can lead to improvements in cardiopulmonary course.[74,75] Thus, based on data from these studies and others, the preterm lung circulation as characterized by a reduced surface area, with increased vascular tone and an enhanced myogenic response, may increase susceptibility for additional vascular injury due to the hemodynamic stress of prolonged exposure to a PDA or ASD, suggesting that early interventions may potentially prevent the presence or severity of BPD-PH in susceptible preterm infants.

SELECTED PHYSIOLOGIC ASPECTS OF BRONCHOPULMONARY DYSPLASIA-PULMONARY HYPERTENSION

Although it is plausible that PH is simply a marker of more advanced lung disease, high pulmonary artery pressure clearly contributes to the disease severity in many infants with severe BPD, causing poor right ventricular function, impaired cardiac output, limited oxygen delivery, worsened pulmonary edema, and perhaps a higher risk of sudden death. Physiologic abnormalities of the pulmonary circulation in BPD include elevated PVR and abnormal vasoreactivity, as evidenced by the exaggerated vasoconstrictor response to acute hypoxia (**Fig. 5**). As studied during cardiac catheterization, acute exposure to hypoxia causes large elevations in pulmonary artery pressure, even in infants with modest basal levels of PH.[76] This study further showed that the degree of hypoxia that increases PH can be fairly modest in many patients, and that achieving oxygen saturations above 92% to 94% was effective in lowering pulmonary artery pressure. The current recommendation for treatment of patients with BPD and PH is to avoid oxygen saturations below 92%, and to maintain levels of 94% to 96%.

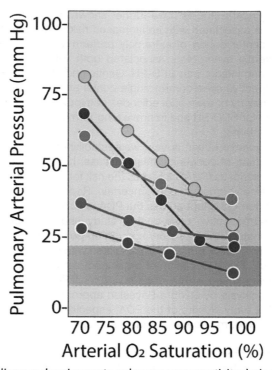

Fig. 5. Schematic diagram showing acute pulmonary vasoreactivity during brief exposure to hypoxia in patients with BPD-PH demonstrating variability in baseline pulmonary arterial pressure and response to hypoxemia.[76]

Whether the risk of attaining higher oxygen saturations is to induce more lung injury remains unconfirmed, but the adverse effects of hypoxemia are clear. Strategies that maintain lower pulmonary artery pressure or limit injury to the pulmonary vasculature during the treatment of acute hypoxemic respiratory failure may attenuate the subsequent development or contribution of PH to BPD.

In addition to PH, clinical studies have also shown that metabolic function of the lung circulation is impaired in BPD-PH, as reflected by the lack of pulmonary clearance of circulating norepinephrine across the lung.[77] The lung circulation normally clears 20% to 40% of circulating norepinephrine during a single passage through the lung, but transpulmonary measurements of circulating norepinephrine levels in infants with severe BPD performed during cardiac catheterization had negligible clearance and a net production of norepinephrine across the pulmonary circulation. Whether impaired metabolic function of the lung contributes to the pathophysiology of BPD by increasing circulating catecholamine levels, or if it is simply a marker of endothelial dysfunction due to pulmonary vascular disease, remains unknown. It has been speculated that high catecholamine levels may lead to LV diastolic dysfunction or hypertrophy (LVH) or systemic hypertension, which are known complications of BPD.

DIAGNOSTIC STRATEGIES FOR BRONCHOPULMONARY DYSPLASIA-PULMONARY HYPERTENSION

Due its non-invasive nature, well-standardized approaches and verified metrics, and the ease of its bedside use, the echocardiogram provides a useful approach for diagnosing PH and defining the severity of disease, identifying anatomic defects, characterizing the presence and nature of shunt lesions and pulmonary vein stenosis (PVS), and assessing left ventricular size and performance. The striking growth of world-wide programs in targeted neonatal echocardiography has provided remarkable opportunities for providing precise and serial physiologic hemodynamic assessments which better define physiologic phenotypes, responses to therapeutic interventions, and long-term outcomes. Specific echocardiographic parameters and their relative utility remain under study as discussed in recent review publications.[78–84] Recommendations of the PPHNet regarding the timing of obtaining diagnostic or screening echocardiograms are summarized in **Fig. 8** below.

Cardiac catheterization is considered the "gold standard" for more precise characterization of PH and cardiac performance by direct measurements of pulmonary hemodynamic to better determine disease severity, assess acute vasoreactivity testing (AVT), and identify associated cardiovascular co-morbidities, such as anatomic cardiac lesions, systemic-pulmonary collateral vessels, pulmonary venous obstruction, and left heart dysfunction. Although in experienced centers, the complication rates of catheterization are relatively low,[85] careful consideration must be given due to its invasive nature and potential risks in sick premature infants and patient selection must be considered carefully. As a result, PH-specific therapy in the BPD-PH population is most often initiated as based on clinical and echocardiogram-based findings of PH without cardiac catheterization. In the setting of BPD-PH, the procedure is generally reserved to enhance clinical decision-making in the following settings: 1) clinical and echocardiogram findings of sustained PH despite optimized respiratory and cardiac care; 2) considerations of adding another agent in patients already under treatment with a single initial PH-targeted drug with or without inhaled NO; 3) clinical suspicions of associated cardiovascular problems, including left ventricular dysfunction, pulmonary venous obstruction, the need to better define the contributions of high flow due to left-to-right shunts due to PDA, ASD, arterio-venous malformations, or other vascular lesions; 4) worsening pulmonary edema and increased diuretic need after the initiation of PH drug therapy, suggesting left ventricular diastolic dysfunction and/or pulmonary PVS; and 5) considerations of the need for chronic use of systemic prostanoid therapy.[20]

Functional studies such as AVT can help guide the selection of drug therapy, as older subjects with positive AVT are often preferentially treated with calcium channel blockade, but experience with AVT is exclusively based on studies in the setting of World Symposium of Pulmonary Hypertension (WSPH) Group 1 disease. In a recent study of BPD-PH, positive AVT was more strongly associated with better late outcomes than baseline pulmonary hemodynamics.[86] Cardiovascular MRI has been used to assess cardiac performance in PH as well, often in conjunction with cardiac catheterization, and is particularly useful as a non-invasive approach to diagnosing PVS.[87–90]

In addition to the use of serial echocardiograms and clinical assessments of cardiovascular and pulmonary disease, circulating changes in brain-type natriuretic peptide (BNP) or N-terminal cleavage product (NT-pro-BNP) levels are useful in monitoring disease course and the response to clinical therapies over time. In some centers, serum BNP or NT-pro-BNP levels are used to screen preterm infants for PH, and if elevated, an echocardiogram is subsequently performed. Most clinicians use changes in these biomarkers to supplement echocardiogram findings to better enable clinical decision-making to fine-tune cardiorespiratory and drug interventions. BNP and NT-pro-BNP are not specific for right ventricular disease alone, however, and may be elevated in the setting of high-flow shunts or with LV stress.

SELECTED ASPECTS OF CARE

The management of BPD-associated PH includes defining the relative contributions of airway, lung, cardiac, and pulmonary vascular disease to the pathophysiology of PH (**Figs. 6 and 7**).

Respiratory

An overall approach for screening and managing BPD-PH as developed by the Pediatric Pulmonary Hypertension Network (PPHNet) is outlined in **Fig. 8** and is related to consensus recommendations from joint AHA and ATS guidelines (see **Fig. 8**).[20] The initial clinical strategy for the management of PH in infants with BPD begins with treating the underlying lung disease, including an extensive evaluation for chronic reflux and aspiration, structural airway abnormalities (such as tonsillar and adenoidal hypertrophy, vocal cord paralysis, subglottic stenosis, tracheomalacia, and other lesions), assessments of bronchial reactivity, improving lung edema, airway function, lung mechanics and lung volumes, assessing the need for non-invasive or invasive support, and any other intervening factors. Periods of acute hypoxemia, whether intermittent or prolonged, can often contribute to late PH in BPD. A sleep study may be necessary to determine the presence of noteworthy episodes of hypoxemia and whether hypoxemia has predominantly obstructive, central, or mixed causes. Additional studies that may be required include flexible bronchoscopy for the diagnosis of anatomic and dynamic airway lesions (such as tracheomalacia) that can contribute to hypoxemia and poor clinical responses to oxygen therapy. Upper gastrointestinal series, pH or impedance probe, and swallow studies may be indicated to evaluate for gastro-esophageal reflux and aspiration that can contribute to ongoing lung injury. For patients with BPD and severe PH who fail to maintain near normal ventilation or require high levels of fraction of inspired oxygen (FiO_2) despite conservative treatment, strong consideration should be given to chronic mechanical ventilatory support to halt progression of PH.

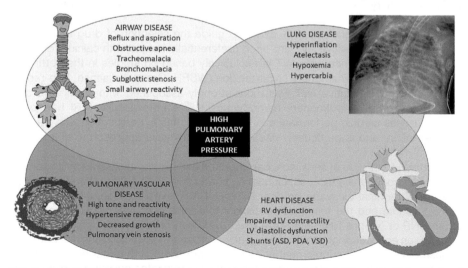

Fig. 6. Pathophysiologic mechanisms underlying BPD-associated PH: potential effects of heart, lung, and vascular interactions on elevated pulmonary artery pressure. (Image Courtesy of Dr. Satyan Lakshminrusimha.)

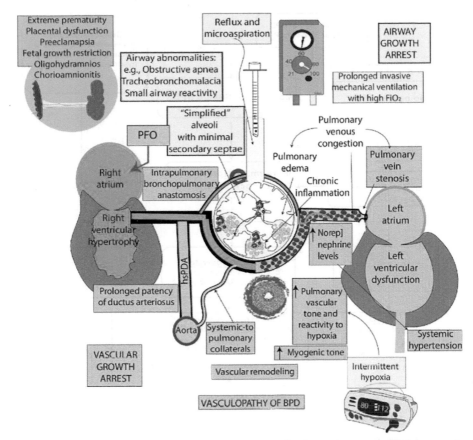

Fig. 7. Schematic illustrating diverse interactive mechanisms that can contribute to the pathophysiology of BPD-PH. Vascular lesions are shown in pink boxes and airway lesions are shown in yellow boxes. (Image courtesy of Dr. Satyan Lakshminrusimha.)

ASSOCIATED CARDIOVASCULAR ABNORMALITIES IN BRONCHOPULMONARY DYSPLASIA-PULMONARY HYPERTENSION

Cardiovascular abnormalities associated with BPD include (LVH, systemic hypertension, and the development of prominent systemic to pulmonary collateral vessels (see **Fig. 7**). An early report described infants with severe BPD and LVH in the absence of right ventricular hypertrophy and suggested that left ventricular dysfunction may contribute to recurrent edema in BPD.[91] Systemic steroid treatment can cause LVH, and in this setting, LVH tends to be transient, resolves with cessation of steroid treatment, and is of uncertain clinical importance. A high incidence of systemic hypertension has also been recognized as a cardiovascular complication of BPD, but its cause remains obscure.[92] Systemic hypertension may be mild, transient, and respond readily to pharmacologic treatment; however, the rise in blood pressure can be striking in some cases. On occasion, further evaluation of such infants shows considerable renal vascular or urinary tract disease. Whether the high incidence of systemic hypertension in BPD reflects altered neurohumoral regulation or increased catecholamines, angiotensin, or antidiuretic hormone levels is not known. Prominent bronchial or other systemic to pulmonary collateral vessels were noted in early morphometric studies of

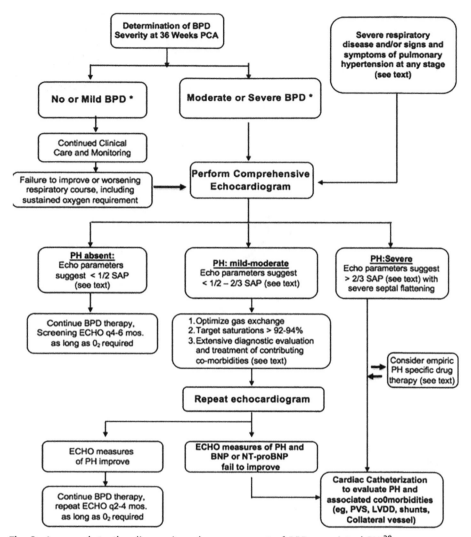

Fig. 8. Approach to the diagnosis and management of BPD-associated PH.[20]

infants with BPD and can be readily identified in many infants during cardiac catheterization. Although these collateral vessels are generally small, large collaterals may contribute to appreciable shunting of blood flow to the lung, causing edema and the need for higher FiO$_2$. Some infants have improved after embolization of large collateral vessels, as reflected by a reduced need for supplemental oxygen, ventilator support, or diuretics, but the actual contribution of collateral vessels to the pathophysiology of BPD is poorly understood.

Although causality cannot be assumed, available data show that prolonged exposure to a post-tricuspid valve high-volume and high-pressure shunt, such as a hemodynamically significant moderate to large left-to-right PDA, ventricular septal defect (VSD), or ASD, increases the likelihood of the development of PH related to high pulmonary flow, over-circulation, and pulmonary vascular remodeling. In these patients, decreasing the PVR by using pulmonary vasodilators can further increase left-to-right shunting and induce systemic hypotension with reduced RV perfusion, which can worsen RV performance. This emphasizes the need for monitoring PH in high-risk preterm infants with prolonged exposure to post-tricuspid valve shunts and incorporating the risk of developing or worsening PH into the clinical decisions regarding the definitive closure by catheter occlusion or surgery.

ASDs are characterized by high-volume and low-pressure pre-tricuspid valve shunts, and may contribute to late PH.[93–95] Some studies have demonstrated improvement in PH and respiratory signs after ASD closure, suggesting that earlier closure of ASDs or PDAs may hasten recovery from BPD-PH and reduce the need for late PH-targeted drug therapies. PVS is an additional cause of late PH in BPD (**Fig. 9**), usually presenting beyond term corrected age in premature infants beyond term corrected age.[96,97]) PVS can present with the onset or worsening of PH by echocardiogram, which may or may not be initially accompanied by progressive pulmonary edema with an increasing need for higher FiO_2 or diuretic requirement, especially in

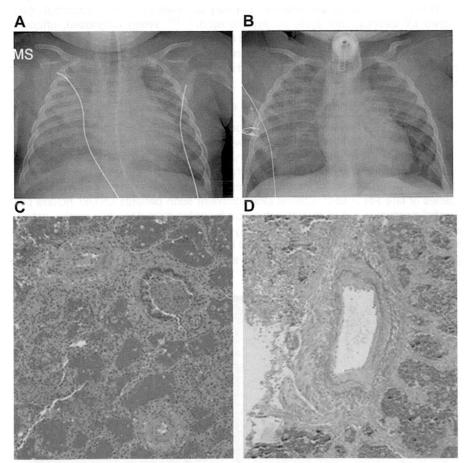

Fig. 9. Radiologic and histopathologic features of pulmonary vein stenosis (PVS) in BPD-associated PH. The upper panel represents CXR signs of pulmonary edema before (A) and after (B) stent placement. The lower panel shows lung histopathology from an infant with PVS that demonstrates striking pulmonary arterial remodeling with acute hemorrhage (C) and muscularization of pulmonary veins (D).

response to PH vasodilator therapy (**Fig. 10**). Diagnosis can be suggested by echocardiogram, followed by cardiac MRI or catheterization, and PH drugs should be used very cautiously due to the risk of worsening respiratory distress. Multiple PVS sites are associated with worse outcomes than single vein involvement.[97] Current treatment approaches include PVS dilation and stenting with close monitoring with serial echocardiograms, imaging scans, and cardiac catheterization to assess disease course. In some centers, sirolimus therapy has been used to abate progressive pulmonary venous obstruction after anatomic interventions.

In addition, there has been a growing recognition regarding the role of left ventricular diastolic dysfunction (LVDD) as a contributor to PH, usually in combination with precapillary disease. LVDD is often clinically suspected in subjects who have persistent or progressive pulmonary edema requiring increasing amounts of diuretic therapy, which is worsened with the addition of PH-targeted drug therapy (see **Fig. 10**). LVDD can also be associated with a more prolonged ventilator course than patients with BPD-PH who do not have a poorly compliant LV. Mechanisms contributing to LVDD in preterm infants are uncertain, but may be related to early myocardial injury, altered LV development systemic hypertension.[98–100] When diagnosed, afterload reduction of the LV with milrinone followed by chronic angiotensin-converting enzyme inhibitors (ACEi) are often used.[101] Close monitoring of renal function is important to avoid acute kidney injury, especially in the setting of aggressive diuretic use with ACEi therapy.

Ambulatory Care Post-Neonatal Intensive Care Unit Discharge

Most patients with "resolving" BPD show progressive increases in growth parameters and follow their growth curves for body weight and length. Patients who show evidence of poor growth, lack of respiratory improvement, intermittent tachypnea or cyanosis, or additional signs of PH by echocardiogram may require more extensive studies. First, prolonged, or intermittent periods of acute hypoxia are often important causes of late PH in BPD. Clinical evaluations of such patients should include prolonged measurements of oxygen saturation by pulse oximeter while awake, asleep, and during feeds. Brief assessments of oxygenation ("spot checks") are not sufficient for decisions on the level of supplemental oxygen needed. As described earlier, targeting oxygen saturations to 92% to 94% should be sufficient to prevent the adverse

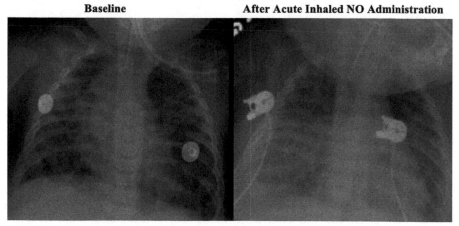

Baseline   **After Acute Inhaled NO Administration**

Fig. 10. Inhaled NO increases pulmonary edema in a BPD patient with LV diastolic dysfunction.

effects of hypoxia in most infants, without increasing the risk of additional lung inflammation and injury. A sleep study may be necessary to determine the presence of noteworthy episodes of hypoxemia and whether apnea has predominantly obstructive, central, or mixed causes. It is not uncommon to uncover unsuspected causes of airway obstruction in patients with BPD and persistent PH, such as tonsillar and adenoidal hypertrophy, vocal cord paralysis, subglottic stenosis, tracheomalacia, and others. Additional studies that may be required include flexible bronchoscopy for the diagnosis of anatomic and dynamic airway lesions (such as tracheomalacia) that may contribute to hypoxemia and poor clinical responses to oxygen therapy. Growth failure during home oxygen therapy may be the result of poor parental compliance or premature discontinuation of supplemental oxygen, as previously reported.[27] In this study, nearly one-third of families in a home oxygen program had prematurely discontinued oxygen therapy. Assessments of PH should generally include serial echocardiograms in infants with the diagnosis of BPD, even if stable or rapidly improving, to enable safe discontinuation of PH medications.

The authors recommend serial echocardiograms in patients with moderate or severe BPD, or with past echocardiograms showing the presence of PH. Previous work suggests that with adequate oxygen therapy and related interventions, PH should progressively improve and resolve in most children by 8 to 12 months of age. Cardiac catheterization is reserved for patients with the most severe disease which has not responded to oxygen therapy. The purpose of cardiac catheterization is to rule out anatomic cardiac lesions, especially associated with high flow due to left to right shunts.

Experience suggests that infants with BPD do not tolerate even relatively small atrial or ventricular level shunting and are at high risk of developing more severe PH than other patients. This may be because of the decrease in vascular surface area relative to body size and cardiac output in BPD, and the fact that even mild increases in pulmonary blood flow may represent relatively high shunt. As a result, the authors advise earlier closure of shunt lesions in patients with BPD, especially with the growing development of non-invasive approaches. In addition, cardiac catheterization is useful for the following: to ensure the absence of pulmonary vein stenosis or veno-occlusion; to define the level and severity of PH; to assess vasoreactivity to increased oxygen tension or to assess the response to vasodilator treatment; and to determine whether large systemic to pulmonary collateral vessels are present. Studies of vasoreactivity are helpful to determine the relative safety—that is, lack of systemic hypotension and impaired cardiac contractility—and potential efficacy of PH-targeted drugs, which would be initiated in patients with exceptional PH despite adequate oxygen therapy. Clearly, cardiac catheterization is invasive and reserved for the most severely ill infants who develop PH despite optimal medical management.

Late Pulmonary Hypertension in Adults Born Prematurely

In addition to the need for close follow-up and monitoring throughout infancy and early childhood, multiple investigators have noted late echocardiographic markers of PH that persist into early adulthood.[102] There is growing evidence for PVD in older children and young adults, or "PVD across the lifespan," in which there has been growing evidence for high risk of development of "borderline" PH and abnormal cardiac structure and function in young adults who were born preterm. In addition, cardiac imaging studies of adults born prematurely have shown small LV and RV chamber size with thickened ventricular walls, along with elevated systemic vascular resistance, and a high proportion of adults who develop congestive heart failure at a younger age[103] Clearly, there is a need for close cardiovascular as well as pulmonary function monitoring throughout the life course. Identification of early risk factors for late cardio-respiratory outcomes is required to design and install personalized preventive treatment strategies.

SUMMARY

In addition to persistent respiratory disease, survivors of premature birth with BPD are at risk of cardiovascular sequelae, including PH, as well as cardiac dysfunction, systemic hypertension, exercise intolerance, and related clinical problems. Early monitoring with serial echocardiograms aids the selection of infants with BPD who are at high risk of cardiovascular morbidity and allows for earlier initiation of treatment after a rigorous diagnostic evaluation. The major treatment of PH in BPD is supplemental oxygen with appropriate levels of respiratory support, but infants with late PH despite adequate treatment require pharmacologic treatment in addition to careful management of underlying respiratory disease. Despite increasing experience with PH-targeted drugs for chronic PH management, strong evidence for selecting specific agents or combinations of agents at diagnosis and for long-term therapy remains limited. Exciting new data suggest that insights into physiologic phenotypes of early PH may provide unique opportunities for clinical trials to address novel interventions to reduce the incidence and severity of BPD and BPD-PH. Finally, better designed and appropriately powered multicenter randomized controlled trials are needed to improve our understanding of disease natural history, response to therapeutic interventions, and optimal endpoints for studies of BPD-PH over the lifespan.

Best Practice Box

- Extremely preterm infants with lung disease requiring late or sustained levels of high respiratory support should be screened early with echocardiograms to detect PH.

- Evaluating airway abnormalities, such as tracheobronchiomalacia, vocal cord paralysis, subglottic stenosis, and small airway hyperreactivity, as well gastroesophageal reflux and aspiration is part of workup for severe BPD with PH.

- Infants with BPD-PH can have intermittent hypoxemia, which may lead to spikes or sustained PH due to increased hypoxic pulmonary vascular reactivity. Targeting SpO_2 in the 92% to 94% with continuous or frequent monitoring to minimize hypoxemia may reduce the risk of PH.

- In addition to strategies that optimize oxygenation, respirator support, and systemic cardiovascular performance, PH-targeted drug therapy, including PDE5 inhibitors and endothelin antagonists, is the mainstay of BPD-PH management. Exacerbations are treated with inhaled nitric oxide and severe and poorly responsive PH despite optimal management may improve with systemic prostanoid therapy.

- Infants with BPD-PH not responding to initial PH-specific drug therapy may require cardiac catheterization to assess severity and phenotype of PH and to evaluate shunts, LVDD, and PVS.

- Preterm infants with BPD-PH have pulmonary vascular disease that persists into adulthood and requires serial pulmonary function testing and cardiovascular monitoring with serial echocardiograms.

DISCLOSURE

The authors report no conflicts of interest related to this chapter.

REFERENCES

1. Northway WH Jr, Rosan RC, Porter DY. Pulmonary disease following respirator therapy of hyaline-membrane disease. Bronchopulmonary dysplasia. N Engl J Med 1967;276(7):357–68.
2. Jobe AJ. The new BPD: an arrest of lung development. Pediatr Res 1999;46(6): 641–3.
3. Abman SH, Bancalari E, Jobe A. The evolution of bronchopulmonary dysplasia after 50 years. Am J Respir Crit Care Med 2017;195(4):421–4.
4. Thébaud B, Goss KN, Laughon M, et al. Bronchopulmonary dysplasia. Nat Rev Dis Prim 2019;5(1):78.
5. Bell EF, Hintz SR, Hansen NI, et al, Eunice Kennedy Shriver National Institute of Child Health and Human Development Neonatal Research Network. Mortality, in-hospital morbidity, care practices, and 2-year outcomes for extremely preterm infants in the US, 2013-2018. JAMA 2022;327(3):248–63.
6. Regin Y, Gie A, Eerdekens A, et al. Ventilation and respiratory outcome in extremely preterm infants: trends in the new millennium. Eur J Pediatr 2022; 181(5):1899–907.
7. Stoll BJ, Hansen NI, Bell EF, et al, Eunice Kennedy Shriver National Institute of Child Health and Human Development Neonatal Research Network. Trends in care practices, morbidity, and mortality of extremely preterm neonates, 1993-2012. JAMA 2015;314(10):1039–51.
8. Mourani PM, Abman SH. Pulmonary hypertension and vascular abnormalities in bronchopulmonary dysplasia. Clin Perinatol 2015;42(4):839–55.
9. Arattu Thodika FMS, Nanjundappa M, Dassios T, et al. Pulmonary hypertension in infants with bronchopulmonary dysplasia: risk factors, mortality and duration of hospitalisation. J Perinat Med 2022;50(3):327–33.
10. Levy PT, Levin J, Leeman KT, et al. Diagnosis and management of pulmonary hypertension in infants with bronchopulmonary dysplasia. Semin Fetal Neonatal Med 2022;27(4):101351.
11. Arjaans S, Zwart EAH, Ploegstra MJ, et al. Identification of gaps in the current knowledge on pulmonary hypertension in extremely preterm infants: a systematic review and meta-analysis. Paediatr Perinat Epidemiol 2018;32(3):258–67.
12. Slaughter JL, Pakrashi T, Jones DE, et al. Echocardiographic detection of pulmonary hypertension in extremely low birth weight infants with bronchopulmonary dysplasia requiring prolonged positive pressure ventilation. J Perinatol 2011;31(10):635–40.
13. Kim DH, Kim HS, Choi CW, et al. Risk factors for pulmonary artery hypertension in preterm infants with moderate or severe bronchopulmonary dysplasia. Neonatology 2012;101(1):40–6.
14. Bhat R, Salas AA, Foster C, et al. Prospective analysis of pulmonary hypertension in extremely low birth weight infants. Pediatrics 2012;129(3):e682–9.
15. Arjaans S, Haarman MG, Roofthooft MTR, et al. Fate of pulmonary hypertension associated with bronchopulmonary dysplasia beyond 36 weeks postmenstrual age. Arch Dis Child Fetal Neonatal Ed 2021;106(1):45–50.
16. Mourani PM, Sontag MK, Younoszai A, et al. Early pulmonary vascular disease in preterm infants at risk for bronchopulmonary dysplasia. Am J Respir Crit Care Med 2015;191(1):87–95.
17. An HS, Bae EJ, Kim GB, et al. Pulmonary hypertension in preterm infants with bronchopulmonary dysplasia. Korean Circ J 2010;40(3):131–6.

18. Abman SH, Mullen M, Sleeper L, et al. Characterization of pediatric pulmonary hypertensive vascular disorders from the pediatric pulmonary hypertension Network registry. Eur Respir J 2021;59(1):2003337.

19. Abman SH, Hansmann G, Archer SL, et al, American Heart Association Council on Cardiopulmonary, Critical Care, Perioperative and Resuscitation; Council on Clinical Cardiology; Council on Cardiovascular Disease in the Young; Council on Cardiovascular Radiology and Intervention; Council on Cardiovascular Surgery and Anesthesia; and the American Thoracic Society. Pediatric pulmonary hypertension: guidelines from the American heart association and American thoracic society. Circulation 2015;132(21):2037–99.

20. Krishnan U, Feinstein JA, Adatia I, et al. Pediatric Pulmonary Hypertension Network PPHNet, Evaluation and management of pulmonary hypertension in children with bronchopulmonary dysplasia. J Pediatr 2017;188:24.

21. Jakkula M, Le Cras TD, Gebb S, et al. Inhibition of angiogenesis decreases alveolarization in the developing rat lung. Am J Physiol Lung Cell Mol Physiol 2000;279(3):L600–7.

22. Abman SH. Bronchopulmonary dysplasia: "a vascular hypothesis". Am J Respir Crit Care Med 2001;164(10 Pt 1):1755–6.

23. Thebaud B, Abman SH. Bronchopulmonary dysplasia: where have all the vessels gone? Roles of angiogenic growth factors in chronic lung disease. Am J Respir Crit Care Med 2007;175(10):978–85.

24. Bhatt AJ, Pryhuber GS, Huyck H, et al. Disrupted pulmonary vasculature and decreased vascular endothelial growth factor, Flt-1, and TIE-2 in human infants dying with bronchopulmonary dysplasia. Am J Respir Crit Care Med 2001; 164(10 Pt 1):1971–80.

25. Zeng X, Wert SE, Federici R, et al. VEGF enhances pulmonary vasculogenesis and disrupts lung morphogenesis in vivo. Dev Dynam 1998;211(3):215–27.

26. Grover TR, Parker TA, Zenge JP, et al. Intrauterine hypertension decreases lung VEGF expression and VEGF inhibition causes pulmonary hypertension in the ovine fetus. Am J Physiol Lung Cell Mol Physiol 2003;284(3):L508–17.

27. Le Cras TD, Markham NE, Tuder RM, et al. Treatment of newborn rats with a VEGF receptor inhibitor causes pulmonary hypertension and abnormal lung structure. Am J Physiol Lung Cell Mol Physiol 2002;283(3):L555–62.

28. Abman SH, Shanley PF, Accurso FJ. Failure of postnatal adaptation of the pulmonary circulation after chronic intrauterine pulmonary hypertension in fetal lambs. J Clin Invest 1989;83:1849–58.

29. Cornfield DN Cornfield DN, Chatfield BA, McQueston JA, et al. Effects of birth-related stimuli on L-Arginine dependent vasodilation in the ovine fetal lung. Am J Physiol 1992;262:H1474–81.

30. McQueston J McQueston JA, Kinsella JP, Ivy DD, et al. Chronic pulmonary hypertension in utero impairs endothelium-dependent vasodilation. Am J Physiol 1995;268:H288–94.

31. Yun EJ, Lorizio W, Seedorf G, et al. VEGF and endothelial-derived retinoic acid regulate lung vascular and alveolar development. Am J Physiol. LCMP. 2015; 310:L287–98.

32. Nagiub M, Kanaan U, Simon D, et al. Risk factors for development of pulmonary hypertension in infants with bronchopulmonary dysplasia: systematic review and meta-analysis. Paediatr Respir Rev 2017;23:27–32.

33. Kim YJ, Shin SH, Park HW, et al. Risk factors of early pulmonary hypertension and its clinical outcomes in preterm infants: a systematic review and meta-analysis. Sci Rep 2022;12(1):14186.

34. Pierro M, Villamor-Martinez E, van Westering-Kroon E, et al. Association of the dysfunctional placentation endotype of prematurity with bronchopulmonary dysplasia: a systematic review, meta-analysis and meta-regression. Thorax 2022;77(3):268–75.

35. Yallapragada SG, Yallapragada SG, Mestan KK, et al. Placental villous vascularity is decreased in premature infants with bronchopulmonary dysplasia-associated pulmonary hypertension. Pediatr Dev Pathol 2016;19(2):101–7.

36. Check J, Gotteiner N, Liu X, et al. Fetal growth restriction and pulmonary hypertension in premature infants with bronchopulmonary dysplasia. J Perinatol 2013; 33(7):553–7.

37. Mestan KK, Check J, Minturn L, et al. Placental pathologic changes of maternal vascular underperfusion in bronchopulmonary dysplasia and pulmonary hypertension. Placenta 2014;35(8):570–4.

38. Watterberg KL, Demers LM, Scott SM, et al. Chorioamnionitis and early lung inflammation in infants in whom bronchopulmonary dysplasia develops. Pediatrics 1996;97(2):210–5.

39. Hansen AR, Barnés CM, Folkman J, et al. Maternal preeclampsia predicts the development of bronchopulmonary dysplasia. J Pediatr 2010;156(4):532–6.

40. Taglauer E, Abman SH, Keller RL. Recent advances in antenatal factors predisposing to bronchopulmonary dysplasia. Semin Perinatol 2018;42(7):413–24.

41. Mandell EW, Abman SH. Fetal vascular origins of bronchopulmonary dysplasia. J Pediatr 2017;185:7–10.e1.

42. Morrow LA, Wagner BD, Ingram DA, et al. Antenatal determinants of bronchopulmonary dysplasia and late respiratory disease in preterm infants. Am J Respir Crit Care Med 2017;196(3):364–74.

43. Tang JR, ETX model, Tang JR, Karumanchi SA, et al. Excess soluble vascular endothelial growth factor receptor-1 impairs lung growth in infant rats: linking preeclampsia with bronchopulmonary dysplasia. Am J Physiol. Lung Cell Molecular. 2011;302:L36–46.

44. Tang JR, Seedorf G, Muehlethaler V, et al. Moderate hyperoxia accelerates lung growth and attenuates pulmonary hypertension in infant rats after exposure to intra-amniotic endotoxin. Am J Physiol: Lung 2010;299:L735–48.

45. Wallance B, Peisl A, Seedorf G, et al. Anti-sFlt-1 monoclonal antibody therapy preserves lung alveolar and vascular growth in antenatal models of BPD. Am J Respir Crit Care Med 2018;197:776–87.

46. Keller RL, Feng R, DeMauro SB, et al, Prematurity and Respiratory Outcomes Program. Prematurity and respiratory outcome program. Bronchopulmonary dysplasia and perinatal characteristics predict 1-year respiratory outcomes in newborns born at extremely low gestational age: a prospective cohort study. J Pediatr 2017;187:89–97.

47. Baker CD, Balasubramaniam V, 48 PM, et al. Cord blood angiogenic progenitor cells are decreased in bronchopulmonary dysplasia. Eur Respir J 2012;40(6): 1516–22.

48. Mestan KK, Gotteiner N, Porta N, et al. Cord blood biomarkers of placental maternal vascular underperfusion predict bronchopulmonary dysplasia-associated pulmonary hypertension. J Pediatr 2017;185:33–41.

49. Mourani PM, Mandell EW, Meier M, et al. Early pulmonary vascular disease in preterm infants is associated with late respiratory outcomes in childhood. Am J Respir Crit Care Med 2019;199(8):1020–7.

50. Mirza H, Ziegler J, Ford S, et al. Pulmonary hypertension in preterm infants: prevalence and association with bronchopulmonary dysplasia. J Pediatr 2014; 165(5):909–914 e1.
51. Arjaans S, Haarman MG, Roofthooft MTR, et al. Fate of pulmonary hypertension associated with bronchopulmonary dysplasia beyond 36 weeks postmenstrual age. Arch Dis Child Fetal Neonatal Ed 2021;106(1):45–50.
52. An HS, Bae EJ, Kim GB, et al. Pulmonary hypertension in preterm infants with bronchopulmonary dysplasia. Korean Circ J 2010;40(3):131–6.
53. Arjaans J, Fries MWF, Schoots MH, et al. Clinical significance of early pulmonary hypertension in preterm infants. J Pediatr 2022 Dec;251:74–81.e3.
54. Abman SH. Characterization of early pulmonary hypertension in preterm newborns: a key step towards improving critical outcomes. J Pediatr 2022;251:44–6.
55. Mirza H, Mandell EW, Kinsella JP, et al. Pulmonary vascular phenotypes of prematurity: the path to precision medicine. J Pediatr 2023;259:113444.
56. Lagatta JM, Hysinger EB, Zaniletti I, et al, Children's Hospital Neonatal Consortium Severe BPD Focus Group. The impact of pulmonary hypertension in preterm infants with severe bronchopulmonary dysplasia through 1 year. J Pediatr 2018;203:218–24.e3.
57. Hirsch K, Taglauer E, Seedorf G, et al. Perinatal stabilization of hypoxia-inducible factor preserves lung alveolar and vascular growth in experimental BPD. Am J Respir Crit Care Med 2020;202(8):1146–58.
58. Seedorf G, Kim C, Wallace B, et al. rhIGF-1/BP3 preserves lung growth and prevents pulmonary hypertension in experimental bronchopulmonary dysplasia. Am J Respir Crit Care Med 2020;201(9):1120–34.
59. Kunig AM, Balasubramaniam V, Markham NE, et al. Recombinant human VEGF treatment transiently increases lung edema but enhances late lung structure in neonatal hypeoxic lung injury. Am J Physiol 2006;291:L1068–98.
60. Thebaud B, Ladha F, Michelakis ED, et al. Vascular endothelial growth factor gene therapy increases survival, promotes lung angiogenesis, and prevents alveolar damage in hyperoxia-induced lung injury: evidence that angiogenesis participates in alveolarization. Circulation 2005;112(16):2477–86.
61. Altit G, Bhombal S, Feinstein J, et al. Diminished right ventricular function at diagnosis of pulmonary hypertension is associated with mortality in bronchopulmonary dysplasia. Pulm Circ 2019;9(3). 2045894019878598.
62. Mirza H, Garcia JA, Crawford E, et al. Natural history of postnatal cardiopulmonary adaptation in infants born extremely preterm and risk for death or bronchopulmonary dysplasia. J Pediatr 2018;198:187–93.e1.
63. Jones R, Zapol WM, Reid LM. Oxygen toxicity and restructuring of pulmonary arteries: a morphometric study. Am J Pathol 1985;121:212–23.
64. Roberts RJ, Weesner KM, Bucher JR. Oxygen-induced alterations in lung vascular development in the newborn rat. Pediatr Res 1983;17:368–75.
65. Wilson Wl, Mullen M, Olley PM, et al. Hyperoxia-induced pulmonary vascular and lung abnormalities in young rats and potential for recovery. Pediatr Res 1985;19:1059–67.
66. Tomashefski JF, Opperman HC, Vawter GF, et al. BPD: a morphometric study with emphasis on the pulmonary vasculature. Pediatr Pathol 1984;2:469–87.
67. Anderson WR, Engel RR. Cardiopulmonary sequelae of reparative stages of BPD. Arch Pathol Lab Med 1983;107:6603–8.
68. Laliberté C, Hanna Y, Ben Fadel N, et al. Target oxygen saturation and development of pulmonary hypertension and increased pulmonary vascular resistance in preterm infants. Pediatr Pulmonol 2019;54(1):73–81.

69. Jensen EA, Edwards EM, Greenberg LT, et al. Severity of bronchopulmonary dysplasia among very preterm infants in the United States. Pediatrics 2021; 148(1).
70. Gentle SJ, Travers CP, Nakhmani A, et al. Intermittent hypoxemia and bronchopulmonary dysplasia with pulmonary hypertension in preterm infants. Am J Respir Crit Care Med 2023;207(7):899–907.
71. Gentle SJ, Travers CP, Clark M, et al. Patent ductus arteriosus and development of bronchopulmonary dysplasia-associated pulmonary hypertension. Am J Respir Crit Care Med 2023;207(7):921–8.
72. Villamor E, van Westering-Kroon E, Bartoš F, et al. Patent ductus arteriosus and bronchopulmonary dysplasia-associated pulmonary hypertension: a systematic review and Bayesian meta-analysis. JAMA Network 2023;6(11):e2345299.
73. Vyas-Read S, Guglani L, Shankar P, et al. Atrial septal defects accelerate pulmonary hypertension diagnoses in premature infants. Front Pediatr 2018;6:342.
74. Choi EK, Jung YH, Kim HS, et al. The impact of atrial left-to-right shunt on pulmonary hypertension in preterm infants with moderate or severe bronchopulmonary dysplasia. Pediatr Neonatol 2015;56(5):317–23.
75. Webb MK, Cuevas Guaman M, Sexson Tejtel SK, et al. Atrial septal defect closure is associated with improved clinical status in patients ≤ 10 kg with bronchopulmonary dysplasia. Pulm Circ 2023 Oct 20;13(4):e12299.
76. Abman SH, Wolfe RR, Accurso FJ, et al. Pulmonary vascular response to oxygen in infants with severe BPD. Pediatrics 1985;75:80–4.
77. Abman SH, Schaffer MS, Wiggins JW, et al. Pulmonary vascular extraction of circulating norepinephrine in infants with BPD. Pediatr Pulmonol 1987;3:386–91.
78. Singh A, Feingold B, Rivera-Lebron B, et al. Correlating objective echocardiographic parameters in patients with pulmonary hypertension due to bronchopulmonary dysplasia. J Perinatol 2019;39:1282–90.
79. Nawaytou H, Steurer MA, Zhao Y, et al. Clinical utility of echocardiography in former preterm infants with bronchopulmonary dysplasia. J Am Soc Echocardiogr 2020;33:378–88.
80. Di Maria MV, Sontag MK, et al. Maturational changes in diastolic longitudinal myocardial velocity in preterm infants. J Am Soc Echocardiogr 2015;28: 1045–52.
81. Murase M, Ishida A. Serial pulsed Doppler assessment of pulmonary artery pressure in very low birth-weight infants. Pediatr Cardiol 2000;21:452–45783.
82. Ehrmann DE, Mourani PM, Abman SH, et al. Echocardiographic measurements of right ventricular mechanics in infants with bronchopulmonary dysplasia at 36 weeks postmenstrual age. J Pediatr 2018;203:210–7.
83. Mourani PM, Sontag MK, Younoszai A, et al. Clinical utility of echocardiography for the diagnosis and management of pulmonary vascular disease in young children with chronic lung disease. Pediatrics 2008;121:317–25.
84. Levy PT, Jain A, Nawaytou H, et al, Pediatric Pulmonary Hypertension Network PPHNet. Risk assessment and monitoring of chronic pulmonary hypertension in premature infants. J Pediatr 2020;217:199–209.
85. Rosenzweig EB, Bates A, Mullen MP, et al. Cardiac catheterization and hemodynamics in a multicenter cohort of children with pulmonary hypertension. Ann Am Thorac Soc 2022 Jun;19(6):1000–12. Rosenzweig.
86. Frank BS, Schäfer M, Grenolds A, et al. Acute vasoreactivity testing during cardiac catheterization of neonates with bronchopulmonary dysplasia-associated pulmonary hypertension. J Pediatr 2019;208:127–33.

87. Higano NS, Bates AJ, Gunatilaka CC, et al. Correction to: bronchopulmonary dysplasia from chest radiographs to magnetic resonance imaging and computed tomography: adding value. Pediatr Radiol 2022;52(12):2442.
88. Critser PJ, Higano NS, Lang SM, et al. Cardiovascular magnetic resonance imaging derived septal curvature in neonates with bronchopulmonary dysplasia associated pulmonary hypertension. J Cardiovasc Magn Reson 2020;22(1):50.
89. Latus H, Kuehne T, Beerbaum P, et al. Cardiac MR and CT imaging in children with suspected or confirmed pulmonary hypertension/pulmonary hypertensive vascular disease. Expert consensus statement on the diagnosis and treatment of paediatric pulmonary hypertension. The European Paediatric Pulmonary Vascular Disease Network, endorsed by ISHLT and DGPK. Heart 2016; 102(Suppl 2):ii30–i35.
90. Moledina S, Pandya B, Bartsota M, et al. Prognostic significance of cardiac magnetic resonance imaging in children with pulmonary hypertension. Circ Cardiovasc Imaging 2013;6(3):407–14.
91. Mourani PM, Ivy DD, Rosenberg AA, et al. Left ventricular diastolic dysfunction in bronchopulmonary dysplasia. J Pediatr 2008;152(2):291–3.
92. Sehgal A, Steenhorst JJ, McLennan DI, et al. The left heart, systemic circulation, and bronchopulmonary dysplasia: relevance to pathophysiology and therapeutics. J Pediatr 2020;225:13–22.e2.
93. Kumar KR, Clark DA, Kim EM, et al. Association of atrial septal defects and bronchopulmonary dysplasia in premature infants. J Pediatr 2018;202: 56–62.e2.
94. Thomas VC, Vincent R, Raviele A, et al. Transcatheter closure of secundum atrial septal defect in infants less than 12 months of age improves symptoms of chronic lung disease. Congenit Heart Dis 2012;7(3):204–11.
95. Lim DS, Matherne GP. Percutaneous device closure of atrial septal defect in a premature infant with rapid improvement in pulmonary status. Pediatrics 2007; 119(2):398–400.
96. Drossner DM, Kim DW, Maher KO, et al. Pulmonary vein stenosis: prematurity and associated conditions. Pediatrics 2008;122(3):e656–61.
97. Mahgoub L, Kaddoura T, Kameny AR, et al. Pulmonary vein stenosis of ex-premature infants with pulmonary hypertension and bronchopulmonary dysplasia, epidemiology, and survival from a multicenter cohort. Pediatr Pulmonol 2017;52(8):1063–70.
98. Reyes-Hernandez ME, Bischoff AR, Giesinger RE, et al. Echocardiography assessment of left ventricular function in extremely preterm infants, born less than 28 weeks gestation, with bronchopulmonary dysplasia and systemic hypertension. J Am Soc Echocardiogr 2023. S0894-7317-7.
99. Bensley JG, Moore L, De Matteo R, et al. Impact of preterm birth on the developing myocardium of the neonate. Pediatr Res 2018;83(4):880–8.
100. de Waal K, Costley N, Phad N, et al. Left ventricular diastolic dysfunction and diastolic heart failure in preterm infants. Pediatr Cardiol 2019;40(8):1709–15.
101. Sehgal A, Krishnamurthy MB, Clark M, et al. ACE inhibition for severe bronchopulmonary dysplasia - an approach based on physiology. Phys Rep 2018;6(17): e13821.
102. Goss KN, Beshish AG, Barton GP, et al. Early pulmonary vascular disease in young adults born preterm. Am J Respir Crit Care Med 2018;198(12):1549–58.
103. Lewandowski AJ, Raman B, Bertagnolli M, et al. Association of preterm birth with myocardial fibrosis and diastolic dysfunction in young adulthood. J Am Coll Cardiol 2021 Aug 17;78(7):683–92.

Pulmonary Hypertension in Developmental Lung Diseases

Olivier Danhaive, MD[a,b,*], Csaba Galambos, MD, PhD[c],
Satyan Lakshminrusimha, MD, MBBS[d], Steven H. Abman, MD[e]

KEYWORDS

- Newborn • Hypoxic respiratory failure • Alveolar capillary dysplasia
- Acinar dysplasia • Trisomy 21 • Genetics

KEY POINTS

- At birth, the pulmonary circulation undergoes a dramatic transition from its low pulmonary flow and high resistant state in utero, to a high flow and progressively decreasing pulmonary vascular resistance (PVR).
- During the next days to weeks of life, pulmonary artery pressure (PAP) and PVR continue to decline, achieving normal postnatal levels within the first weeks to months.
- In some newborns, PAP and PVR remain elevated and fail to respond to the normal birth-related stimuli of loss of fetal lung liquid, increases in inspired oxygen, and rhythmic distension of the lung with normal breathing efforts.

BACKGROUND

At birth, the pulmonary circulation undergoes a dramatic transition from its low pulmonary flow and high resistant state in utero, to a high flow and progressively decreasing pulmonary vascular resistance (PVR).[1] During the next days to weeks of life, pulmonary artery pressure (PAP) and PVR continue to decline, achieving normal postnatal levels within the first weeks to months.[2] In some newborns, PAP and PVR remain elevated and fail to respond to the normal birth-related stimuli of loss of fetal lung

[a] Division of Neonatology, Saint-Luc University Hospital, UCLouvain, Avenue Hippocrate 10, B-1200 Brussels, Belgium; [b] Department of Pediatrics, University of California San Francisco, 530 Parnassus Avenue, San Francisco, CA 94143, USA; [c] Department of Pathology and Laboratory Medicine, University of Colorado Anschutz School of Medicine, 13001 East 17th Place, Aurora, CO 80045, USA; [d] Department of Pediatrics, University of California, UC Davis Children's Hospital, 2516 Stockton Boulevard, Sacramento CA 95817, USA; [e] Department of Pediatrics, The Pediatric Heart Lung Center, University of Colorado Anschutz Medical Campus, Mail Stop B395, 13123 East 16th Avenue, Aurora, CO 80045, USA
* Corresponding author. Division of Neonatology, Saint-Luc University Hospital, Avenue Hippocrate 10, B-1200 Brusssels, Belgium.
E-mail address: olivier.danhaive@saintluc.uclouvain.be

Clin Perinatol 51 (2024) 217–235
https://doi.org/10.1016/j.clp.2023.12.001
0095-5108/24/© 2023 Elsevier Inc. All rights reserved.
perinatology.theclinics.com

liquid, increase in inspired oxygen, and rhythmic distension of the lung with normal breathing efforts. In many of these infants, high PVR leads to extrapulmonary right-to-left shunt across the patent ductus arteriosus or foramen ovale, leading to striking hypoxemia.

This condition, known as persistent pulmonary hypertension of the newborn (PPHN), often contributes to hypoxemia associated with diverse cardiac or respiratory disorders, including meconium aspiration syndrome, sepsis, perinatal stress or idiopathic, requiring aggressive clinical strategies, including mechanical ventilation, pulmonary hypertension-targeted drug therapies, such as inhaled nitric oxide, pulmonary vasodilators, and extracorporeal membrane oxygenation (ECMO) therapy in severe cases.[3]

In some cases, PPHN can be the initial clinical manifestation of a genetic disorder of lung development. With an incidence in the range of 1 to 2 per 1000 live births, PPHN is a "nonrare disease" with an incidence similar to early-onset sepsis in population-based studies.[4–6] Yet, the incidence of genetic diseases underlying pediatric pulmonary hypertension, if largely unknown, is estimated to be of a much smaller magnitude, in the order of 1 to 10 per million.[7] In addition, PPHN due to genetic developmental lung diseases (DLDs) can often be refractory to clinical interventions, requiring prolonged ECMO treatment and slow or poor resolution of high PVR, cardiac dysfunction and hypoxemia, which likely reflects underlying lung hypoplasia and structural lung interstitial and vascular disease.[8]

In addition, neonatal PH associated with diverse genetic DLDs is often severe with many clinical concerns, has high early mortality, and can have uncertain late outcome. Thus, a major challenge is the recognition of these diseases among neonates presenting with hypoxic respiratory failure and PPHN. Early identification is important because it may lead to a precise diagnosis, allow for targeted management and follow-up, inform decisions for care orientation, provide families with definitive answers and counseling, and generate questions and advance research, among other benefits.

DLDs have been historically discovered and classified based on their histopathological phenotype.[9] However, the expanding discovery of molecular etiologies underlying these diseases increasingly reveals that genotypes and phenotypes do not strictly overlap. Classifying DLD based on their genetic cause offers the advantage of connecting to specific molecular mechanisms, which is of great importance for the development of targeted therapies and future curative approaches.[10,11] In this review, we present a genotype-based approach of the main genetic disorders and syndromes associated with primary or secondary neonatal hypoxic respiratory failure, review their clinical and histopathological phenotypes, and provide clinicians with indications for early recognition, diagnostic workup, and targeted management (**Table 1**).

DISORDERS OF THE *FOXF1* GENE AND CLUSTER

The first description of a DLD causing lethal hypoxic respiratory failure in neonates dates back to 1948[12] (**Fig. 1**). Since then, more than 200 cases were reported, allowing to define a specific histopathological phenotype coined alveolar capillary dysplasia with misaligned pulmonary veins (ACDMPV). Mono-allelic inactivating mutations (missense, nonsense, and frameshift indels) and genomic deletions of the FOXF1 gene at the 16q24.1 locus were identified as the main molecular cause of ACDMPV.[13] The vast majority of FOXF1 variants are de novo and originate from the maternal chromosome, supporting lung paternal imprinting of the 16q24.1 locus.[14] Some familial cases are reported, suggesting complex inheritance mechanisms.[15]

Table 1
Correlations among clinical presentation, phenotypic classification, genetic causes, and inheritance in primary lung diseases associated with PPHN or infantile PAH

Phenotypic Classification	Clinical Presentation	Rare Variants Associated	Inheritance
ACDMPV	Refractory PPHN	*FOXF1*, del16q24.1 LINC01081 LINC01082	Autosomal dominant, mostly de novo
AD CAD	Refractory PPHN, stillborn PPHN, infantile PAH	*TBX4*, del17q23.2 *FGF10* *FGFR2*	Autosomal dominant, mostly de novo, occasionally inherited
Idiopathic pulmonary arterial hypertension	Mostly pediatric or adult onset Rarely, neonatal or infantile onset	*BMPR2, ACVRL1/ALK1, SMAD9, SOX17, ENG, GDF2, ABCC8, KNCA5, KCNA1, ATP13A1, CAV1, EIF2AK4**	Autosomal dominant except EIF2AK4 (autosomaal recessive)
Surfactant dysfunction diseases	Neonatal RDS	*SFTPB*	Autosomal recessive, mostly inherited; 121ins2 >75% cases
		ABCA3	Autosomal recessive, inherited or de novo, mostly private variants
		SFTPC	Autosomal dominant, inherited (I73 T) or de novo.
		NKX2.1, del14q13.3	Autosomal dominant, inherited or de novo
	chILD	*SFTPC*	Autosomal dominant, inherited (I73 T) or de novo
		NKX2.1, del14q13.3	Autosomal dominant, inherited or de novo
		ABCA3	Autosomal recessive or dominant (E292 V), inherited or de novo; rarely, compound ABCA3/SFTPC heterozygosity
		Ultrarare: RAB5B, SFTPA1, SFTPA2, FLNA, MUCSB	Autosomal dominant
	Alveolar proteinosis	*CSF2RA*, CSFR2B, MARS1*	Autosomal dominan except MARS1(autosomal recessive)

(continued on next page)

Table 1
(continued)

Phenotypic Classification	Clinical Presentation	Rare Variants Associated	Inheritance
PIG NEHI	Persistent tachypnea of infancy, chILD	unknown	Unknown
Down syndrome	PPHN, hypoxic respiratory failure, chronic PAH	**Trisomy 21** 21q22.3 duplication	Mostly sporadic

In bold, most typical molecular defects.

Abbreviations: ACDMPV, alveolar capillary dysplasia with misaligned pulmonary veins; AD, acinar dysplasia; CAD, congenital alveolar dysplasia; chILD, childhood interstitial lung disease; NEHI, neuroendocrine cell hyperplasia of infancy; PAH, pulmonary arterial hypertension; PIG, pulmonary interstitial glycogenosis; PPHN, persistent pulmonary hypertension of the newborn; RDS, respiratory distress syndrome.

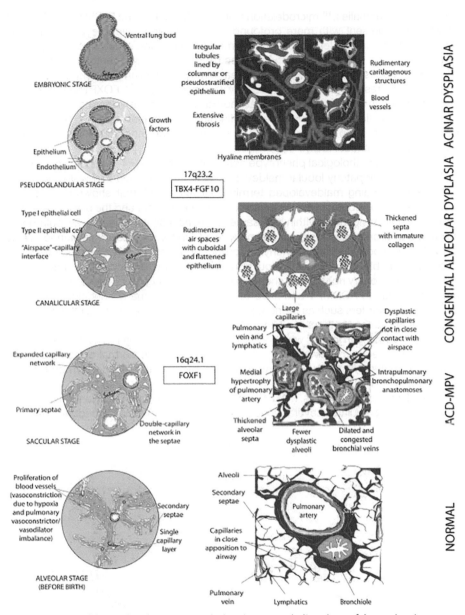

Fig. 1. Stages of lung development and developmental disorders of lung development. Embryonal, pseudoglandular, canalicular, saccular, and alveolar stages of lung development are shown. Mutations of the TBX4 gene and deletions in the 17q23.2 locus result in acinar dysplasia or congenital alveolar dysplasia. Typical histologic features of these conditions are shown in the illustration. (Image Courtesy of Dr. Satyan Lakshminrusimha.)

ACDMPV is almost uniformly lethal in the first weeks of life; however, some infants have few or no respiratory symptoms at birth and present with pulmonary arterial hypertension (PAH) during the first months or years of life.[16,17] Although point mutations in FOXF1 are occasionally associated with gastrointestinal (bowel malrotation) and urinary tract anomalies,[18] microdeletions of the FOX cluster (MTHFSD, FOXC2, and FOXL1) may present with more profound syndromic anomalies beyond ACDMPV, such as hypoplastic left heart syndrome or gastrointestinal and esophageal atresia.[13,19] Less severe clinical phenotypes reported in family members of ACDMPV pedigrees suggest that FOXF1-related disease may have a variable penetrance and a spectrum of presentations that is possibly underestimated.[14] FOXF1 variants have been identified in subjects with Vertebral anomalies, Anorectal malformations, Cardiovascular anomalies, Tracheoesophageal fistula, Esophageal atresia, Renal and/or radial anomalies, Limb defects (VACTERL) syndrome and other digestive and urinary malformations without ACDMPV.[20]

The lung histopathological phenotype associated with FOXF1 variants is characterized by diffuse or patchy lobular maldevelopment, an expanded thin-walled vascular network surrounding maldeveloped terminal airway/alveoli that shows a paucity of capillaries making contact with the alveolar basal membrane, and the presence of pulmonary veins mislocated within the same bronchovascular sheaths as pulmonary arteries and bronchioles reside, a hallmark of ACDMPV.[21] These "misaligned" veins actually correspond to intraparenchymal bronchopulmonary anastomoses that allow deoxygenated blood to bypass the pulmonary bed via the bronchial circulation, leading to intrapulmonary right-to-left shunt and hypoxemia (**Fig. 2**).[22] These anastomoses are not specific to ACDMPV and have been described in many conditions including severe lung disorders such as bronchopulmonary dysplasia and congenital diaphragmatic hernia among others.[22–25] In ACDMPV, the histopathological features are diffusely distributed in infants who die shortly after birth, whereas a patchy distribution of deficient alveolar/microvessel formation alternating with normal-appearing areas characterizes lung histology of infants with late presentation, milder symptoms and a prolonged survival[26] (**Fig. 3**).

During lung morphogenesis, FOXF1 is expressed throughout the splanchnic mesenchyme, where it regulates several signaling pathways, such as sonic hedgehog (SHH),

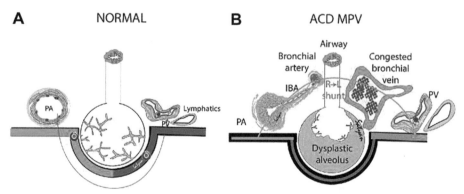

Fig. 2. Physiology of alveolar capillary dysplasia (ACDMPV). (*A*) Normal alveolar and capillary relationship is shown in A. PA, pulmonary artery; PV, pulmonary vein. The pink arrow refers to normal transit of blood through the pulmonary capillaries engaging in gas exchange with the alveoli. (*B*) Physiology of ACDMPV showing remodeled pulmonary arteries, intrapulmonary bronchopulmonary anastomoses (IBA), dilated and congested bronchial veins (often confused as malaligned pulmonary veins), normally located PV and lymphatics along with dysplastic capillaries and dysplastic alveoli. The blue arrow shows a right-to-left shunt (R → L) through the anastomoses between PA → IBA → bronchial artery → bronchial vein → PV bypassing the alveoli, leading to hypoxemia. (Image Courtesy of Dr. Satyan Lakshminrusimha.)

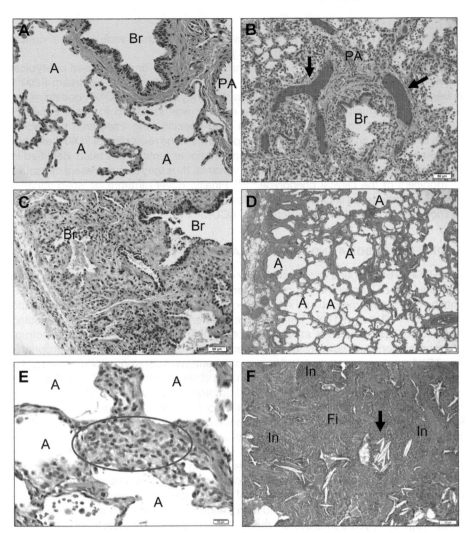

Fig. 3. Histologic spectrum of neonatal lung disease (*A*) normal lung (20×) with delicate interstitium separating alveoli (A) and a thinned pulmonary artery (PA) accompanies a small bronchiole (Br). (*B*) Alveolar capillary dysplasia (20×) shows underdeveloped acini with thickened PA and adjacent thin walled congested blood vessels (*arrows*) of intrapulmonary bronchopulmonary anastomosis (formally known as misaligned pulmonary veins or MPV). (*C*) Congenital alveolar dysplasia (20×) with markedly thickened interstitium separating dysplastic Br structures. (*D*) Down syndrome lung (10×) is characterized by markedly enlarged and simplified alveolar structures. (*E*) PIG (40×) shows that alveoli are separated by markedly cellular interstitium that contains numerous immature mesenchymal cells with pale and bubbly cytoplasm (*circled*). (*F*) Surfactant deficiency syndrome (10×) is characterized markedly remodeled acini showing extensive inflammation (In), fibrosis (Fi), and cholesterol clefts (*arrow*).

critical for normal alveolar and vascular development.[27] In ACDMPV, FOXF1 variants disrupt gene expression in endothelial cell progenitors, inhibit pulmonary vasculogenesis, and increase VEGF signaling, resulting in deficient alveolar microvasculature and aberrant expansion of systemic (bronchial) microvessels.[26] FOXF1 variants also disrupt bone morphogenetic protein (BMP)/transforming growth factor beta (TGFβ) signaling in endothelial and pulmonary vascular smooth muscle cells, a critical pathway in pulmonary hypertension pathogenesis.[27,28]

Complex posttranscriptional mechanisms may account for unexplained or atypical phenotypes in certain cases of ACDMPV. Hypermethylation of an upstream FOXF1 enhancer may contribute to FOXF1 haploinsufficiency caused by FOXF1 coding mutations, and hypermethylation of FOXF1's exon 1 was identified in some cases of ACDMPV without coding variants.[29] The lung-specific long intergenic noncoding RNAs LINC01081 and LINC01082 are of importance in the regulation of FOXF1 expression, and deletions disrupting this upstream enhancer region have been identified in cases both with and without FOXF1 coding variants, thus they may represent causative or modifiers of the clinical phenotype.[30,31] Finally, novel ultrarare de novo variants emerge in other genes such as ESRP1, a downstream gene in the FOXF1 pathway,[31,32] as more genomic studies are performed in ACDMPV cases.[33,34]

DISORDERS OF T-BOX 4 AND THE FIBROBLAST GROWTH FACTOR 10 PATHWAY

The TBX4 (T-box 4) gene encodes a highly conserved transcription factor acting as a key regulator of lung branching morphogenesis and hind limb formation. TBX4 variants have recently emerged as the most frequent genetic cause of PAH in the pediatric population.[35] Because TBX4 variants have different organ manifestations, including foot anomalies and the small patella syndrome (OMIM 147891), and a broad spectrum of manifestations and severity, using the term "TBX4 syndrome" may be appropriate. The TBX4 syndrome is caused by de novo or inherited (<10%) monoallelic small nucleotide variants (SNVs) and genomic deletions on chromosome 17q23.2, most of which encompass both TBX4 and TBX2 genes. Functional assessment of SNVs in a large cohort showed that these variants, mostly private, were missense, nonsense, or frameshift mutations resulting either in partial/complete loss-of-function or in gain-of-function, the latter being associated with later onset and lesser severity.[36]

Clinical manifestations associated with TBX4 variants include severe PPHN, but TBX4-associated PH can also present later during infancy, childhood, and even in adulthood.[37,38] In these cases, the clinical course is often similar to idiopathic or other forms of PAH, often with mild or no signs of chronic respiratory disease.[39] About 20% will declare in the perinatal period, 40% in childhood, and 40% in adulthood, with a median age of 14 years (interquartile range: 2–48).[36] Skeletal manifestations are found either isolated or in association with lung disease but are inconsistently reported, thus their prevalence is difficult to estimate. In a pediatric cohort of TBX4 carriers with PAH, 11 out of 14 infants showed characteristic foot anomalies.[40] Other associated anomalies include congenital heart defects (persistent patent ductus arteriosus, atrial and ventricular septal defects) and neurologic anomalies (hearing loss, developmental delay, and other), the latter being more prevalent in deletion carriers compared with SNVs.[40] We and others have shown that TBX4 variant carriers may present with PPHN in the neonatal period, which apparently resolves upon discharge, then relapses as PAH in the first months or years of life.[40] The prevalence of TBX4 variants in PPHN subjects is unknown. TBX4 variants may also underlie a lethal form of DLD presenting as critical hypoxic respiratory failure at birth, refractory to ventilation, pulmonary vasodilators, and ECMO[41] (**Fig. 4**).

Histopathological studies in TBX4 carriers with neonatal hypoxic respiratory failure have demonstrated a spectrum of developmental anomalies of the lung, which seems to be arrested at the pseudoglandular stage in the acinar dysplasia phenotype, or at the canalicular/early saccular stage in congenital alveolar dysplasia (see **Fig. 1**).[41,42] Lung biopsies and autopsy samples obtained at a later age showed a progression of distal

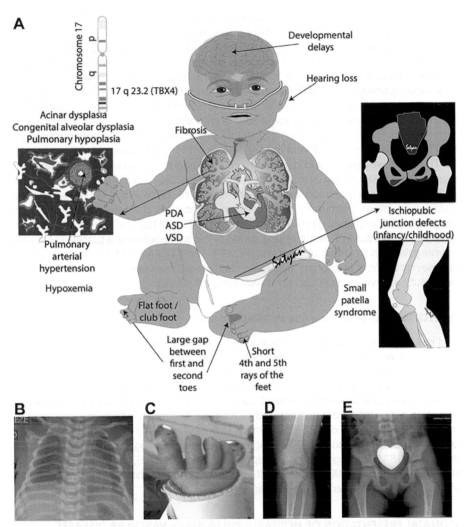

Fig. 4. (*A*) Clinical features associated with TBX4 variants. Developmental lung disorders ranging from pulmonary hypoplasia to acinar dysplasia, skeletal, cardiac, and neurologic anomalies can occur in these infants. (*B*) Chest x-ray of a 1-day-old TBX4 variant carrier with PPHN, showing small clear lungs with few vascular markings. (*C*) Foot caption of a newborn with TBX4 variant sowing suggestive first toe anomalies. (*D*) Knee x-ray of a 10-year-old child with no identifiable patella. (*E*) Pelvis x-ray of the same infant showing small iliac wings and wide ischiopubic junction. ([A] Image Courtesy of Dr. Satyan Lakshminrusimha; [C] Image Courtesy of Dr. Steven Abman; and [D and E] Image Courtesy of Dr. N. Ullmann.)

lung anomalies, with simplified alveolar structures, pulmonary arterial hypertensive remodeling and plexiform lesions, intrapulmonary bronchopulmonary anastomoses, and airway wall thickening[40] (see **Fig. 3**). In addition, mesenchymal maldevelopment including ectopic vessels, smooth muscle and bone formations characterize the lung histopathology in late-stage TBX4 syndrome.[43] These studies reveal the complex pathophysiology of pulmonary hypertension in the TBX4 syndrome, in association with a diffuse lung disease involving both the airways and the vasculature (see **Fig. 3**).

TBX4 is expressed in lung mesenchyme from the earliest phases of development and is a key regulator of branching morphogenesis in the distal lung through several pathways, including the fibroblast growth factor 10 (FGF10) pathway. TBX4 orchestrates the mesenchymal-epithelial cross talk though complex interactions with important epithelial factors such as NK2 homeobox 1 (NKX2.1), sex determining region Y -box transcription factor 9 (SOX9), and vascular endothelial growth factor A (VEGFA).[44] Ultrarare mutations and deletions of the downstream TBX4 effectors, FGF10 and FGFR2, have been described in some infants with acinar dysplasia and other primary forms of PAH.[45,46] In addition, noncoding variants in regulatory elements upstream of the TBX4 locus have been found in association with hypomorphic coding variants in the TBX4 pathway genes and may play a role in modulating disease expression and severity.[47] TMEM100 is a critical factor in lung vascular development and maintenance, acting as a common downstream target of TBX4 and FGF10, as well as FOXF1 and other pulmonary hypertension-associated pathways such as bone morphogenetic protein 9 (BMP9).[48] Although no TMEM100 variants have been reported so far as cause of neonatal lung disease, this transmembrane protein is critically downregulated in DLDs associated with FOXF1[27] and TBX4/FGF10 variants,[33] as well as in severe bronchopulmonary dysplasia,[49] thus could represent a potential target for therapeutic interventions in various developmental disorders.

DEVELOPMENTAL LUNG DISEASE IN TRISOMY 21

PAH is a frequent comorbidity in Down syndrome, with a prevalence as high as 6% at the age of 1 year and 15% at 10 years of age.[50] Even though PAH is associated with congenital heart disease in the majority of affected infants, past postmortem studies have shown evidence of decreased alveolarization, peripheral lung cysts, persistence of the double-capillary network and intrapulmonary bronchopulmonary anastomoses, indicating a disruption of vascular and airway development, which may suggest an implication of this form of DLD in Down syndrome's mortality and morbidity.[51] Overexpression of chromosome 21 antiangiogenic factors collagen, type XVIII, alpha 1 chain (COL18A1), collagen, type IV, alpha 3 chain (COL4A3), and tissue inhibitor of metalloproteinases 3 (TIMP3) represents a plausible mechanism for impaired vascular and alveolar development in these infants.[52]

NEONATAL PRESENTATION OF HERITABLE PULMONARY VASCULAR DISEASES

Variants in several genes in the BMP/TGFβ pathway regulating cell proliferation and apoptosis in pulmonary vessels (bone morphogenetic protein receptor type II [BMPR2], activin A receptor type II-like 1/activin receptor-like kinase 1 [ACVRL1/ ALK1], mothers against decapentaplegic homolog 9 [SMAD9], sex determining region Y -box transcription factor 17 [SOX17], endoglin [ENG], growth/differentiation factor 2 [GDF2] and other) account for a large subset of heritable PAH in adult cohorts, the most frequent being BMPR2.[35] Transmembrane channel genes such as ABCC8, KNCA5, and ATP13A1, and transmembrane receptors such as KDR (encoding the VEGFR2 receptor) and the caveolin-encoding gene CAV1 also account for a minor subset of cases. EIF2AK4 variants underlie a rare form of PAH known as pulmonary veno-occlusive disease or pulmonary capillary hemangiomatosis.[53] Rare variants of some of these genes are enriched in the pediatric PAH population, particularly TBX4 and BMPR2, but the contribution of these variants to PPHN or infantile PAH has been poorly studied to date. De novo variants account for a large proportion of pediatric PAH, due to severity-related negative selection.[54] Overall, the contribution of "adult" and "pediatric" PAH genes in PPHN is currently unknown, and large registries and population-based studies are warranted in order to elucidate this question.

DIFFERENTIAL DIAGNOSIS: DISORDERS OF THE SURFACTANT SYSTEM AND CHILDHOOD INTERSTITIAL LUNG DISEASES

Genetic disorders of surfactant homeostasis, also designated as surfactant dysfunction diseases, may present as hypoxic respiratory failure at birth or early onset interstitial lung disease, most typically those caused by surfactant protein B (SFTPB)[55] and ABCA3 biallelic variants,[56] and more rarely by monoallelic variants of the surfactant protein C (SFTPC)[57] and NKX2.1 genes, the latter encoding thyroid transcription factor-1 (TTF-1).[58] In these infants, the prominent parenchymal disease is often accompanied by pulmonary hypertension, secondary to hypoxia or chronic lung disease. TTF-1 is a transcription factor regulating several surfactant-related proteins but also involved in lung, brain, and thyroid development, and the clinical phenotype of NKX2.1 mutants include variable degrees of pulmonary, neurologic, and endocrine symptoms (the "brain-lung-thyroid syndrome"). NKX2.1 plays a key role in fetal alveolar development.[59] Features such as alveolar simplification have been described in certain infants carrying NKX2.1 variants[60,61] and NKX2.1 has recently been identified as one of the causal genes of acinar dysplasia,[62] suggesting that NKX2.1-related respiratory manifestations may be regarded as the expression of a developmental lung disorder beyond surfactant deficiency. Additional ultrarare variants in other genes (including RAB5B,[63] SFTPA1/2,[64] CSF2RA/B,[65] FLNA,[66] MARS,[67] and MUC5B[68]) have been described in infants with a surfactant dysfunction disease phenotype but no data are currently available on the prevalence of these disorders and their relevance in PPHN. Overall, surfactant dysfunction diseases may mimic the neonatal and infantile presentations of DLD and should be considered in the genetic workup of neonatal PH, even in the absence of striking lung parenchymal disease.

Childhood interstitial lung diseases (chILD) are a heterogeneous group of uncommon disorders characterized by impaired gas exchange and diffuse infiltrates on lung imaging.[9] Among these, pulmonary interstitial glycogenosis (PIG) and neuroendocrine cell hyperplasia of infancy (NEHI) are two disorders of elusive etiology with an onset in infancy.[69] Immature interstitial cells of PIG, thought to have functions similar to those of mesenchymal stem cells[70] or lipofibroblasts[71], have been described in lung samples of infants and children with a wide variety of DLD[72] including TBX4 syndrome, suggesting a possible, yet unexplored overlap between these 2 entities.[40]

DLD associated with lung hypoplasia and thoracic malformations such as congenital diaphragmatic hernia[73] is beyond the scope of this review and discussed in a different article in this issue.

THE CONTRIBUTION OF PATHOLOGY AND GENETICS IN PRECISION DIAGNOSIS

Genetic analyses and lung histopathology are two mainstems for the diagnosis of DLDs. They yield complementary but distinct information and should be integrated in the diagnostic workflow based on clinical presentation and time course, deep phenotyping, and available resources. Rapid precision diagnosis may be critical for care orientation in infants with hypoxic respiratory failure unresponsive to treatment.

Lung histopathology is critical for initial diagnosis and precision phenotyping of DLDs.[9] Distinct entities described historically have constituted a basis for classification. However, advances in genetic and genomic testing have allowed to classify DLD based on their molecular etiologies, more accurate and relevant for precision therapies. The ACDMPV phenotype has a strong correlation with FOXF1 disorders. However, acinar dysplasia and congenital alveolar dysplasia likely represent a continuum of developmental anomalies and have been described in DLDs of different genetic etiologies, thus lack specificity for precision diagnosis. Histopathology phenotypes in surfactant dysfunction diseases are also heterogeneous, and multiple labeling may be necessary for identification of specific disorders.

Electron microscopy may be contributive for diagnosis, as specific lamellar bodies anomalies have been described[56,74] but this technique requires specific technology and pathologist's expertise, and its availability is limited. Histopathology diagnosis encounters some limitations. Surgical lung biopsy is an invasive procedure with potential risks of complications. Biopsy samples provide limited amounts of peripheral lung tissue; however, radiology guidance significantly increases the likelihood of sampling the diseased areas and current surgical techniques limit these inconveniences. Given their mostly diffuse nature, nonuniformity is not a significant issue in DLD.[75] Since lung sample processing and labelling takes time and the interpretation of biopsies requires pathologists with a specific expertise in neonatal lung diseases,[75] histopathology may have less utility for acute care decisions in critically ill infants, but is still essential for retrospective diagnosis and for the interpretation of genetic findings, even if postmortem.

Genetic testing will ultimately allow for precision diagnosis and, potentially, orient targeted management. Targeted gene testing by Sanger sequencing of the main DLD genes (FOXF1, TBX4, and FGF10) is a valid and, possibly, fast approach, and may be an effective strategy in suggestive presentations, such as unexplained neonatal hypoxic respiratory failure, even more so when associated with typical extrapulmonary malformations. Extended gene panels by next-generation sequencing, allowing testing for rarer causes of DLD and disorders mimicking DLD (surfactant disorders, primary PAH), may be a time-effective and cost-effective approach according to available resources. Comparative genomic hybridization or similar array testing for genomic copy number variations should be performed in any case, given the established role of genomic deletions in DLDs. Whole exome sequencing (WES), possibly applied to family trio, broadens further the capacity of detecting ultrarare gene variants, assessing their potential pathogenicity, and elucidating complex inheritance. Finally, testing for noncoding variants either selectively of by whole-genome sequencing (WGS) can be necessary in unexplained cases. The sequence and timing of these tests will be determined by the clinical requests and resource availability. Fast next generation sequencing (NGS) tests (panels, WES, and WGS) with a daylong or weeklong turnover are emerging in selected academic institutions, with a high yield for the identification of rare genetic diseases, and may become a preferred model for rapid, noninvasive precision diagnosis in DLD.[76,77] Given the complexity of molecular mechanisms at play, these tests may require advanced resources to be performed and a deep expertise for interpretation.

Rapid, systematic, and comprehensive genomic diagnoses have demonstrated a high diagnostic yield and a substantial benefit in assisting acute and long-term clinical decisions in neonatal and pediatric intensive care units.[77] However, many questions remain open regarding limitations, accessibility, and appropriateness of resource use for NGS-based techniques. The key difference between current and next-generation sequencing techniques is the targeted enrichment step: gene panels focus on a limited number of genes, WES include all protein-coding regions (~1%–2% of the genome), and WGS does not involve targeted enrichment. WGS has a marginally higher yield than WES in identifying disease-causing variants and can be used as a single test to capture nearly all known genetic variations, including single-nucleotide variants, small insertions/deletions (indels), and large copy-number variants. Conversely, WES has a lower cost per sample, a greater depth of coverage in target regions, fewer storage requirements, and is easier to analyze.[78] Time may be a limiting factor, especially in critically ill infants for whom a precision diagnosis is needed for care decisions. Gene panels, targeting a set number of genes at a higher sequencing depth and lower cost when compared with WES and WGS, may be completed in a few days in selected laboratories, allowing for molecular diagnosis in a matter of weeks; however, the number and specificity of genes included in the panel influences its success rate.

NGS technology generates considerable numbers of false positives, and the differentiation of sequencing errors from true mutations is not a straightforward task. Sanger sequencing is often necessary for the confirmation of novel variations. Moreover, the identification of disease-causing variants among tens of thousands of sequence changes requires annotation drawn from various sources and advanced filtering capabilities, using software tools often designated as "pipelines." Trio analyses—including the proband's parents—facilitate variant calling and improve diagnostic yield. Ultimately, precise phenotype correlations are important for assessing variant pathogenicity,[79] hence the importance of lung histology in the field of DLD. Overall, genetics and histopathology provide essential, often complementary information for precision diagnosis, clinical management, and research.

ACUTE AND LONG-TERM MANAGEMENT

Until recently, DLDs were mostly regarded as lethal, and a diagnosis of ACDMPV or acinar dysplasia would often lead to redirection of care on an ethical basis, in order to alleviate the burden on affected infants, their families, caregivers, and neonatal intensive care resources.[80] However, the emergence of atypical cases with prolonged survival for months or years with or without lung transplant challenges this vision.[16] Decisions of care should consider aggressive medical management and lung transplantation as a possible option in selected cases. More recently, a recent cohort study on TBX4 syndrome has shown that a substantial number of subjects presenting with critical hypoxic respiratory failure in the neonatal period have a biphasic clinical course, showing an initial resolution or improvement of symptoms with PH-targeted therapy, often allowing for discharge from the neonatal intensive care units (NICU), followed by relapsing PAH in the first months or years of life.[40] The majority of these infants will evolve with a more chronic course and may have a prolonged survival with medical therapies, only some of which require lung transplant at a later age. Hence, early precision diagnosis and prolonged multidisciplinary follow-up by expert teams may offer these patients the chance of a better prognosis.

Advances in genetic engineering bring new perspectives for the cure of genetic diseases by replacing or repairing the gene to correct cellular and organ function. Tools and techniques allowing to deliver genes, RNAs, or proteins using a variety of vehicles (vectors) allowing to deliver targeted cargoes to specific cells involved in the disorder. Disorders involving nuclear transcription factors such as TBX4 and FOXF1 pose a particular challenge as cell type, subcellular location, dosage, and timing are all critical for proper gene function. Comprehensive lung transcriptome analyses in newborns with histopathologically confirmed DLDs and genomically identified causative FOXF1[27] and TBX4[33] variants have contributed to elucidate the complex signaling pathways at play. Novel three-dimensional spatial transcriptomic approaches allow in-situ examinations of signaling between diseased vessels and airspaces and their environment in human samples.[81] Clustered regularly interspaced short palindromic repeats (CRISPR) technology for gene editing offer new possibilities for the correction of gene variants at specific sites in the human genome. Viral vectors have potentialities for transient or permanent gene correction but need to be engineered in order to target cell types of interest and avoid triggering undesirable host responses. Alternative vectors such as RNA, plasmid, or nanoparticles exist but have limited half-life and require repeated administration. Cell-based therapies with progenitor cells permanently integrating elective lung tissues and multiplying may represent a durable approach in the future. An alternative strategy is to use highly specific pharmacologic compounds to restore physiologic levels of transcription factors and correct the effect of haploinsufficiency. In a recent preclinical study, TanFe (Transcellular activator of nuclear FOXF1 expression), a small molecule compound that specifically increases FOXF1 protein concentrations in pulmonary endothelial cells by antagonizing FOXF1 degradation, was shown to restore proper angiogenesis in a human ACDMPV lung organoid model and to prevent mortality in a mouse model of FOXF1 haploinsufficiency.[82] The same investigators showed that nanoparticle-based STAT3 delivery in mice carrying a FOXF1 mutation affecting its binding capacity to STAT3—a downstream effector of angiogenesis—allowed to restore angiogenesis and alveologenesis, paving the way for future mutation-specific therapies.[83] Overall, these pioneering preclinical works offer concrete hope for developing pharmacologic precision therapies for ACDMPV and other DLDs.

SUMMARY

DLDs are rare and complex genetic syndromes that mostly present in the neonatal period with hypoxic respiratory failure and PPHN but have a broad spectrum of clinical manifestations, course, and severity. Identifying them and reaching a precision diagnosis is essential and requires advanced resources and expertise. Infants with refractory PPHN should preferentially be managed in level IV NICUs,[84] undergo fast genetic testing and possibly a lung biopsy in order to rapidly recognize DLD and identify the genetic cause, and an autopsy should be proposed in nonsurvivors. Neonates with PPHN amenable to therapy should undergo echocardiographic evaluation of pulmonary hypertension before and possibly after discharge, in particular if apparently idiopathic and/or associated with suggestive anomalies. Acute and long-term management of such infants should ideally be conducted in—or coordinated by—multidisciplinary teams in centers with extended diagnostic resources and appropriate expertise. Exciting preclinical work from basic science will likely lead to more precise interventions that are directed toward the targeted correction of specific genetic abnormalities and related downstream molecular signaling pathways to improve outcomes.

Best Practice Box

- Neonates and infants with atypical or persistent PPHN may need a genetic evaluation to rule out developmental disorders of lung development associated with hypoxemia and pulmonary hypertension.

- FOXF1 gene abnormalities are associated with ACD-MPV and can present with neonatal hypoxemia and pulmonary hypertension not responding to medical management with prolonged dependence on ECMO.

- TBX4 gene mutations are increasingly being recognized as cause for pulmonary hypertension and can be associated with lower limb abnormalities with variable age at presentation.

- Trisomy 21 with or without congenital heart disease is commonly associated with pulmonary hypertension.
- A combination of clinical findings, histopathology, and genetic studies may be needed for early diagnosis and prognostication.

DISCLOSURE

The authors have nothing to disclose.

REFERENCES

1. Steinhorn RH. Advances in neonatal pulmonary hypertension. Neonatology 2016; 109(4):334–44.
2. Rudolph AM. The changes in the circulation after birth. Their importance in congenital heart disease. Circulation 1970;41(2):343–59.
3. Fortas F, Di Nardo M, Yousef N, et al. Response to: life-threatening PPHN refractory to NO: therapeutic algorithm. Eur J Pediatr 2022;181(1):425–6.
4. Angus DC, Linde-Zwirble WT, Clermont G, et al. Epidemiology of neonatal respiratory failure in the United States: projections from California and New York. Am J Respir Crit Care Med 2001;164(7):1154–60.
5. Steurer MA, Jelliffe-Pawlowski LL, Baer RJ, et al. Persistent pulmonary hypertension of the newborn in late preterm and term infants in California. Pediatrics 2017; 139(1):e20161165.
6. Kuzniewicz MW, Puopolo KM, Fischer A, et al. A quantitative, risk-based approach to the management of neonatal early-onset sepsis. JAMA Pediatr 2017;171(4):365–71.
7. Li L, Jick S, Breitenstein S, et al. Pulmonary arterial hypertension in the USA: an epidemiological study in a large insured pediatric population. Pulm Circ 2017;7(1):126–36.
8. Kamp JC, Neubert L, Ackermann M, et al. A morphomolecular approach to alveolar capillary dysplasia. Am J Pathol 2022;192(8):1110–21.
9. Deutsch GH, Young LR, Deterding RR, et al. Diffuse lung disease in young children: application of a novel classification scheme. Am J Respir Crit Care Med 2007;176(11):1120–8.
10. Wambach JA, Nogee LM. A step toward treating a lethal neonatal lung disease. STAT3 and alveolar capillary dysplasia. Am J Respir Crit Care Med 2019;200(8): 961–2.
11. Cornfield DN, Nogee LM. Rare to "ubiquitous": alveolar capillary dysplasia, FOXF1, and a sly approach to angiogenesis. Am J Respir Crit Care Med 2023; 207(8):969–71.
12. Mac MH. Congenital alveolar dysplasia; a developmental anomaly involving pulmonary alveoli. Pediatrics 1948;2(1):43–57.
13. Stankiewicz P, Sen P, Bhatt SS, et al. Genomic and genic deletions of the FOX gene cluster on 16q24.1 and inactivating mutations of FOXF1 cause alveolar capillary dysplasia and other malformations. Am J Hum Genet 2009;84(6):780–91.
14. Sen P, Yang Y, Navarro C, et al. Novel FOXF1 mutations in sporadic and familial cases of alveolar capillary dysplasia with misaligned pulmonary veins imply a role for its DNA binding domain. Hum Mutat 2013;34(6):801–11.
15. Sen P, Gerychova R, Janku P, et al. A familial case of alveolar capillary dysplasia with misalignment of pulmonary veins supports paternal imprinting of FOXF1 in human. Eur J Hum Genet 2013;21(4):474–7.

16. Towe CT, White FV, Grady RM, et al. Infants with atypical presentations of alveolar capillary dysplasia with misalignment of the pulmonary veins who underwent bilateral lung transplantation. J Pediatr 2018;194:158–164 e151.

17. Edwards JJ, Murali C, Pogoriler J, et al. Histopathologic and genetic features of alveolar capillary dysplasia with atypical late presentation and prolonged survival. J Pediatr 2019;210:214–219 e212.

18. Jourdan-Voyen L, Touraine R, Masutti JP, et al. Phenotypic and genetic spectrum of alveolar capillary dysplasia: a retrospective cohort study. Arch Dis Child Fetal Neonatal Ed 2020;105(4):387–92.

19. Shaw-Smith C. Genetic factors in esophageal atresia, tracheo-esophageal fistula and the VACTERL association: roles for FOXF1 and the 16q24.1 FOX transcription factor gene cluster, and review of the literature. Eur J Med Genet 2010; 53(1):6–13.

20. Thiem CE, Stegmann JD, Hilger AC, et al. Re-sequencing of candidate genes FOXF1, HSPA6, HAAO, and KYNU in 522 individuals with VATER/VACTERL, VACTER/VACTERL-like association, and isolated anorectal malformation. Birth Defects Res 2022;114(10):478–86.

21. Bishop NB, Stankiewicz P, Steinhorn RH. Alveolar capillary dysplasia. Am J Respir Crit Care Med 2011;184(2):172–9.

22. Galambos C, Sims-Lucas S, Abman SH. Three-dimensional reconstruction identifies misaligned pulmonary veins as intrapulmonary shunt vessels in alveolar capillary dysplasia. J Pediatr 2014;164(1):192–5.

23. Galambos C, Sims-Lucas S, Abman SH. Histologic evidence of intrapulmonary anastomoses by three-dimensional reconstruction in severe bronchopulmonary dysplasia. Ann Am Thorac Soc 2013;10(5):474–81.

24. Galambos C, Sims-Lucas S, Ali N, et al. Intrapulmonary vascular shunt pathways in alveolar capillary dysplasia with misalignment of pulmonary veins. Thorax 2015;70(1):84–5.

25. Acker SN, Mandell EW, Sims-Lucas S, et al. Histologic identification of prominent intrapulmonary anastomotic vessels in severe congenital diaphragmatic hernia. J Pediatr 2015;166(1):178–83.

26. Guo M, Wikenheiser-Brokamp KA, Kitzmiller JA, et al. Single cell multiomics identifies cells and genetic networks underlying alveolar capillary dysplasia. Am J Respir Crit Care Med 2023;208(6):709–25.

27. Karolak JA, Gambin T, Szafranski P, et al. Perturbation of semaphorin and VEGF signaling in ACDMPV lungs due to FOXF1 deficiency. Respir Res 2021;22(1):212.

28. Wang G, Wen B, Deng Z, et al. Endothelial progenitor cells stimulate neonatal lung angiogenesis through FOXF1-mediated activation of BMP9/ACVRL1 signaling. Nat Commun 2022;13(1):2080.

29. Slot E, Boers R, Boers J, et al. Genome wide DNA methylation analysis of alveolar capillary dysplasia lung tissue reveals aberrant methylation of genes involved in development including the FOXF1 locus. Clin Epigenetics 2021;13(1):148.

30. Szafranski P, Dharmadhikari AV, Wambach JA, et al. Two deletions overlapping a distant FOXF1 enhancer unravel the role of lncRNA LINC01081 in etiology of alveolar capillary dysplasia with misalignment of pulmonary veins. Am J Med Genet 2014;164A(8):2013–9.

31. Szafranski P, Herrera C, Proe LA, et al. Narrowing the FOXF1 distant enhancer region on 16q24.1 critical for ACDMPV. Clin Epigenetics 2016;8:112.

32. Szafranski P, Gambin T, Dharmadhikari AV, et al. Pathogenetics of alveolar capillary dysplasia with misalignment of pulmonary veins. Hum Genet 2016;135(5): 569–86.

33. Karolak JA, Deutsch G, Gambin T, et al. Transcriptome and immunohistochemical analyses in TBX4- and FGF10-deficient lungs imply TMEM100 as a mediator of human lung development. Am J Respir Cell Mol Biol 2022;66(6):694–7.

34. Yildiz Bolukbasi E, Karolak JA, Szafranski P, et al. High-level gonosomal mosaicism for a pathogenic non-coding CNV deletion of the lung-specific FOXF1 enhancer in an unaffected mother of an infant with ACDMPV. Mol Genet Genomic Med 2022;10(11):e2062.

35. Zhu N, Gonzaga-Jauregui C, Welch CL, et al. Exome sequencing in children with pulmonary arterial hypertension demonstrates differences compared with adults. Circ Genom Precis Med 2018;11(4):e001887.

36. Prapa M, Lago-Docampo M, Swietlik EM, et al. First genotype-phenotype study in TBX4 syndrome: gain-of-function mutations causative for lung disease. Am J Respir Crit Care Med 2022;206(12):1522–33.

37. Eyries M, Montani D, Nadaud S, et al. Widening the landscape of heritable pulmonary hypertension mutations in paediatric and adult cases. Eur Respir J 2019;53(3):1801371.

38. Kerstjens-Frederikse WS, Bongers EM, Roofthooft MT, et al. TBX4 mutations (small patella syndrome) are associated with childhood-onset pulmonary arterial hypertension. J Med Genet 2013;50(8):500–6.

39. Thore P, Girerd B, Jais X, et al. Phenotype and outcome of pulmonary arterial hypertension patients carrying a TBX4 mutation. Eur Respir J 2020;55(5):1902340.

40. Galambos C, Mullen MP, Shieh JT, et al. Phenotype characterisation of TBX4 mutation and deletion carriers with neonatal and paediatric pulmonary hypertension. Eur Respir J 2019;54(2):1801965.

41. Vincent M, Karolak JA, Deutsch G, et al. Clinical, histopathological, and molecular diagnostics in lethal lung developmental disorders. Am J Respir Crit Care Med 2019;200(9):1093–101.

42. Suhrie K, Pajor NM, Ahlfeld SK, et al. Neonatal lung disease associated with TBX4 mutations. J Pediatr 2019;206:286–292 e281.

43. Doughty ES, Norvik C, Levin A, et al. Long-Term Effect of *TBX4* Germline Mutation on Pulmonary Clinico-Histopathologic Phenotype. Pediatr Dev Pathol 2023. 10935266231199933.

44. Karolak JA, Welch CL, Mosimann C, et al. Molecular function and contribution of TBX4 in development and disease. Am J Respir Crit Care Med 2023;207(7):855–64.

45. Schutz K, Schmidt A, Schwerk N, et al. Variants in FGF10 cause early onset of severe childhood interstitial lung disease: a detailed description of four affected children. Pediatr Pulmonol 2023.

46. Bzdega K, Karolak JA. Phenotypic spectrum of FGF10-related disorders: a systematic review. PeerJ 2022;10:e14003.

47. Karolak JA, Vincent M, Deutsch G, et al. Complex compound inheritance of lethal lung developmental disorders due to disruption of the TBX-FGF pathway. Am J Hum Genet 2019;104(2):213–28.

48. Pan J, Liu B, Dai Z. The role of a lung vascular endothelium enriched gene TMEM100. Biomedicines 2023;11(3):937.

49. Galambos C, Logan JW, Stankiewicz P, et al. Histologic features and decreased lung FOXF1 gene expression in severe bronchopulmonary dysplasia without a genetic diagnosis of alveolar capillary dysplasia. Pediatr Pulmonol 2023;58(10):2746–9.

50. Bush D, Galambos C, Ivy DD, et al. Clinical characteristics and risk factors for developing pulmonary hypertension in children with down syndrome. J Pediatr 2018;202:212–219 e212.

51. Bush D, Abman SH, Galambos C. Prominent intrapulmonary bronchopulmonary anastomoses and abnormal lung development in infants and children with down syndrome. J Pediatr 2017;180:156–162 e151.
52. Galambos C, Minic AD, Bush D, et al. Increased lung expression of anti-angiogenic factors in down syndrome: potential role in abnormal lung vascular growth and the risk for pulmonary hypertension. PLoS One 2016;11(8):e0159005.
53. Welch CL, Austin ED, Chung WK. Genes that drive the pathobiology of pediatric pulmonary arterial hypertension. Pediatr Pulmonol 2021;56(3):614–20.
54. Welch CL, Chung WK. Genetics and other omics in pediatric pulmonary arterial hypertension. Chest 2020;157(5):1287–95.
55. Somaschini M, Nogee LM, Sassi I, et al. Unexplained neonatal respiratory distress due to congenital surfactant deficiency. J Pediatr 2007;150(6):649–53, 653 e641.
56. Peca D, Cutrera R, Masotti A, et al. ABCA3, a key player in neonatal respiratory transition and genetic disorders of the surfactant system. Biochem Soc Trans 2015;43(5):913–9.
57. Peca D, Boldrini R, Johannson J, et al. Clinical and ultrastructural spectrum of diffuse lung disease associated with surfactant protein C mutations. Eur J Hum Genet 2016;24(5):780.
58. Peca D, Petrini S, Tzialla C, et al. Altered surfactant homeostasis and recurrent respiratory failure secondary to TTF-1 nuclear targeting defect. Respir Res 2011;12(1):115.
59. Lim K, Donovan APA, Tang W, et al. Organoid modeling of human fetal lung alveolar development reveals mechanisms of cell fate patterning and neonatal respiratory disease. Cell Stem Cell 2023;30(1):20–37 e29.
60. Hamvas A, Deterding RR, Wert SE, et al. Heterogeneous pulmonary phenotypes associated with mutations in the thyroid transcription factor gene NKX2-1. Chest 2013;144(3):794–804.
61. Galambos C, Levy H, Cannon CL, et al. Pulmonary pathology in thyroid transcription factor-1 deficiency syndrome. Am J Respir Crit Care Med 2010;182(4):549–54.
62. Soreze Y, Nathan N, Jegard J, et al. Acinar Dysplasia in a Full-Term Newborn with a NKX2.1 Variant. Neonatology 2023;1–4.
63. Huang H, Pan J, Spielberg DR, et al. A dominant negative variant of RAB5B disrupts maturation of surfactant protein B and surfactant protein C. Proc Natl Acad Sci U S A 2022;119(6). e2105228119.
64. Nathan N, Giraud V, Picard C, et al. Germline SFTPA1 mutation in familial idiopathic interstitial pneumonia and lung cancer. Hum Mol Genet 2016;25(8):1457–67.
65. Suzuki T, Sakagami T, Young LR, et al. Hereditary pulmonary alveolar proteinosis: pathogenesis, presentation, diagnosis, and therapy. Am J Respir Crit Care Med 2010;182(10):1292–304.
66. Carlens J, Johnson KT, Bush A, et al. Heterogenous disease course and long-term outcome of children's interstitial lung disease related to filamin A gene variants. Ann Am Thorac Soc 2022;19(12):2021–30.
67. Hadchouel A, Wieland T, Griese M, et al. Biallelic mutations of methionyl-tRNA synthetase cause a specific type of pulmonary alveolar proteinosis prevalent on reunion island. Am J Hum Genet 2015;96(5):826–31.
68. Alsamri MT, Alabdouli A, Alkalbani AM, et al. Genetic variants of small airways and interstitial pulmonary disease in children. Sci Rep 2021;11(1):2715.
69. Rauch D, Wetzke M, Reu S, et al. Persistent tachypnea of infancy. Usual and aberrant. Am J Respir Crit Care Med 2016;193(4):438–47.

70. Galambos C, Wartchow E, Weinman JP, et al. Pulmonary interstitial glycogenosis cells express mesenchymal stem cell markers. Eur Respir J 2020;56(4):2000853.
71. Deutsch GH, Young LR. Lipofibroblast phenotype in pulmonary interstitial glycogenosis. Am J Respir Crit Care Med 2016;193(6):694–6.
72. Cutz E, Chami R, Dell S, et al. Pulmonary interstitial glycogenosis associated with a spectrum of neonatal pulmonary disorders. Hum Pathol 2017;68:154–65.
73. Lingappan K, Olutoye OO 2nd, Cantu A, et al. Molecular insights using spatial transcriptomics of the distal lung in Congenital Diaphragmatic Hernia. Am J Physiol Lung Cell Mol Physiol 2023;325(4):L477–86.
74. Citti A, Peca D, Petrini S, et al. Ultrastructural characterization of genetic diffuse lung diseases in infants and children: a cohort study and review. Ultrastruct Pathol 2013;37(5):356–65.
75. Deutsch GH, Young LR. Lung biopsy in the diagnosis and management of chILD. Pediatr Pulmonol 2023.
76. Wojcik MH, D'Gama AM, Agrawal PB. A model to implement genomic medicine in the neonatal intensive care unit. J Perinatol 2023;43(2):248–52.
77. French CE, Delon I, Dolling H, et al. Whole genome sequencing reveals that genetic conditions are frequent in intensively ill children. Intensive Care Med 2019; 45(5):627–36.
78. Alfares A, Aloraini T, Subaie LA, et al. Whole-genome sequencing offers additional but limited clinical utility compared with reanalysis of whole-exome sequencing. Genet Med 2018;20(11):1328–33.
79. Richards S, Aziz N, Bale S, et al. Standards and guidelines for the interpretation of sequence variants: a joint consensus recommendation of the American college of medical genetics and genomics and the association for molecular pathology. Genet Med 2015;17(5):405–24.
80. Lazar DA, Olutoye OO, Cass DL, et al. Outcomes of neonates requiring extracorporeal membrane oxygenation for irreversible pulmonary dysplasia: the Extracorporeal Life Support Registry experience. Pediatr Crit Care Med 2012;13(2): 188 90.
81. Rao A, Barkley D, Franca GS, et al. Exploring tissue architecture using spatial transcriptomics. Nature 2021;596(7871):211–20.
82. Pradhan A, Che L, Ustiyan V, et al. Novel FOXF1-stabilizing compound TanFe stimulates lung angiogenesis in alveolar capillary dysplasia. Am J Respir Crit Care Med 2023;207(8):1042–54.
83. Pradhan A, Dunn A, Ustiyan V, et al. The S52F FOXF1 mutation inhibits STAT3 signaling and causes alveolar capillary dysplasia. Am J Respir Crit Care Med 2019;200(8):1045–56.
84. Stark AR, Pursley DM, Papile LA, et al. Standards for Levels of Neonatal Care: II, III, and IV. Pediatrics 2023;151(6):e2023061957.

Etiology, Diagnosis and Management of Persistent Pulmonary Hypertension of the Newborn in Resource-limited Settings

Prathik Bandiya, MD, DM[a],
Rajeshwari Madappa, MBBS, DCH, DNB (Pead)[b],*,
Ajay Raghav Joshi, MBBS, DCH, DNB (Pead)[b]

KEYWORDS

- Hypoxia • Respiratory failure • Pneumonia • Nitric oxide • Sildenafil

KEY POINTS

- Although the exact prevalence is not known, persistent pulmonary hypertension of the newborn (PPHN) is common (~2–4 out of 1000 live births) in low-and-middle-income countries (LMICs).
- Meconium aspiration syndrome, asphyxia and pneumonia/sepsis are common causes of PPHN in LMICs.
- Clinical diagnosis can be made in neonates with hypoxemic respiratory failure with labile hypoxemia and differential cyanosis but confirmation requires echocardiography.
- Supplemental oxygen, ventilator and hemodynamic support followed by sildenafil are common therapeutic strategies for PPHN in LMICs.
- Mortality can be as high as ~20% with PPHN in LMICs.

INTRODUCTION

Persistent pulmonary hypertension of the newborn (PPHN) is a syndrome of failed circulatory adaptation at birth and is relatively common in low-and-middle income countries (LMICs). PPHN in LMICs can be secondary to lung disease such as pneumonia or

a Department of Neonatology, Neonatal Unit, 1st Floor, Indira Gandhi Institute of Child Health, South Hospital complex, Dharmaram college Post, Bangalore - 560029; b Department of Pediatrics, SIGMA Hospital, P8/D, Thonachikoppal -Saraswathipuram Road, Mysore -570009 Karnataka, India
* Corresponding author. Thonachikoppal, Saraswathipuram Road, Mysore, Karnataka 570 009, India.
E-mail address: rajeesubbaiah@gmail.com

Clin Perinatol 51 (2024) 237–252
https://doi.org/10.1016/j.clp.2023.11.002
0095-5108/24/© 2023 Elsevier Inc. All rights reserved.
perinatology.theclinics.com

due to abnormal transition resulting in birth asphyxia often associated with meconium aspiration syndrome (MAS). This review focuses on the estimated incidence of PPHN, etiology and diagnostic and therapeutic challenges faced in LMICs. Although access to diagnostic modalities such as echocardiography may be limited in some regions of LMICs leading to underdiagnosis of PPHN, in some urban areas, overdiagnosis and unnecessary use of pulmonary vasodilators such as sildenafil may occur. We review diagnostic challenges faced in LMICs and provide an algorithm for the management of PPHN in these settings.

EPIDEMIOLOGY

The incidence of PPHN is considered to be 1.9 to 2 per 1000 live births in the United States.[1,2] There are no comprehensive registries in LMICs such as South Asia and sub-Saharan Africa to know the exact prevalence of PPHN.

The common antenatal factors associated with PPHN are prepregnancy and mid-pregnancy smoking, hypertension, diabetes, gestational age less than 37 weeks, maternal age greater than 30 years, high maternal body mass index, cesarean delivery, asthma, urinary tract infections, and anemia.[3–5] Antenatal exposure to certain medications increase the risk of PPHN. The common implicated medications are aspirin and other nonsteroidal anti-inflammatory drugs and selective serotonin reuptake inhibitors.[5]

Neonates born to mothers with lower socioeconomic status have higher incidence of PPHN. MAS and perinatal asphyxia contribute to majority of cases of secondary PPHN in LMICs. These are seen in populations of LMICs with poor access to antenatal and perinatal care.[6,7]

Fetal growth restriction (FGR) is an important cause of PPHN in developing countries. FGR accounts for nearly two-thirds of all low-birth-weight babies in India and nearly 75% of all FGR s are born in Asian continent followed by Africa and south America. FGR is also an important cause for MAS and perinatal asphyxia, which in turn increase the risk of PPHN.[8,9]

The Asian Persistent Pulmonary Hypertension of the Newborn Study (APPHN study), a multicenter retrospective study involving 7 level-III neonatal intensive care units (NICUs) from 6 Asian countries reported an incidence ranging from 1.2 to 4.6 per 1000 live births. Mortality rate from all the causes was 20.6%. MAS was the most common cause of PPHN (24.1% of cases).[10]

In a survey-based study conducted in India, majority of neonatal units (65%) admitted an average of 1 to 3 patients with PPHN per month. The surveyors reported the 3 most common noncardiac causes of PPHN. These were parenchymal lung diseases (97%), birth asphyxia (75%), and sepsis (52%); followed by respiratory distress syndrome (RDS; 44%), congenital diaphragmatic hernia (CDH; 16%) and pulmonary hypoplasia (2%). The most common clinical predictor of PPHN was labile oxygen saturations (86%) followed by preductal and postductal saturation difference (77%) and high fraction of inspired oxygen (Fio_2) requirements on respiratory support (73%). The mortality rate of PPHN observed was less than 10% at 58% NICUs, 10% to 30% at 30% NICUs, 30% to 50% at 10% NICUs and greater than 50% at 2% NICUs. The commonest causes of mortality with PPHN were birth asphyxia (45%), MAS (35%) and associated cardiac disease (33%). CDH (19%), primary or idiopathic PPHN (11%), sepsis (3%) and hypoplastic lungs (2%) were other causes.[11]

Arshad and colleagues evaluated cases of PPHN in Pakistan. Patients were predominantly (66.3%) male, with 64% being term (gestational age above 37 weeks). MAS (42.6%), birth asphyxia (39.3%), RDS (18.8%) and sepsis (27.0%) were found to be the common causes of PPHN. Morality was noted among 21.3% of cases.[12] In another study from Pakistan, common associated factors for PPHN were male sex (72.1%), cesarean section delivery (54.2%), positive pressure ventilation during resuscitation (44.2%), birth asphyxia (40.4%) and MAS (35.4%). Among premature infants, male sex (88.8%), cesarean-section delivery (77.7%), RDS (44.8%) and sepsis (44.4%) were commonly associated with PPHN. Mortality was 26.6% and was associated with cesarean section (71.4%) and birth asphyxia (57.1%).[13] Similarly, 2 studies from Thailand have reported the incidence of PPHN to be 2.8 per 1000 live births and between 0.38 and 0.99 per 1000 live births, respectively.[14,15]

In many studies from LMICs, asphyxia and MAS seem to be common precipitating causes of PPHN. In a study conducted in Rajasthan, 100 neonates with MAS were evaluated by echocardiography and 19% of these infants had PPHN.[16]

In an unpublished survey conducted by authors from 56 NICUs from LMICs including India, Brazil, Columbia, Belarus, Malaysia, Zimbabwe, and Guatemala, the median incidence of PPHN was 3.15%. The most common cause of PPHN was MAS (71.4%), pneumonia (14.3%) and perinatal asphyxia (7.1%) followed by transient tachypnea of newborn, CDH and prematurity (1.8% each) (**Fig. 1**). Echocardiography was available in 89.3% of the centers.

Data from the above studies suggest that the incidence of PPHN may be common in LMICs with a wide range (0.38–4.6 per 1000 live births), although lack of clear definition and lack of population-based studies make the determination of prevalence difficult. However, it is likely that given the high prevalence of sepsis and MAS along with birth asphyxia in LMICs, the prevalence of PPHN is likely higher in these countries compared with United States. Mortality seems to range from 21% to 27%.

CLINICAL FEATURES

Similar to high-income countries, neonates with PPHN present with labile hypoxemia and cyanosis disproportionate to lung disease in LMICs (**Fig. 2**). Not uncommonly, many of these infants are delivered at home or In community hospitals and referred

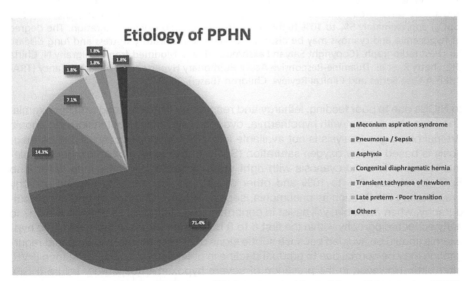

Etiology of PPHN

- Meconium aspiration syndrome
- Pneumonia / Sepsis
- Asphyxia
- Congenital diaphragmatic hernia
- Transient tachypnea of newborn
- Late preterm - Poor transition
- Others

Fig. 1. Common etiologies of PPHN among a survey conducted by authors among NICUs from LMICs. MAS and pneumonia are the most common causes of PPHN.

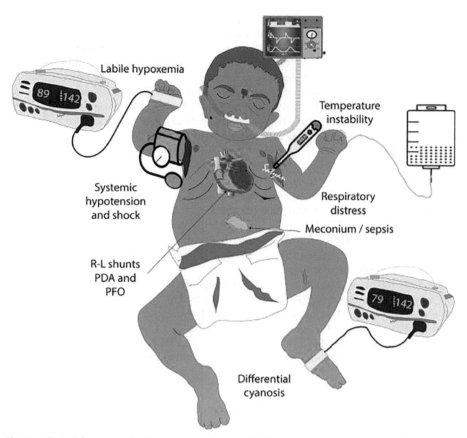

Fig. 2. Clinical features of PPHN among infants in LMICs. Asphyxia, meconium aspiration, and sepsis can be associated with labile hypoxemia, temperature instability, systemic hypotension, and shock. Differential cyanosis with right upper limb oxygen saturation by pulse oximetry (SpO$_2$) approximately 5% to 10% higher than the lower limb oxygen saturation. The degree of hypoxemia and cyanosis may be disproportionate to respiratory distress and lung disease on chest radiograph. (Copyright Satyan Lakshminrusimha. Modified from Panigrahy N, Chirla DK, Shetty R, et al. Thiamine-Responsive Acute Pulmonary Hypertension of Early Infancy (TRA-PHEI)-A Case Series and Clinical Review. Children (Basel). 2020;7(11).)

to NICUs due to poor feeding, lethargy and respiratory distress along with hypoxemia. They can also present with hypothermia, cyanosis, systemic hypotension and shock. Arterial blood gas analysis is not available in many community centers, hence diagnosis is based on low oxygen saturation (SpO$_2$) or cyanosis despite oxygen supplementation, differential cyanosis with right upper limb SpO$_2$ greater than lower limb SpO$_2$ by at least 5% to 10% and other symptoms secondary to primary etiology precipitating PPHN such as pneumonia, sepsis, or MAS. Chest x-ray and echocardiography, when available, will assist in confirming the diagnosis. Overdiagnosis due to early echocardiography within the first 6 to 8 hours after birth in infants with mild hypoxemia should be avoided because subtle signs of PPHN such as mild tricuspid regurgitation may be normal due to gradual decline in pulmonary vascular resistance (PVR) after birth. However, in the presence of severe hypoxemic respiratory failure (HRF), echocardiographic evidence of elevated PVR and absence of cyanotic congenital heart disease can confirm the diagnosis of PPHN.

The severity of HRF is often estimated by calculating oxygenation index (OI = Fio_2 × 100 × Paw / Pao_2), where Paw is mean airway pressure measured in cm H_2O and Pao_2 is measured in mm Hg. HRF is classified into mild (OI ≤ 15), moderate (15 to ≤ 25), severe (>25–40) and very severe or critical (>40).[17] In the absence of arterial blood gases, oxygen saturation index (OSI = Fio_2 × 100 × Paw / SpO_2) may be a potential alternative.[18,19] The advantage of OSI is that it is noninvasive, and it can be measured continuously by the assessment of preductal oxygenation (if pulse oximeter probe can be placed on the right upper limb). The disadvantage is that at extremes of oxygen saturation (<90% and >98%), it is not reliable because the slope of the oxygen dissociation curve is altered. OI can be approximately estimated from OSI by using the equation, OI = 0.745 + 1.783 × OSI.[18] For practical purposes, some clinicians use OI = OSI × 2.[19,20]

MANAGEMENT

The management can be broadly classified into supportive management, ventilation and oxygenation, pulmonary vasodilator therapy (including ildenafil and inhaled nitric oxide [iNO], if available) and other medications. In resource-limited settings in LMICs, availability of advanced ventilator modalities and iNO is limited, requiring long distance transfers for such therapy. Access to extracorporeal membrane oxygenation (ECMO) is extremely limited and available in select tertiary centers.

In the unpublished survey conducted by the authors regarding management of PPHN in LMICs, iNO requirement was present in 29.1% and ECMO in 3.6%. Oral sildenafil (80.4%) was the first-line medication in the majority of centers. Other medications used among these NICUs included IV milrinone (76.8%), IV sildenafil (60.7%), bosentan (25%) and IV prostaglandin E1 (PGE1) (23.2%).

Neonates without cardiac dysfunction commonly received norepinephrine (32%) or dopamine (25%) as the first-line vasopressor medication followed by epinephrine (23%), vasopressin (2%), dobutamine (11%) and milrinone (7%). Among neonates with hypotension and cardiac dysfunction by echocardiography, milrinone (54%) was the first drug of choice followed by dobutamine (22%) and epinephrine (14%). The average length of stay was around 14 days with a mortality rate of 18%.

Supportive Management

General supportive care is important in the management of PPHN. This includes maintenance of temperature, glucose, electrolytes such as sodium, calcium, and magnesium, hemoglobin, pH, blood pressure, fluid status, and oxygenation in normal range. With high prevalence of infections, appropriate cultures and antibiotic therapy is important. Avoiding acidosis and temperature management is critical to improve outcomes in asphyxia and MAS. There should be minimal handling with covering of eyes and ears and clustering of care should be practiced in these neonates. Sedation and analgesia can be considered in moderate-to-severe PPHN. There is no role of muscle relaxants in these cases, and its use has been shown to increase mortality.[21]

Oxygenation Target

In neonates with PPHN, oxygen saturation should be continuously monitored by placing the pulse oximeter probe in right upper limb (Preductal saturation). Saturation in the right upper limb should be in the low to mid 90s (see **Fig. 2**). Postductal saturation should be more than 80% provided there is no metabolic or lactic acidosis with good urine output. Hyperoxia should be avoided because it has shown to cause pulmonary vasoconstriction, increase the oxidative stress, and reduce the response to iNO.[21] However, availability of blenders may be limited increasing the risk of exposure to hyperoxia.[22]

In many special newborn care units (SNCUs) in India, oxygen is primarily administered through oxygen hood at higher rates of 5 to 10 L/min.[23] In a large cross-sectional cluster survey done across medical college hospitals (MCH) and district hospitals (DH) across India, 68% of MCH and 36% of DH had facility of continuous positive airway pressure (CPAP), and among the units who used CPAP, only 50% had facility of air-oxygen blenders to deliver CPAP.[22]

Many neonates with mild-to-moderate distress, especially with transient tachypnea of newborn are managed without CPAP and mostly with oxygen hood at high flow rates. Apart from wastage of oxygen and other oxygen-related toxicities, provision of 100% oxygen via hood without CPAP results in worsening of PPHN due to atelectasis by nitrogen wash out.[23,24] In the presence of parenchymal lung disease, end-expiratory pressure by CPAP or peak end expiratory pressure (PEEP) should be provided and providing high concentrations of oxygen without airway pressure should be avoided.

Ventilation

Many cases of PPHN secondary to MAS and pneumonia can be managed by CPAP or noninvasive ventilation. If intubation is necessary, hyperinflation and underinflation should be avoided because it leads to increase in PVR. PVR is least at functional residual capacity (FRC); hence, optimum PEEP/MAP to achieve FRC is essential to reduce PVR. Gentle ventilation strategies with optimal PEEP/MAP with moderate tidal volume and permissive hypercapnia should be followed. This will ensure optimal ventilation with minimizing ventilator-induced lung injury. Among neonates with parenchymal lung disease such as MAS and pneumonia, 8 to 9 rib expansion is considered optimal. Limited access to portable x-ray machines may limit frequent radiological monitoring. Increased adaptation of lung ultrasound techniques at the bedside in LMICs may potentially decrease the need for x-rays in the future.

Role of Surfactant

In neonates with PPHN due parenchymal lung disease, surfactant therapy has been shown to reduce the death or need for ECMO.[25] Surfactant deficiency can be either a primary deficiency as seen in RDS or secondary deficiency or an inactivation as seen in MAS or congenital pneumonia.

In neonates with parenchymal lung disease, there will be areas of atelectasis and overinflation. Collapse of alveoli results in constriction of extra alveolar vessels and overdistension results in compression of alveolar vessels. These together result in an increased PVR. Administration of surfactant along with sufficient PEEP results in adequate lung recruitment and uniform distension of all the alveoli (**Fig. 3**). In centers where iNO is not available, surfactant alone might be effective in improving hypoxemia. If nitric oxide is available, surfactant assists in an effective delivery of iNO leading to pulmonary vasodilatation and decrease in PVR and improvement in oxygenation.[26]

In developing countries, the incidence of PPHN secondary parenchymal lung diseases such as meconium aspiration remains highest followed by perinatal asphyxia and sepsis.[11,12] Surfactant replacement in MAS plays a major role in decreasing the progressive respiratory failure and need for ECMO.[27]

Inhaled Nitric Oxide Therapy

Inhaled nitric oxide is only available in a few centers in LMICs. It is a selective pulmonary vasodilator with minimal effect on systemic blood pressure. It is the only therapy

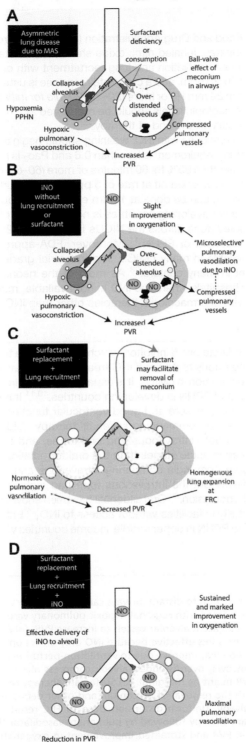

Fig. 3. Beneficial effects of surfactant in newborn infants with parenchymal lung disease such as MAS and PPHN. (*A*) Meconium induces chemical pneumonitis and surfactant

approved by the US Food and Drug Administration (FDA) for the treatment of PPHN in term or near-term neonates. Inhaled nitric oxide should be initiated when OI is more than 20 despite adequate ventilation and lung recruitment with or without surfactant. The initial dose is usually 20 ppm, and a complete response is usually defined as Pao_2/Fio_2 ratio of greater than 20 mm Hg or more *(20–20–20 rule for initiation of iNO)*.[21] Once iNO is initiated, methemoglobin levels should be monitored at 2 hours and 8 hours after initiation and then daily till the end of therapy.[25]

After achieving good response with iNO, weaning should begin approximately 30 minutes after initiation if Fio_2 requirement is less than 0.6 and Pao_2 is more than 60 mm Hg or preductal SpO_2 greater than 90% for 60 minutes or more *(60–60–60 rule for weaning)*. Inhaled nitric oxide can be weaned off at rate of 5 ppm, 2 to 4 hourly and once dose of 5 ppm is reached weaning can be done at 1 ppm every 2 to 4 hourly.[21]

The major constraint in developing countries is nonavailability of iNO in most of the centers. In a large survey done across the NICUs in India, only 25% of the units had iNO facility for the treatment of PPHN.[11] Moreover, FDA-approved medical grade iNO is not readily available in many LMICs, and industrial grade iNO is being used with parental consent in many centers.[28] As most of the neonates with PPHN are born in public sector hospitals where the iNO is not available, majority of these neonates are managed with pharmacologic therapies other than iNO.

Sildenafil

Sildenafil is a phosphodiesterase 5 inhibitor, which is used in the treatment of PPHN in neonates who respond poorly to iNO or if iNO treatment is not available. Because the latter scenario is more common in LMICs, it is usually the first pulmonary vasodilator of choice for the treatment of PPHN in developing countries.[10,11] It has to be used in neonates with normal blood pressure and good ventricular function; hence, echocardiography is essential before commencing sildenafil therapy. Sildenafil in developing countries is available in both intravenous and oral forms, and the intravenous form is more commonly used in acute stages than the oral formulation.[11]

In an RCT conducted from India comparing intravenous and oral forms, both the forms had similar efficacy but the intravenous form had higher complication rate in the form of systemic hypotension.[29] Oral sildenafil has been shown to improve oxygenation and reduce mortality in facilities without access to iNO.[25] Enteral sildenafil is also cost effective for severe PPHN in upper middle-income countries where ECMO and iNO is not available.[30]

◄――――――――――――――――――――――――――――――――――――

inactivation. Partial obstruction to distant airways can lead to atelectasis or overdistension. Collapsed alveoli are associated with regional hypoxic pulmonary vasoconstriction. Overdistended alveoli compress adjacent alveolar vessels to increase PVR. (*B*) Administration of iNO without lung recruitment is less effective because iNO only enters open alveoli and dilates blood vessels. Oxygenation may improve due to ventilation-perfusion matching (microselective effect of iNO). However, overdistended alveoli compress alveolar pulmonary vessels, and the decrease in PVR might be marginal. (*C*) Surfactant therapy reduces surface tension and also may assist with the removal of meconium and other debris leading to more symmetric expansion of alveoli. Uniform distension close to FRC results in the reduction in PVR. (*D*) Initial surfactant therapy followed by pulmonary vasodilator therapy (iNO) results in maximal reduction in PVR and sustained improvement in oxygenation. (*Modified from Lakshminrusimha S, Keszler M. Diagnosis and management of persistent pulmonary hypertension of the newborn. In: Keszler M, Suresh GK, eds. Assisted Ventilation of the Neonate. Vol 1. 7 ed. Philadelphia: Elsevier; 2022. Copyright Satyan Lakshmirusimha.*)

Recommended dose for IV—Loading dose of 0.4 mg/kg over 3 hours (0.14 mg/kg/h) followed by 1.6 mg/kg/d as a continuous infusion (0.07 mg/kg/h). Sildenafil (oral): 1 to 2 mg/kg/dose every 6 hours. A minimum dose of 1 mg/kg is recommended by the enteral route based on pharmacokinetic data and comparison of plasma sildenafil levels between neonates and adults.[31]

Animal studies have shown that sildenafil decreases pulmonary arterial pressure in sepsis-induced PH.[32] However, significant systemic hypotension is observed with sildenafil use in this model. Hence, we recommend caution with the use of IV and enteral sildenafil in sepsis-induced PPHN. Close monitoring of systemic blood pressure is critical during sildenafil therapy among patients with sepsis.

Milrinone

Milrinone is a phosphodiesterase 3A inhibitor, which causes pulmonary vasodilatation by increasing cyclic adenosine monophosphate (cAMP) levels. It is an inotropic agent as well as systemic and pulmonary vasodilator.[25] It is the preferred agent in the treatment of PPHN with left ventricular dysfunction.[21] Echocardiographic evaluation in these neonates will reveal presence of left to right shunt across the PFO and right to left shunt across PDA. In these situations, iNO is contraindicated because it may result in pulmonary edema and worsen the respiratory condition.[21] This kind of scenario in developing countries is usually observed in neonates with perinatal asphyxia with meconium aspiration. Milrinone is also used in iNO nonresponders and as a second-line agent as an alternative to sildenafil.

Echocardiography may not be readily available bedside in all the units in developing countries. In such situations, systolic blood pressure can be used as a surrogate for the assessment of cardiac function before initiating pulmonary vasodilators such as milrinone.[33]

In most of the units in developing countries, it is the second-line intravenous pulmonary vasodilator of choice after sildenafil.[10,11] In a large survey conducted on PPHN across 118 NICUs in India, it was the first-line inotrope of choice in neonates with PPHN.[11] The typical dose of milrinone includes a loading dose of 50 mcg/kg during 60 minutes followed by a maintenance dose of 0.33 mcg/kg/min to a maximum of 1 mcg/kg/min. A fluid bolus can be considered before the loading dose to reduce the risk of systemic hypotension. Milrinone is excreted by the kidneys. Acute tubular necrosis and other forms or renal compromise are commonly associated with perinatal asphyxia and can exacerbate systemic hypotension with milrinone.[34] In these instances, we recommend avoiding the loading dose and starting maintenance at a lower dose of 0.2 to 0.25 mcg/kg/min and titrate based on response and blood pressure.

In a randomized controlled trial form Egypt, comparing milrinone with sildenafil, milrinone was superior in improving oxygenation without lowering blood pressure.[35] In a similar study from the same country, combination of oral sildenafil with milrinone (IV) was more effective in improving oxygenation than monotherapy alone. Milrinone was more effective in the initial part of the treatment course and sildenafil in latter part. This effect was probably due to the development of tolerance due to prolonged therapy with milrinone.[36] In neonates with severe PPHN from resource-limited settings, with lack of access to iNO and ECMO and where intravenous sildenafil may not be readily available, a combination of oral sildenafil with IV milrinone can be considered.

Prostaglandins

In neonates with PPHN who have poor right ventricular contractility, opening a constricting PDA can act as a "pop off" to relieve the high pulmonary pressure and decrease the right ventricular afterload by facilitating right to left shunt across the patent ductus arteriosus (PDA). In such a situation consisting of failing right ventricle (RV) and constricting duct, infusion of PGE1 can open the constricting PDA and decrease the RV after load.[25] This approach should be ideally guided by echocardiography. Prostaglandin E1 also has pulmonary vasodilator properties. It has been used both in intravenous form and nebulized form[37] in PPHN although neither approach has been evaluated in a multicenter RCT. The typical dose of Prostaglandin E1 (IV) is between 0.025 and 0.1 mcg/kg/min.

Bosentan

Bosentan is an endothelin receptor antagonist, which is used as an adjuvant medication in the treatment of PPHN. In a recent metanalysis of 8 RCTs, bosentan use has been shown to cause significant reduction in pulmonary arterial pressure in neonates with PPHN.[38] In a study from India, conducted in neonates and infants aged younger than 3 months with PPHN, combination of bosentan and sildenafil resulted in a significant reduction in pulmonary pressures compared with sildenafil alone.[39] Bosentan is also associated with many adverse effects such as abnormal liver function, anemia, and edema. Hence, it is not primarily used in the management of PPHN.

Even though Bosentan is easily available in developing countries such as India, its current role is limited as an adjuvant therapy along with other medications in the treatment of PPHN. A typical dose of Bosentan is 1 mg/kg per dose given twice a day with close monitoring of liver function tests.

Vasopressin

Vasopressin is a useful adjunct as a rescue therapy in refractory cases of PPHN with systemic hypotension despite iNO and other medications.[40] The mechanism of reduction in pulmonary pressure is due to stimulation of oxytocin endothelin receptors and activation of nitric oxide pathway.[41]

Hydrocortisone

Hydrocortisone has been shown to improve blood pressure and oxygenation in neonates with PPHN. An additional benefit is secondary to the inhibitory effect of hydrocortisone on the phosphodiesterase 5 enzyme activity with subsequent increase in cyclic guanosine monophosphate (cGMP) levels.[41] Neonates with MAS seem to benefit the most because it has shown to reduce oxygen need and duration of hospitalization without increase in infection.[42] A commonly used dose is 1 mg/kg/dose 12 hourly for 48 hours. Higher doses (4 mg/kg loading dose followed by maintenance as described above) have been used in infants with PPHN and systemic hypotension in the absence of sepsis.[43]

A simple algorithm for the management of PPHN in resource-limited settings is depicted in **Fig. 4**. This algorithm is based on echocardiographic availability to assess ventricular function. In the absence of echocardiographic access, systemic hypotension not responding to fluid bolus or worsening with a fluid bolus may be seen as a sign of cardiac dysfunction.

Thiamine Responsive Pulmonary Hypertension

In developing countries, thiamine responsive acute pulmonary hypertension is one of the common causes of acute pulmonary hypertension with right heart failure in early infancy.[44] Most of the babies are from low socioeconomic status, who are exclusively breastfed with normal growth and male preponderance (**Fig. 5**).[45] The most common presenting symptoms are fast breathing, vomiting, and change in voice

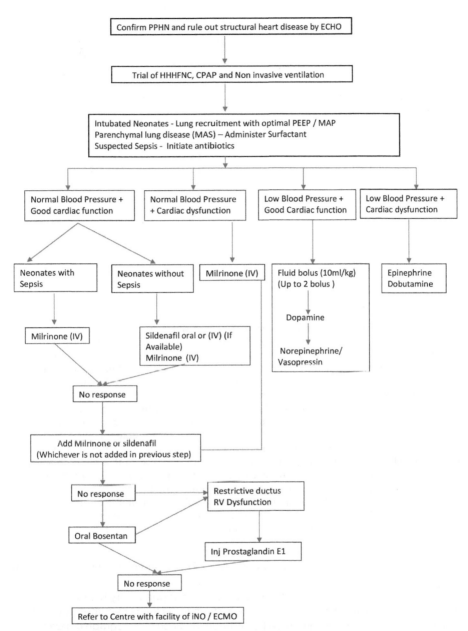

Fig. 4. Suggested algorithm for managing PPHN in centers with access to echocardiography but without access to iNO or ECMO. If echocardiography is not available to confirm the diagnosis of PPHN and assess cardiac shunts and function, a modified approach where systemic hypotension not responding to a fluid bolus can be considered to be a sign of cardiac dysfunction.

during crying. Tachypnea, tachycardia, and hepatomegaly are the common findings on examination. Blood gas analysis reveals metabolic acidosis with elevated lactate. They have severe pulmonary hypertension that cannot be usually explained by cardiac or pulmonary cause.[44,45] The striking history is consumption of polished rice

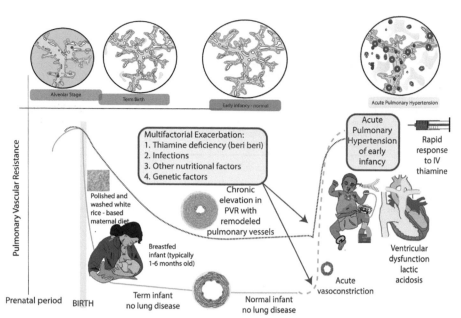

Fig. 5. Early infantile pulmonary hypertension possibly due to thiamine deficiency commonly seen in the Indian subcontinent and other LMICs. Two hypothetical pathways of change in PVR during birth and postnatal periods are shown. (i) The solid green line shows the normal reduction in PVR at birth and early infancy. The dashed green line depicts acute exacerbation in an infant with normal PVR before presentation. (ii) The blue dotted line shows the possible trajectory with incomplete reduction in PVR during early neonatal period leading to clinically unrecognized chronic pulmonary hypertension with possible pulmonary vascular remodeling and subsequent acute exacerbation. We suspect that a combination of both these processes with multifactorial cause is responsible for acute pulmonary hypertension of early infancy seen in Indian children. A common association with maternal polished rice intake, exclusive breastfeeding, and rapid response to thiamine replacement suggests that vitamin deficiency along with other factors may play a role. (*Modified from* Lakshminrusimha S, Madappa R. Acute Pulmonary Hypertension of Early Infancy – Is Thiamine Deficiency the Only Cause? Indian Pediatrics. 2023; E-pub and Panigrahy N, Chirla DK, Shetty R, et al. Thiamine-Responsive Acute Pulmonary Hypertension of Early Infancy (TRAPHEI)-A Case Series and Clinical Review. Children (Basel). 2020;7(11).Copyright Satyan Lakshmirusimha.)

with very minimal lentils and milk by the mothers. The outer layers of cereals are rich in thiamine.[44]

Echocardiogram in these neonates shows features of pulmonary hypertension with right heart failure. The response to thiamine is dramatic in these neonates. Most of the clinical signs and symptoms improve by 24 hours and echocardiographic parameters start improving by 24 to 48 hours. Aphonia usually takes 3 to 4 days to resolve.[44,45]

Biochemical tests to diagnose thiamine deficiency are not widely available in resource-limited settings, and a therapeutic thiamine challenge is an easier way of diagnosis.

In developing countries, diets in the postpartum period have very less diversity in food intake with predominant intake of polished rice. The process of milling, polishing, and repeated washing of the rice with discarding excess water reduces the thiamine content drastically. The consumption of such rice during the postpartum period results in thiamine deficiency.

Health-care providers should be aware of this condition in developing countries and a high index of suspicion should be kept in any infant presenting with newly diagnosed pulmonary hypertension without preexisting cardiac or pulmonary condition with metabolic acidosis and elevated lactate. A trial of IV thiamine should be promptly given.

Outcome

The mortality rate in neonates with PPHN in developing countries varies from 10% to 50% with an average mortality rate of 20%.[10,11] The common causes of mortality in PPHN is due to associated conditions such as birth asphyxia, MAS, and associated cardiac disease.[10] These neonates also have long-term consequences such as cognitive, hearing, and neurodevelopmental abnormalities.[21] Among the neonates who received iNO, approximately 25% of the neonates have neurodevelopmental and hearing impairment.[46] In a study by Rohana and colleagues from Malaysia, mental developmental index and physical developmental index scores were 85 and 87, respectively, with approximately 18% of the neonates having developmental disability.[47] Hence early intervention and close follow-up is absolutely essential in reducing the morbidities in these neonates.

Many countries have developed their own health programs to improve maternal health and reduce neonatal mortality. One such initiative by the government of India is Janani Shishu Suraksha Karyakaram offering care for pregnant women and neonates. These services are offered free of cost.

Under a 3-tier system, different units have been set up, including, Newborn Care Corners at all delivery units, Newborn Stabilization Units at community health centers, and special newborn Care Units with facilities of CPAP and ventilation at all centers with more than 3000 deliveries per year.[48] This has ensured a proper "hub and spoke model" for immediate management and referral of sick neonates including neonates with PPHN.

SUMMARY

In resource-limited settings meconium aspiration, asphyxia, and sepsis still remain the common cause of PPHN, and most of these neonates are managed by supportive care, ventilation, and pulmonary vasodilators. Early referral and close follow-up are essential to improve the outcome of these neonates.

Best Practice Box

- Infection and birth asphyxia are common causes of PPHN in LMICs.

- An assessment of resources available and creation of algorithm for managing PPHN with these resources is needed at every setting. This algorithm should include indications for transfer of these patients.

- Oral sildenafil remains an effective first line of therapy for PPHN in resource-limited settings. Close monitoring of systemic blood pressure is needed while managing PPHN with sildenafil.

DISCLOSURE

The authors have no financial disclosures or relevant conflicts of interest pertaining to the topics discussed in this article.

REFERENCES

1. Walsh-Sukys MC, Tyson JE, Wright LL, et al. Persistent pulmonary hypertension of the newborn in the era before nitric oxide: practice variation and outcomes. Pediatrics 2000;105(1 Pt 1):14–20.

2. Steurer MA, Jelliffe-Pawlowski LL, Baer RJ, et al. Persistent pulmonary hypertension of the newborn in late preterm and term infants in California. Pediatrics 2017; 139(1):e20161165.

3. Mohsen AA, Amin A. Risk factors and outcomes of persistent pulmonary hypertension of the newborn in neonatal intensive care unit of al-minya university hospital in Egypt. J Clin Neonatol 2013;2(2):78.

4. Zhou R, Zheng YN, Zhang XY, et al. A meta-analysis of the risk factors of persistent pulmonary hypertension in newborns. Front Pediatr 2021;9(October):1–6.

5. Delaney C, Cornfield DN. Risk factors for persistent pulmonary hypertension of the newborn. Pulm Circ 2012;2(1):15–20.

6. Silvani P, Camporesi A. Drug-induced pulmonary hypertension in newborns: a review. Curr Vasc Pharmacol 2007;5(2):129–33.

7. Abate E, Alamirew K, Admassu E, et al. Prevalence and factors associated with meconium-stained amniotic fluid in a tertiary hospital, northwest Ethiopia: a cross-sectional study. Obstet Gynecol Int 2021;2021:5520117.

8. Malhotra A, Allison BJ, Castillo-Melendez M, et al. Neonatal morbidities of fetal growth restriction: pathophysiology and impact. Front Endocrinol 2019;10:55.

9. Sankar MJ, Neogi SB, Sharma J, et al. State of newborn health in India. J Perinatol 2016;36(s3):S3–8.

10. Nakwan N, Jain S, Kumar K, et al. An Asian multicenter retrospective study on persistent pulmonary hypertension of the newborn: incidence, etiology, diagnosis, treatment and outcome. J Matern Neonatal Med 2020;33(12):2032–7.

11. Singh P, Deshpande S, Nagpal R, et al. Management of neonatal pulmonary hypertension-a survey of neonatal intensive care units in India. BMC Pediatr 2023;23(1):149.

12. Arshad MS, Adnan M, Anwar-ul-Haq HM, et al. Postnatal causes and severity of persistent pulmonary Hypertension of Newborn. Pakistan J Med Sci 2021;37(5): 1387–91.

13. Razzaq A, Iqbal Quddusi A, Nizami N. Risk factors and mortality among newborns with persistent pulmonary hypertension. Pak J Med Sci 2013;29(5): 1099–104.

14. Khorana M, Yookaseam T, Layangool T, et al. Outcome of oral sildenafil therapy on persistent pulmonary hypertension of the newborn at Queen Sirikit National Institute of Child Health. J Med Assoc Thai 2011;94(Suppl 3):S64–73.

15. Nakwan N, Pithaklimnuwong S. Acute kidney injury and pneumothorax are risk factors for mortality in persistent pulmonary hypertension of the newborn in Thai neonates. J Matern Fetal Neonatal Med 2016;29(11):1741–6.

16. Choudhary M, Meena MK, Chhangani N, et al. To study prevalence of persistent pulmonary hypertension in newborn with meconium aspiration syndrome in western Rajasthan, India: a prospective observational study. J Matern Fetal Neonatal Med 2016;29(2):324–7.

17. Golombek SG, Young JN. Efficacy of inhaled nitric oxide for hypoxic respiratory failure in term and late preterm infants by baseline severity of illness: a pooled analysis of three clinical trials. Clin Ther 2010;32(5):939–48.

18. Muniraman HK, Song AY, Ramanathan R, et al. Evaluation of oxygen saturation index compared with oxygenation index in neonates with hypoxemic respiratory failure. JAMA Netw Open 2019;2(3):e191179.

19. Rawat M, Chandrasekharan PK, Williams A, et al. Oxygen saturation index and severity of hypoxic respiratory failure. Neonatology 2015;107(3):161–6.

20. Lakshminrusimha S, Keszler M, Kirpalani H, et al. Milrinone in congenital diaphragmatic hernia - a randomized pilot trial: study protocol, review of literature

and survey of current practices. Maternal health, neonatology and perinatology 2017;3:27.

21. Lakshminrusimha S, Keszler M. Persistent pulmonary hypertension of the newborn. NeoReviews 2015;16(12):e680–92.

22. Dewez JE, Nangia S, Chellani H, et al. Availability and use of continuous positive airway pressure (CPAP) for neonatal care in public health facilities in India: a cross-sectional cluster survey. BMJ Open 2020;10(2):e031128.

23. Parmar J, Pawar V, Warathe A, et al. Rationalising oxygen usage in a level II special newborn care unit in Madhya Pradesh, India. BMJ Open Qual 2021;10(Suppl 1):e001386.

24. Lakshminrusimha S, Saugstad OD. The fetal circulation, pathophysiology of hypoxemic respiratory failure and pulmonary hypertension in neonates, and the role of oxygen therapy. J Perinatol 2016;36(S2):S3–11.

25. Singh Y, Lakshminrusimha S. Pathophysiology and management of persistent pulmonary hypertension of the newborn. Clin Perinatol 2021;48(3):595–618.

26. Konduri GG, Lakshminrusimha S. Surf early to higher tides: surfactant therapy to optimize tidal volume, lung recruitment, and iNO response. J Perinatol 2021; 41(1):1–3.

27. El Shahed AI, Dargaville PA, Ohlsson, et al. Surfactant for meconium aspiration syndrome in term and late preterm infants. Cochrane Database Syst Rev 2014; 14(12):CD002054.

28. Razak A, Nagesh NK, Venkatesh HA, et al. Inhaled nitric oxide in neonates with severe hypoxic respiratory failure-early indian experience. J Neonatol 2013; 27(2):1–3.

29. Chetan C, Suryawanshi P, Patnaik S, et al. Oral versus intravenous sildenafil for pulmonary hypertension in neonates: a randomized trial. BMC Pediatr 2022; 22(1):1–7.

30. Evers PD, Critser PJ, Hoelle S, et al. Cost-utility of sildenafil for persistent pulmonary hypertension of the newborn. Am J Perinatol 2021;38(14):1505–12.

31. Rhee S, Shin SH, Oh J, et al. Population pharmacokinetic analysis of sildenafil in term and preterm infants with pulmonary arterial hypertension. Sci Rep 2022; 12(1):7393.

32. Kemper DAG, Otsuki DA, Maia DRR, et al. Sildenafil in endotoxin-induced pulmonary hypertension: an experimental study. Braz J Anesthesiol 2021; S0104-0014(21):00239–46.

33. Mullaly R, El-Khuffash AF. Haemodynamic assessment and management of hypotension in the preterm. Arch Dis Child - Fetal Neonatal 2023;2022:324935, fetalneonatal-.

34. Bischoff AR, Habib S, McNamara PJ, et al. Hemodynamic response to milrinone for refractory hypoxemia during therapeutic hypothermia for neonatal hypoxic ischemic encephalopathy. J Perinatol 2021;41(9):2345–54.

35. Imam SS, El-Farrash RA, Taha AS, et al. Milrinone versus sildenafil in treatment of neonatal persistent pulmonary hypertension: a randomized control trial. J Cardiovasc Pharmacol 2022;80(5):746–52.

36. El-Ghandour M, Hammad B, Ghanem M, et al. Efficacy of milrinone plus sildenafil in the treatment of neonates with persistent pulmonary hypertension in resource-limited settings: results of a randomized, double-blind trial. Pediatr Drugs 2020; 22(6):685–93.

37. Sood BG, Keszler M, Garg M, et al. Inhaled PGE1 in neonates with hypoxemic respiratory failure: two pilot feasibility randomized clinical trials. Trials 2014; 15(1):486.

38. Li LX, Wei B, Yang M, et al. Efficacy and safety of bosentan in the treatment of persistent pulmonary hypertension of the newborn: a Metaanalysis. Zhong Guo Dang Dai Er Ke Za Zhi 2022 Mar 15;24(3):319–25.

39. Vijay Kumar JR, Natraj Setty HS, Jayaranganath M, et al. Efficacy, safety and tolerability of bosentan as an adjuvant to sildenafil and sildenafil alone in persistant pulmonary hypertension of newborn (PPHN). Interv Med Appl Sci 2021;11(4): 216–20.

40. Shah S, Dhalait S, Fursule A, et al. Use of vasopressin as rescue therapy in refractory hypoxia and refractory systemic hypotension in term neonates with severe persistent pulmonary hypertension—a prospective observational study. Am J Perinatol 2022. https://doi.org/10.1055/a-1969-1119.

41. Siefkes HM, Lakshminrusimha S. Management of systemic hypotension in term infants with persistent pulmonary hypertension of the newborn: an illustrated review. Arch Dis Child Fetal Neonatal Ed 2021;106(4):446–55.

42. Aleem S, Robbins C, Murphy B, et al. The use of supplemental hydrocortisone in the management of persistent pulmonary hypertension of the newborn. J Perinatol 2021;41(4):794–800.

43. Alsaleem M, Malik A, Lakshminrusimha S, et al. Hydrocortisone improves oxygenation index and systolic blood pressure in term infants with persistent pulmonary hypertension. Clin Med Insights Pediatr 2019;13. 117955651988891.

44. Sastry UMK, Jayranganath M, Kumar RK, et al. Thiamine-responsive acute severe pulmonary hypertension in exclusively breastfeeding infants: a prospective observational study. Arch Dis Child 2021;106(3):241–6.

45. Panigrahy N, Chirla DK, Shetty R, et al. Thiamine-responsive acute pulmonary hypertension of early infancy (TRAPHEI)-a case series and clinical review. Children 2020;7(11):199.

46. Konduri GG, Vohr B, Robertson C, et al. Early inhaled nitric oxide therapy for term and near-term newborn infants with hypoxic respiratory failure: neurodevelopmental follow-up. J Pediatr 2007;150(3):235–40.e1.

47. Rohana J, Boo NY, Chandran V, et al. Neurodevelopmental outcome of newborns with persistent pulmonary hypertension. Malays J Med Sci 2011;18(4):58–62.

48. National health mission. Facility based newborn care. Available at: https://nhm.gov.in/index4.php?lang=1&level=0&linkid=484&lid=754. Accessed June 28, 2023.

Randomized Controlled Trials of Pulmonary Vasodilator Therapy Adjunctive to Inhaled Nitric Oxide for Persistent Pulmonary Hypertension of the Newborn: A Systematic Review

Check for updates

Kristen Coletti, MD[a],*, K. Taylor Wild, MD[a,b],
Elizabeth E. Foglia, MD, MSCE[a,b],
Suzan Cochius-den Otter, MD, PhD[c], Haresh Kirpalani, BM, MSc[d,e]

KEYWORDS

- Persistent pulmonary hypertension of the newborn • Inhaled nitric oxide
- Pulmonary vasodilator • Randomized controlled trial • Term and late-preterm infants

KEY POINTS

- Inhaled nitric oxide (iNO) is one of only 2 pulmonary vasodilators with a body of randomized controlled trial (RCT) evidence supporting its use in late-preterm and term infants with persistent pulmonary hypertension of the newborn (PPHN).
- Neonatal RCTs studying iNO plus an additional pulmonary vasodilator faced recruitment challenges, limiting conclusions regarding therapeutic efficacy and safety.
- Heterogeneity in eligibility criteria and outcomes assessed in RCTs alongside potential variation in clinical care across study sites suggest consensus recommendations would benefit future trials.
- Alternative trial methodologies to study pulmonary vasodilators as well as nonvasodilator therapies for critically ill infants with PPHN may help obtain evidence.

[a] Department of Pediatrics, Division of Neonatology, The Children's Hospital of Philadelphia, 3401 Civic Center Boulevard, Philadelphia, PA 19104, USA; [b] Perelman School of Medicine, University of Pennsylvania, 8th Floor Ravdin Building, 3400 Spruce Street, Philadelphia, PA 19104, USA; [c] Department of Neonatal and Pediatric Intensive Care, Division of Pediatric Intensive Care, Erasmus MC University Medical Center, Wytemaweg 80, Rotterdam 3015CN, The Netherlands; [d] Emeritus, Perelman School of Medicine, University of Pennsylvania, 3400 Civic Center Boulevard, Philadelphia, PA 19104, USA; [e] Emeritus, Pediatrics, McMaster University, 1200 Main Street West, Hamilton, Ontario L8N3Z5, Canada
* Corresponding author.
E-mail address: colettik@chop.edu

Clin Perinatol 51 (2024) 253–269
https://doi.org/10.1016/j.clp.2023.11.009   perinatology.theclinics.com
0095-5108/24/© 2023 Elsevier Inc. All rights reserved.

BACKGROUND

Persistent pulmonary hypertension of the newborn (PPHN) occurs in approximately 1.8 to 1.9 per 1000 live births in infants $\geq$ 34 weeks gestational age.[1,2] It is characterized by delayed or inadequate transition from a state of high pulmonary vascular resistance (PVR) in utero to low PVR after birth. Clinical severity of PPHN varies, ranging from mild hypoxemia to cardiopulmonary collapse requiring extracorporeal membrane oxygenation (ECMO). Mortality is estimated between 7% and 11% of affected infants.[1–3]

Inhaled nitric oxide (iNO) and ECMO are evidence-based therapies for PPHN. Their efficacy has been confirmed by high-quality, moderately large randomized controlled trials (RCTs).[4–8] As such, iNO remains the first-line therapy recommended by the American Heart Association and American Thoracic Society's Pediatric Pulmonary Hypertension Guideline Statement to treat PPHN. ECMO is reserved for infants with disease refractory to iNO (class 1, level of evidence A).[9] Unfortunately, approximately 40% of infants treated with iNO are "non-responders," often requiring ECMO.[5,8,10–12] For these infants, data regarding efficacy and safety of additional pulmonary vasodilator therapies are needed.

Other medications targeting known enzymatic pathways in the pulmonary vascular smooth muscle include sildenafil, bosentan, milrinone, and prostacyclin and its analogs. As iNO is expensive and not always easily accessible, sildenafil and bosentan have been trialed as first-line therapies in resource-poor settings. In RCTs, these medications improved oxygenation and mortality compared to placebo.[13,14] Data on prostacyclin and its analogs are limited to small case series and retrospective studies. There are limited RCTs studying the use of such drugs as second tier after iNO initiation. This systematic review took the perspective that iNO is 'standard of care' in highly resourced countries. In settings without access to iNO, RCTs of other therapies compared to iNO or without iNO remain appropriate.

The current systematic review sought to determine whether there is RCT evidence to guide pulmonary vasodilator therapy for infants with PPHN nonresponsive to iNO and preceding ECMO cannulation. The authors aimed to consider methodologic quality and challenges of these RCTs. Thus, they characterized the degree of heterogeneity in trials, including in the enrollment process and patterns, eligibility criteria, and outcomes. The authors assessed calculated target sample sizes and whether these were attained. Finally, they aimed to pool data on efficacy and potential harm, if possible.

METHODS
Search Strategy

RCTs published in English between 1997 and May 1, 2023 were identified. The Neonatal Inhaled Nitric Oxide Study publication[8] in 1997 serves to date the modern era of PPHN management. The authors searched the following electronic resources: PubMed, Embase, clinicaltrials.gov, euclinicaltrials.eu, anzctr.org.au, ISRCTN (International Standard Randomized Controlled Trial Number) registry, and the International Clinical Trials registry platform for trials that met the inclusion criteria. The specific search terms are listed in Appendix 1. The authors searched reference lists of found papers and also publications from the Cochrane Library for additional sources.

Inclusion/Exclusion Criteria

The authors included trials with the following eligibility criteria: (1) neonates with PPHN or hypoxemic respiratory failure, (2) late-preterm or term (born$\geq$34 weeks gestational age), (3) less than 28 days old; (4) randomized into a placebo-controlled RCT examining a pulmonary vasodilator with iNO compared to iNO alone. The authors excluded studies examining infants with significant congenital heart disease (CHD) except ventricular septal defect, atrial septal defect, or patent ductus arteriosus (PDA); infants with congenital diaphragmatic hernia (CDH); and nonrandomized studies. The authors included all eligible trials regardless of the specified outcomes.

Abstract and Article Review Process

Two authors (KC, KTW) reviewed each abstract for inclusion and exclusion criteria to determine eligibility for full review. Disagreements were resolved by a third author (EEF). Data extraction included study author, publication year, study title, journal, published versus unpublished status, details regarding patient characteristics and demographics, inclusion criteria, exclusion criteria, primary and secondary outcomes, pulmonary vasodilator therapy studied, enrollment patterns, safety events, harms identified, study results and conclusions, as well as details about study methodologic quality and trial design. The published journal article was the primary source for data collection. Source of bias was collected (KC, KTW) and standardized with the Cochrane risk of bias tool. Disagreements were resolved (EEF). The authors focused on the primary trial design when assessing risk of bias. Trial methodologic quality was assessed using a neonatal adaptation of the Consolidated Standards of Reporting Trials guidelines.[15]

Statistical Analysis

Descriptive analyses were performed on study variables. All analyses were performed with Excel.

Definitions

The authors accepted the terminology investigators used to describe their own trials, which may have overlaps. For example, investigators used the terms "pilot" and "feasibility" interchangeably. The authors used the term "early stopping" based on nonachievement of formal, calculated target sample sizes.

RESULTS

The authors' search yielded 197 articles, of which 5 were eligible for study inclusion (**Fig. 1**). The trials were published between 2014 and 2023 and study characteristics are shown in **Table 1**. Different medications were studied: sildenafil (n = 2), bosentan (n = 1), milrinone (n = 1), and inhaled prostaglandin E_1 (n = 1). In all studies, infants were randomized to treatment with a pulmonary vasodilator or to a placebo medication. Four trials (80%) were self-categorized as 'feasibility,' 'pilot,' or 'exploratory' by study investigators. Study durations ranged from 0.5 to 5.4 years (median 3 years, interquartile range [IQR]: 2–4). All but 1 trial were multicenter, ranging from 3 to 25 sites. The median number of subjects recruited per year was 11 (IQR: 8–12). All trials required parental consent.

Inclusion Criteria

All infants were born late preterm or term and were of postnatal age ranging from 2 to 10 days. Each trial specified oxygenation index (OI) entry criteria, though the exact OI values differed by study. Two trials required 2 OI values 15 to 30 minutes apart within the specified criteria for trial eligibility. All other trials required 1 eligible value. Duration and dose requirements of iNO therapy differed by trial. One study specified that infants must be treated with iNO for at least 4 hours, another stated that OI response must be 'suboptimal,' and a third specified a dosing range of 10 to 20 ppm for eligibility. Additional inclusions criteria details are displayed in **Table 2**.

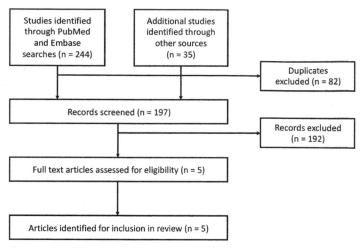

Fig. 1. Study identification and selection for inclusion.

Use of Echocardiography

Echocardiography was performed in all 5 trials; however, only 2 (40%) required diagnosis of echocardiogram-based PPHN as an inclusion criterion. One study assessed the presence of pulmonary hypertension on echocardiogram but did not specify defining measurements. One study diagnosed PPHN based on any of the following: the tricuspid regurgitant jet with pressure gradient ≥ two-thirds systemic systolic blood pressure, interventricular septal flattening or bowing into the left ventricular cavity, PDA with bidirectional or right to left shunt, or a pulmonary artery acceleration time of less than 40 milliseconds.

Exclusion Criteria

There was heterogeneity in exclusion criteria (**Table 3**). A total of 21 different exclusion criteria were specified across all studies. All studies excluded 'congenital anomalies' in some capacity. Three studies (60%) excluded CDH. Four studies (80%) excluded "significant CHD." Four studies excluded "major," "lethal," or "significant" congenital anomalies, which were not comprehensively defined. One study excluded infants with "obvious syndromes." Other common exclusion criteria were laboratory abnormalities, where thrombocytopenia and impaired renal function were most frequent. Markers of severe critical illness such as hypotension or the immediate need for cardiopulmonary resuscitation (CPR) or ECMO were also excluded.

Sample Size Targets

All studies stated sample size goals ranging from 20 to 150 participants. However, only 3 trials (60%) based target enrollment on a priori formal sample size calculations, taking into account an expected baseline event rate. The other 2 studies were self-classified as 'feasibility' or 'pilot' trials and did not formally calculate sample size goals. When calculated, studies were powered to detect a difference in treatment effect for the primary outcome ranging from 16% to 30% between control and intervention groups.

Screening and Eligibility

Across all trials, 241 infants were screened, and 122 (51%) infants were randomized, of which 98% were included in the final analysis. In 1 study, infants were consented

Table 1
Study characteristics

Author, Year, Randomization Arms	Study Drug Dose(s)	Trial Designation	Number of Sites	Regions Included	Enrollment Duration (Years)	Number of Patients Screened	Patients Enrolled (% of Screened)	Funding Source(s)	Primary Outcome(s)
Sood et al,[17] 2014 Inhaled PGE1 vs placebo	150 ng/kg/min; 300 ng/kg/min	Pilot feasibility randomized controlled trial	10	United States	0.5	46	7 (15)	National Institutes of Health, Eunice Kennedy Shriver National Institute of Child Health and Human Development, National Center for Research Resources, and National Center for Advancing Translational Sciences	Ability to recruit 50 patients in 9 mo without>20% protocol violations
Steinhorn et al,[27] 2016 Enteral bosentan vs placebo	2 mg/kg twice daily	Randomized controlled exploratory trial	25	United States, Europe, Australia, and Asia	2	27[a]	23[b] (85)	Actelion Pharmaceuticals Ltd	Treatment failure defined as the need for ECMO or initiation of alternative pulmonary vasodilator; time to complete weaning from iNO; time to complete weaning from mechanical ventilation
Al Omar et al,[44] 2016 Oral sildenafil + iNO vs placebo + iNO	2 mg/kg every 6 h	Randomized controlled feasibility trial	1	Qatar	3	51	24 (47)	None/ unknown	Oxygenation index absolute value and change from baseline measured after the first dose, every 6 h for 7 d or until infant extubates

(continued on next page)

Table 1
(continued)

Author, Year, Randomization Arms	Study Drug Dose(s)	Trial Designation	Number of Sites	Regions Included	Enrollment Duration (Years)	Number of Patients Screened	Patients Enrolled (% of Screened)	Funding Source(s)	Primary Outcome(s)
Pierce et al,[16] 2021 IV sildenafil vs placebo	Load: 0.1 mg/kg over 30 min; Maintenance: 0.03 mg/kg/h	Randomized controlled trial	25[c]	Belgium, Canada, Denmark, France, Germany, Netherlands, Norway, Spain, Sweden, United Kingdom, and United States	5.4	87	59 (68)	Pfizer	Treatment failure defined as the need for ECMO, additional treatment targeting PPHN, or death; time on iNO after initiation of IV study drug for infants without treatment failure
El-Khuffash et al,[34] 2023 IV milrinone vs placebo	Load: 50 μg/kg over 60 min; Maintenance: 0.375–0.75 μg/kg/min	Randomized controlled pilot study	3	Ireland, and Netherlands	4	30	9 (30)	Irish Health Research Board	Duration of iNO treatment; ability to recruit and maintain infants; parental acceptability and adherence to intervention administration; feasibility of randomization; identification of optimal recruitment methods; estimate of effect size to be used to power a definitive trial

Abbreviations: ECMO, extracorporeal membrane oxygenation; iNO, inhaled nitric oxide; IV, intravenous; PGE1, prostaglandin E1; PPHN, persistent pulmonary hypertension of the newborn.

[a] Screened patients were reported after parental informed consent was already obtained.
[b] 2 post-randomization exclusions occurred; 21 infants received study drug and were included in the analysis.
[c] Authors report opening more than 50 additional sites during trial.

Table 2
Inclusion criteria for trials

Criterion (if Listed in>1 Study)	Number of Studies (%)	Value Median (Range)
Gestational age ≥ 34 wk	5 (100)	
Postnatal age (days)	5 (100)	7 (2–10)
Oxygenation index minimum	5 (100)	15 (10–20)
Specifications of iNO in trial	3 (60)	
Clinical diagnosis of hypoxemic respiratory failure	3 (60)	
Presence of PPHN on echocardiogram	2 (40)	
Presence of arterial line	2 (40)	

Abbreviations: iNO, inhaled nitric oxide; PPHN, persistent pulmonary hypertension of the newborn.

before screening and the number of patients screened prior to consent was not reported. The most common reasons for not meeting eligibility criteria were the presence of a congenital anomaly, not meeting OI criteria, and the immediate need for CPR or ECMO (**Fig. 2**). The baseline median OI was 26 (IQR: 14–26.8) in the control group and 25.1 (IQR: 23.8–27) in the intervention group.

Enrollment in Trials

No trial reached target enrollment (**Fig. 3**). The trial duration was extended in 1 study, which was the only trial to approximate the projected target.[16] In another study, the trial was terminated prior to the planned end date due to slow recruitment over 6 months.[17] Of the 4 multisite trials, only 1 trial recruited at all sites, one recruited at 80% of sites, and one recruited from 36% of sites. One study did not report the number of sites recruited from but had fewer participants (n = 59) than study sites (25 initially, then opened>50 new sites to boost recruitment).

Outcomes

Primary outcomes varied and no study had the same primary outcome, though there was overlap (see **Table 1**). "Need for ECMO," need for alternative pulmonary hypertension treatment, and time to wean from iNO were the clinical primary outcomes

Table 3
Exclusion criteria

Criterion (if Listed in>1 Study)	Number of Studies (%)
Congenital anomaly	5 (100)
Congenital heart disease (explicitly excluded)	4 (80)
Congenital diaphragmatic hernia (explicitly excluded)	3 (60)
Laboratory abnormality	3 (60)
Thrombocytopenia	3 (60)
Impaired renal function	2 (40)
Markers of severe critical illness	3 (60)
Mechanical ventilation anticipated<48 h	2 (40)
Intraventricular hemorrhage	2 (40)

Common Reasons for Ineligibility (n = number of infants)[a]
- Congenital anomaly (n = 27; 2 studies)
  - CDH (n = 6)
  - Trisomy 21 (n = 5)
  - Surfactant protein deficiency (n = 2)
  - Syndrome, malformation or CHD (n = 14)
- OI criteria not met (n = 19; 3 studies)
- Immediate need for ECMO/CPR (n = 9; 2 studies)
- Hypoxic ischemic encephalopathy (n = 7; 2 studies)
- Parental refusal (n = 7; 2 studies[b])
- Investigator availability (n = 5; 1 study)

Fig. 2. Most common reasons for study ineligibility. [a]Data from 4 studies and 87 infants; data from the fifth study excluded 32 infants but did not specify which eligibility criteria were not met. [b]One study screened patients after parental consent was obtained.

studied in more than 1 trial. Although "need for ECMO" was a common outcome, it was not uniformly defined. Four studies performed statistical analysis of the primary outcome(s) without achieving statistical significance. One study was too small for formal statistical analysis (n = 7 subjects).

Secondary outcomes varied widely among the studies with the most common listed in **Table 4**. Several other secondary outcomes were only assessed in 1 trial. Four of the 5 studies reported ECMO cannulation as a primary or secondary outcome. Only 15 of 96 patients (15.6%) were cannulated onto ECMO, including 6 of 46 (13%) of control infants and 9 of 50 (18%) of intervention infants. Four of the 5 studies reported mortality data. Three of 96 patients died (3.1%).

Study Drug

All 5 trials cited published pharmacologic data justifying the choice of study drug dosage(s), and 3 cited studies regarded neonates. Ancillary pharmacologic data were

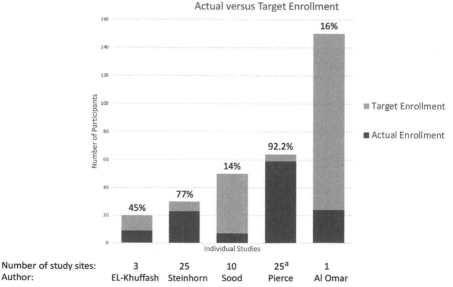

Fig. 3. Enrollment. [a]Study duration was extended, and authors reported adding greater than 50 additional sites to the 25 originally reported.

Table 4
Most common secondary outcomes

Criterion (if Listed in>1 Study)	Number of Studies (%)
Mortality	4 (80)
Need for ECMO	3 (60)
Duration of mechanical ventilation	3 (60)
Duration of hospitalization	3 (60)
Physiologic or hemodynamic factors during study drug treatment	3 (60)
Change in oxygenation (OI, arterial partial pressure of oxygen, peripheral oxygen saturation, alveolar-arterial gradient, and/or fraction of inspired oxygen)	2 (40)
Echocardiogram measurements	2 (40)
Duration of supplemental oxygen	2 (40)
Hypotension	2 (40)

Abbreviations: ECMO, extracorporeal membrane oxygenation; OI, oxygenation index.

reported in 2 trials. A harm assessment was performed in every trial. One trial reported a serious adverse event (SAE) of hypotension with sildenafil treatment. Otherwise, no SAEs were reported as different between the intervention and control groups. No other trial attributed a SAE to the study drug.

Trial Methodology and Bias Analysis

Overall, the trials had high methodologic quality (**Table 5**) with relatively low risk of bias (**Table 6**). In the bias assessment, the study authors had 2 disagreements in their assessments which were reconciled by the third study author. All studies had incomplete enrollment, which increased the risk of bias.

DISCUSSION

This systematic review assessed design and outcomes of RCTs focused on pharmacologic therapies adjunctive to iNO for PPHN. The authors identified 5 trials, and all

Table 5
Trial methodologic quality

Reporting of Each Quality Criterion	n/N (%)
Eligibility criteria are listed	5/5 (100)
Primary outcome is stated	5/5 (100)
Sample size estimate is provided	3/5 (60)
Method of randomization is described	3/5 (60)
Method of allocation concealment is described	2/5 (40)
Blinding of study team members is mentioned, unless study is unblinded	5/5 (100)
If study is multicenter, the number of participating centers is stated	4/4 (100)
Study flow diagram is published	5/5 (100)
Number of study participants is stated	5/5 (100)
Number of participants analyzed is stated	5/5 (100)
Result of the primary outcome is included, if a primary outcome is identified	5/5 (100)

Abbreviations: n, number of trials reporting the specified quality criterion; N, total number of items.

Table 6 Risk of bias					
	Random sequence generation bias (selection bias)	Allocation concealment (selection bias)	Blinding (performance bias and detection bias)	Incomplete outcome data (attrition bias)	Selective reporting (reporting bias)
Sood 2014	+	?	+	+	+
Steinhorn 2016	?	?	?	+	+
Al Omar 2016	?	+	+	+	?
Pierce 2021	+	?	?	+	+
EL-Khuffash 2023	+	+	+	+	+
+ designates low risk of bias; ? designates unclear risk of bias					

were unable to meet predefined target recruitment goals. Naturally, this hinders the ability to draw conclusions regarding therapeutic efficacy, safety, and pharmacology of adjunctive therapies. The authors also found important heterogeneity in trial design related to eligibility criteria (representing potential generalizability) and outcomes (representing clinical relevance). Paradoxically, these trials were of overall high methodologic quality with low risk of bias. These findings demonstrate that several areas warrant attention in future PPHN RCT design.

Enrollment challenges were the largest barrier to trial completion and resulted in early termination prior to recruitment goals being met in all trials. This phenomenon is not isolated to PPHN and has plagued critical care research in neonatal, pediatric, and adult populations.[18–23] Low enrollment increases the risk of bias from early stopping and may yield underpowered sample sizes, so addressing barriers is critical.

Despite a long history of PPHN trials, heterogeneity in eligibility criteria remains, including when defining PPHN itself. While OI was part of the inclusion criteria in all studies, the degree and duration of hypoxemia differed. The minimum eligible OI ranged from 10 to 20, and 2 studies required 2 eligible OI values prior to enrollment. Only 2 studies required echocardiogram evidence of pulmonary hypertension for eligibility, though echocardiogram was performed in all trials. Variability was similarly present in early iNO trials.[4] These findings demonstrate that operationalizing a consensus definition of PPHN for RCTs is required.

The primary outcomes studied across trials were also heterogeneous. Each trial chose a different primary outcome, though reassuringly there was overlap that fell within 3 categories: treatment failure (death, ECMO, or additional vasodilator therapy), oxygenation, or feasibility. This suggests that authors agree about the importance of specific clinical themes but with differing priority, again highlighting a need for community-wide agreement. Trial outcome consensus is particularly important because variability limits data pooling for PPHN meta-analyses, which are crucial given the high early termination rates and small sample sizes within the current body of work.

The primary outcomes chosen must be feasible to achieve, especially given that PPHN is a relatively rare diagnosis. A population-based sample from 2007 to 2011 reported PPHN incidence at 1.8/1000 infants, which likely overestimates an eligible population for RCTs. Approximately 6% of these infants had CDH, and only 1.2/1000 had severe PPHN, defined as the need for positive pressure ventilation.[1] Compounding its rarity, therapies such as iNO and high-frequency oscillatory ventilation are more widely available, skewing referral patterns to regional centers. This could have detrimental effects on trial recruitment. Infants arriving at referral units may be sicker requiring definitive therapies quickly, while milder cases are successfully treated and never transferred. Thought should be given to involving peripheral units in trial conduct. This is a difficult challenge, mandating simpler designs, excellent coordination, easier online randomization and data collection, and not least adequate perceived rewards.

In addition, obtaining agreement on concurrent therapies will be challenging. One example regards ventilation strategies, since the interaction of ventilation parameters and vascular perfusion has not been fully addressed.[24] Whether there has been sufficient ventilator support for the underlying lung disease or left heart dysfunction is not clearly documented. To obtain larger trials than even the largest ones here, such issues need simplification.

Despite outcome heterogeneity, ECMO rates were commonly reported, including as part of the sample size calculation in 2 trials. Notably, "need for ECMO" was not uniformly defined across study sites, though guidelines regarding indications for cannulation may have been followed.[25] The authors found that 16% of infants required ECMO, infrequent compared to early iNO trials that found ~40% ECMO rates.[4,5,8,10] Relatedly, ECMO cannulation worldwide for PPHN has decreased over time.[26] The reason for this improvement is probably multifactorial. The investigators of trials included in this review recognize advances in medical care,[16,17,27] and newer trials may be enrolling less severe PPHN. In support of this hypothesis, the enrollment OI in this review was ~25, in contrast to ~40 in early iNO RCTs.[28] When Konduri and colleagues[6] recruited infants with similar OIs of 15 to 25, they found comparable, low ECMO rates of only 10.7% to 12.1%. As these rates are frequently utilized in sample size calculations, accurate estimates are imperative.

The authors found that several trials used historic event rates in sample size calculations. For example, one specified a baseline primary outcome control event rate of 40% treatment failure. The actual control rate was found to be only 20%.[16] Such discrepancy between anticipated versus actual event rates in the control population is problematic. Overestimating the effect size yields small, underpowered sample size targets. This may lull prospective trialists into overconfident recruitment goals, presenting false reassurance that a study is feasible. More conservative estimates based on contemporary data would be prudent for future trials.

The authors identified several aspects of trial design that may limit enrollment. First, neonates with PPHN are critically ill with a short time window for trial enrollment. The authors found that ~10% of infants across trials were screened but not randomized due to illness severity. Strict trial eligibility criteria may further delay enrollment. For example, 1 study required infants to be treated with iNO for ≥ 4 hours and 2 studies required more than 1 OI value. In practice, that led to a 2.4-hour to 4.7-hour interval between the first and second values and a 4.2-hour to 12.2-hour delay between the first eligible OI and receipt of the study drug.[17] In this same study, 29% of eligible infants were not randomized due to illness severity. The calculation of OI, which was used by all studies, requires arterial blood. Alternative noninvasive oxygenation criteria, such as oxygenation saturation index or oxygen saturation to fraction of inspired oxygen ratio, may make eligibility criteria easier to manage in trial settings. Furthermore, strategies aimed at earlier recruitment, possibly near the time of iNO initiation, may help. One such approach involves deferred proxy consent, which has been successful in critically ill adult and pediatric populations.[29,30] Evidence supports acceptance by families and clinicians of this strategy, particularly in situations of low-risk interventions or narrow therapeutic windows.[31,32]

Second, while aimed at homogeneity, strict exclusion criteria sometimes eliminate diagnoses that could benefit from pulmonary vasodilator therapy. In the authors' review, 7 infants were excluded for hypoxic ischemic encephalopathy, 5 for trisomy 21, and 2 for intraventricular hemorrhage. This likely underestimates excluded infants, since 1 study did not report reasons for screened but not randomized infants, and another excluded syndromic infants without additional specification. Their inclusion may augment recruitment yielding "real-world," generalizable results. Again, consensus recommendations regarding study population eligibility criteria may help guide new trials. In multinational iNO studies, infants with CDH were enrolled in a distinct parallel trial,[33] which is another strategy to consider.

Third, future considerations of including echocardiogram diagnosis to define PPHN must grapple with imposing added recruitment challenges. For EL-Khuffash and colleagues,[34] only few investigators could perform echocardiograms, reducing recruitment to daytime hours. This resulted in investigator unavailability accounting for 24% of infants who were unable to be randomized. However, eliminating echocardiographic inclusion criteria is problematic as clinical markers of oxygenation, such as OI and Fio_2 need, are nonspecific for PPHN. Lung parenchymal disease or low cardiac output may lead to hypoxemia that does not improve or even worsens with initiation of pulmonary vasodilator therapy. This may result from worsening ventilation-perfusion matching or systemic hypotension worsening right-to-left shunts.[24]

Echocardiogram was included in all trial protocols, often to exclude CHD. Future trials with more lenient echocardiogram timing surrounding recruitment and study drug initiation may facilitate exact PPHN diagnoses while decreasing recruitment challenge. Community-wide discussion could help reconcile these priorities.

Simply enrolling more study sites may not be an adequate strategy. Steinhorn and colleagues[27] demonstrated that only 9 of the initial 25 large referral study sites enrolled patients. Moreover, even after adding 50 additional sites to the 25 originals, Pierce and colleagues[16] did not achieve target recruitment. Overall, only 1 of the 4 multisite trials in this review recruited from all sites. Site eligibility characteristics to join trials might include familiarity with the complexity of trial conduct (including Institutional Review Board submissions), sufficient support staff, and monitoring for an adequate number of eligible patients. Alternatively, allocating more resources to fewer sites may increase efficiency.

All trials utilized pharmacologic data to determine study drug dosing; 60% used data from neonatal studies. Determining the most valid dosing regimen may add to the complexity of trial design but is important for accurate efficacy results.[23] Pierce and colleagues[16] used a sildenafil dose lower than the maximum effective dose in neonates[35] in order to minimize hypotension. They found that its steady state concentration was less than half that found to be effective in the original dose escalation trial, potentially falsely invalidating sildenafil's efficacy.[35,36] Dose-escalation RCTs may minimize this challenge and have been employed successfully in iNO research for PPHN in the past.[8]

The authors were aware of a related trial that has remained unpublished (NCT01409031), though it did not meet the authors' inclusion criteria. However, it highlights that publication bias in pharmacy-funded trials is becoming widely appreciated in several fields.[37,38] In addition, when industry-funded trials specify strict entry criteria for patent reasons, they further increase problems for trial enrollment.[39]

Overall, this review identifies immense challenges inherent to performing RCTs in critically ill neonates with PPHN. Overcoming these barriers is ethically necessary to assess the efficacy and safety of therapies increasingly used without an adequate evidence base. The authors believe that consensus agreement is critical for moving this field forward. This should address heterogeneity in eligibility criteria and outcomes, including what clinical, laboratory, and echocardiogram parameters constitute the definition of PPHN itself. Meaningful yet pragmatic primary outcomes should enable data pooling for meta-analysis. While ECMO is commonly studied, acknowledging a declining incidence must be reflected in sample size calculations.

Alternative methodologies including large observational cohort studies may be needed as classic RCT design has proven challenging in recent years. A PPHN consortium, such as in other critical illnesses,[40,41] may assist. The identified problems stem from recruiting a critically ill population with an increasingly rare disease. The use of deferred consent and eligibility criteria allowing for enrollment closer to iNO initiation may address the former. Using real-world controls, including infants who could not be recruited for logistical reasons or whose parents refuse consent, or alternatively, nonrandomized database assessments could decrease recruitment burden. Cluster randomization by study site may reduce each site's workload. Should there be further multiple drug innovations, a Bayesian approach may determine any potential benefit without incurring penalty from multiple looks. This might allow a faster concurrent evaluation of new drugs.

The authors' review has limitations. First, given that several different study drugs were examined, it was not possible to pool results to determine their efficacy. Second, only 5 studies were identified for inclusion, limiting the conclusions that could be drawn. Third, the authors only included data in published journal articles. It is possible that additional information would be clarified by a study protocol. Last, the authors' review only assessed the efficacy of pulmonary vasodilators adjunctive to iNO as compared to iNO alone. In resource-limited countries, iNO may not be available and studying pulmonary vasodilator medications as compared to placebos is important. These trials exist and have promising findings but were outside the scope of the current review.[42,43]

SUMMARY

This systematic review demonstrates that recruitment challenges limit the ability to draw conclusions regarding the efficacy and safety of pulmonary vasodilator therapy adjunctive to iNO for PPHN. The results demonstrate several complexities inherent to recruiting critically ill neonates with an increasingly rare disease. Overcoming these barriers is ethically necessary. The authors suggest that a PPHN consortium may address issues of heterogeneity in eligibility criteria and outcomes and propose that alternative trial design strategies are necessary. These may include deferred consent, real-world controls, nonrandomized database assessments, and Bayesian statistical approaches.

Best Practice Box

What is the current practice for?

- PPHN.

Best practice/guideline/care path objective(s):

- iNO is standard of care in highly resourced settings to treat PPHN.

What changes in current practice are likely to improve outcomes?

- Alternative trial designs and consortium agreement are needed in order to assess the efficacy and safety of pulmonary vasodilator adjunctive to iNO. These strategies may include deferred consent, real-world controls, nonrandomized database assessments, and Bayesian statistical approaches.

ACKNOWLEDGMENTS

Jennifer Lege-Matsuura, MSLIS, AHIP for assisting with search strategy.

DISCLOSURE

The authors have nothing to disclose.

REFERENCES

1. Steurer MA, Jelliffe-Pawlowski LL, Baer RJ, et al. Persistent pulmonary hypertension of the newborn in late preterm and term infants in California. Pediatrics 2017; 139(1):e20161165.
2. Walsh-Sukys MC, Tyson JE, Wright LL, et al. Persistent pulmonary hypertension of the newborn in the era before nitric oxide: practice variation and outcomes. Pediatrics 2000;105(1):14–20.
3. Steurer MA, Baer RJ, Oltman S, et al. Morbidity of persistent pulmonary hypertension of the newborn in the first year of life. J Pediatr 2019;213:58–65.e4.
4. Barrington KJ, Finer N, Pennaforte T, et al. Nitric oxide for respiratory failure in infants born at or near term. Cochrane Database Syst Rev 2017;1(1): CD000399.
5. Roberts JD, Fineman JR, Morin FC, et al. Inhaled nitric oxide and persistent pulmonary hypertension of the newborn. N Engl J Med 1997;336(9):605–10.
6. Konduri GG, Solimano A, Sokol GM, et al. A randomized trial of early versus standard inhaled nitric oxide therapy in term and near-term newborn infants with hypoxic respiratory failure. Pediatrics 2004;113(3):559–64.
7. UK collaborative randomised trial of neonatal extracorporeal membrane oxygenation. Lancet 1996;348(9020):75–82.
8. Inhaled nitric oxide in full-term and nearly full-term infants with hypoxic respiratory failure. N Engl J Med 1997;336(9):597–604.
9. Abman SH, Hansmann G, Archer SL, et al. Pediatric pulmonary hypertension: guidelines from the American heart Association and American Thoracic Society. Circulation 2015;132(21):2037–99.
10. Clark RH, Kueser TJ, Walker MW, et al. Low-dose nitric oxide therapy for persistent pulmonary hypertension of the newborn. N Engl J Med 2000;342(7):469–74.
11. Morel AA, Shreck E, Mally PV, et al. Clinical characteristics and factors associated with term and late preterm infants that do not respond to inhaled nitric oxide (iNO). J Perinat Med 2016;44(6):663–8.
12. Goldman AP, Tasker RC, Haworth SG, et al. Four patterns of response to inhaled nitric oxide for persistent pulmonary hypertension of the newborn. Pediatrics 1996;98(4):706–13.
13. He Z, Zhu S, Zhou K, et al. Sildenafil for pulmonary hypertension in neonates: an updated systematic review and meta-analysis. Pediatr Pulmonol 2021;56(8):2399–412.
14. Mohamed WA, Ismail M. A randomized, double-blind, placebo-controlled, prospective study of bosentan for the treatment of persistent pulmonary hypertension of the newborn. J Perinatol 2012;32(8):608–13.
15. DeMauro SB, Giaccone A, Kirpalani H, et al. Quality of reporting of neonatal and infant trials in high-impact journals. Pediatrics 2011;128(3):e639–44.
16. Pierce CM, Zhang MH, Jonsson B, et al. Efficacy and safety of IV sildenafil in the treatment of newborn infants with, or at risk of, persistent pulmonary hypertension of the newborn (PPHN): a multicenter, randomized, placebo-controlled trial. J Pediatr 2021;237:154–61.e3.

17. Sood BG, Keszler M, Garg M, et al. Inhaled PGE1 in neonates with hypoxemic respiratory failure: two pilot feasibility randomized clinical trials. Trials 2014; 15(1):486.

18. Dempsey EM, Barrington KJ, Marlow N, et al. Hypotension in preterm infants (HIP) randomised trial. Arch Dis Child Fetal Neonatal Ed 2021;106(4):398–403.

19. Watterberg KL, Fernandez E, Walsh MC, et al. Barriers to enrollment in a randomized controlled trial of hydrocortisone for cardiovascular insufficiency in term and late preterm newborn infants. J Perinatol Off J Calif Perinat Assoc 2017;37(11): 1220–3.

20. Hoffman TM, Taeed R, Niles JP, et al. Parental factors impacting the enrollment of children in cardiac critical care clinical trials. Pediatr Cardiol 2007;28(3):167–71.

21. Doyle R, Williams T, Schibler A, et al. Challenges to prospective consent in an interventional clinical trial in a paediatric intensive care unit. Aust Crit Care 2020; 33:S5.

22. Burns KEA, Zubrinich C, Tan W, et al. Research recruitment practices and critically ill patients. A multicenter, cross-Sectional study (the consent study). Am J Respir Crit Care Med 2013;187(11):1212–8.

23. Cochius - den Otter S, Deprest JA, Storme L, et al. Challenges and pitfalls: performing clinical trials in patients with congenital diaphragmatic hernia. Front Pediatr 2022;10:852843.

24. Timberline S, Bhatt A, Sunderji S, et al. Novel scoring tool of hypoxemic respiratory failure and pulmonary hypertension for defining severity of persistent pulmonary hypertension of newborn. J Perinatol 2023;43(10):1281–7.

25. MacLaren G, Conrad S, Peek G. Indications for Pediatric Respiratory Extracorporeal Life Support. Published online 2015.

26. Extracorporeal life support organization (ELSO) registry report. International Summary; 2021.

27. Steinhorn RH, Fineman J, Kusic-Pajic A, et al. Bosontan as adjunctive therapy for persistent pulmonary hypertension of the newborn: results of the randomized multicenter placebo-controlled exploratory trial. J Pediatr 2016;177:90–6.e3.

28. Porta NFM, Steinhorn RH. Pulmonary vasodilator therapy in the NICU: inhaled nitric oxide, sildenafil, and other pulmonary vasodilating agents. Clin Perinatol 2012;39(1):149–64.

29. Jansen TC, Kompanje EJO, Bakker J. Deferred proxy consent in emergency critical care research: ethically valid and practically feasible. Crit Care Med 2009; 37(1):S65.

30. Fivez T, Kerklaan D, Mesotten D, et al. Early versus late parenteral nutrition in critically ill children. N Engl J Med 2016;374(12):1111–22.

31. Furyk J, McBain-Rigg K, Renison B, et al. A comprehensive systematic review of stakeholder attitudes to alternatives to prospective informed consent in paediatric acute care research. BMC Med Ethics 2018;19:89.

32. Fitzpatrick A, Wood F, Shepherd V. Trials using deferred consent in the emergency setting: a systematic review and narrative synthesis of stakeholders' attitudes. Trials 2022;23:411.

33. The Neonatal Inhaled Nitric Oxide Study Group (NINOS). Inhaled nitric oxide and hypoxic respiratory failure in infants with congenital diaphragmatic hernia. Pediatrics 1997;99(6):838–45.

34. EL-Khuffash A, McNamara PJ, Breatnach C, et al. The use of milrinone in neonates with persistent pulmonary hypertension of the newborn - a randomised controlled trial pilot study (MINT 1). J Perinatol 2023;43(2):168–73.

35. Steinhorn RH, Kinsella JP, Pierce C, et al. Intravenous sildenafil in the treatment of neonates with persistent pulmonary hypertension. J Pediatr 2009;155(6): 841–7.e1.
36. Cochius-den Otter S, de Hoog M, Koch BCP, et al. RE: efficacy and safety of IV sildenafil in the treatment of newborn infants with, or at risk of persistent pulmonary hypertension of the newborn (PPHN): a multicenter, randomized, placebo-controlled trial. J Pediatr 2022;246:284–5.
37. Saugstad OD, Kirpalani H. Searching for evidence in neonatology. Acta Paediatr 2023;112(8):1648–52.
38. Binko MA, Reitz KM, Chaer RA, et al. Selective Publication within Vascular Surgery: Characteristics of Discontinued and Unpublished Randomized Clinical Trials. Ann Vasc Surg 2023;95:251–61.
39. Neubert A, Baarslag MA, van Dijk M, et al. The CLOSED trial; CLOnidine compared with midazolam for SEDation of paediatric patients in the intensive care unit: study protocol for a multicentre randomised controlled trial. BMJ Open 2017;7(6):e016031.
40. Newman JH, Elliott GC, Haworth GS, et al. Clinical trials in pulmonary hypertension: time for a consortium. Pulm Circ 2013;3(1):245–51.
41. NHLBI ARDS network | about http://ardsnet.org/. Accessed August 3, 2023.
42. Baquero H, Soliz A, Neira F, et al. Oral sildenafil in infants with persistent pulmonary hypertension of the newborn: a pilot randomized blinded study. Pediatrics 2006;117(4):1077–83.
43. Vargas-Origel A, Gómez-Rodríguez G, Aldana-Valenzuela C, et al. The use of sildenafil in persistent pulmonary hypertension of the newborn. Am J Perinatol 2010;27(3):225–30.
44. Al Omar S, Salama H, Al Hail M, et al. Effect of early adjunctive use of oral sildenafil and inhaled nitric oxide on the outcome of pulmonary hypertension in newborn infants. A feasibility study. J Neonatal Perinat Med 2016;9(3):251–9.

APPENDIX 1: SPECIFIC SEARCH TERMS
Embase

((infant*:ti,ab OR newborn*:ti,ab OR neonat*:ti,ab OR 'infant'/exp) AND ('pulmonary hypertension':ti,ab OR pphn:ti,ab OR 'pulmonary hypertension'/exp OR 'persistent pulmonary hypertension':ti,ab OR 'persistent pulmonary hypertension'/exp OR 'meconium aspiration':ti,ab OR 'meconium aspiration'/exp OR 'hypoxemic respiratory failure':ti,ab OR 'respiratory failure'/exp) AND ('pulmonary vasodilat*':ti,ab OR 'vasodilator agent'/exp OR bosentan:ti,ab OR 'bosentan'/exp OR milrinone:ti,ab OR 'milrinone'/exp OR treprostinil:ti,ab OR 'treprostinil'/exp OR prostacyclin:ti,ab OR 'prostacyclin'/exp OR prostaglandin:ti,ab OR 'prostaglandin'/exp OR sildenafil:ti,ab OR 'sildenafil'/exp OR 'pulmonary vasodilation'/exp) AND (ino:ti,ab OR 'nitric oxide':-ti,ab OR 'nitric oxide'/exp)) AND [randomized controlled trial]/lim AND [1997–2023]/py.

Pubmed

(("infant*"[Title/Abstract] OR "newborn*"[Title/Abstract] OR "neonat*"[Title/Abstract] OR "Infant"[Mesh]) AND ("pulmonary hypertension"[Title/Abstract] OR "PPHN"[Title/Abstract] OR "Hypertension, Pulmonary"[Mesh] OR "Persistent fetal circulation"[Title/Abstract] OR "Persistent Fetal Circulation Syndrome"[Mesh] OR "Meconium aspiration syndrome"[Title/Abstract] OR "Meconium Aspiration Syndrome"[Mesh] OR "Hypoxemic respiratory failure"[Title/Abstract] OR "Respiratory Insufficiency"[Mesh]) AND ("pulmonary vasodilat*"[Title/Abstract] OR "Vasodilator Agents" [Pharmacologic

Action] OR "bosentan"[Title/Abstract] OR "Bosentan"[Mesh] OR "milrinone"[Title/Abstract] OR "Milrinone"[Mesh] OR "treprostenil"[Title/Abstract] OR "flolan"[Title/Abstract] OR "Epoprostenol"[Mesh] OR "prostaglandin*"[Title/Abstract] OR "Prostaglandins"[Mesh] OR "sildenafil"[Title/Abstract] OR "Sildenafil Citrate"[Mesh]) AND ("iNO"[Title/Abstract] OR "nitric oxide"[Title/Abstract] OR "Nitric Oxide"[Mesh])) AND ((randomizedcontrolledtrial[Filter]) AND (1997:2023[pdat]))

Comorbidities and Late Outcomes in Neonatal Pulmonary Hypertension

Emily S. Stieren, MD, PhD*, Deepika Sankaran, MD[1],
Satyan Lakshminrusimha, MD[1], Catherine A. Rottkamp, MD, PhD[1]

KEYWORDS

- Neurodevelopmental outcomes • Congenital diaphragmatic hernia
- Bronchopulmonary dysplasia • Hypoxic-ischemic encephalopathy • Nitric oxide
- Extracorporeal membrane oxygenation • Hearing loss

KEY POINTS

- Neonatal pulmonary hypertension (PH) and various diseases associated with PH are linked to increased mortality and long-term morbidities, including sensorineural hearing loss and neurodevelopmental impairment.
- Neonatal extracorporeal membrane oxygenation (ECMO) for neonatal hypoxemic respiratory failure is associated with worse outcomes. Outcomes can be influenced by etiology of persistent pulmonary hypertension of the newborn (PPHN), severe hypoxemia, hyperventilation, hypocapnia, interventions, and complications of ECMO.
- Despite reduction in the need for ECMO therapy, inhaled nitric oxide does not impact neurodevelopmental outcomes in term newborns with PPHN.
- Congenital diaphragmatic hernia with PPHN still has a mortality rate of approximately 30%, and neurodevelopmental outcomes are influenced by disease severity, mechanical ventilation duration, and other factors.
- PH in preterm infants is associated with increased mortality and neurodevelopmental impairment, particularly when it is associated with bronchopulmonary dysplasia.

INTRODUCTION

Persistent pulmonary hypertension of the newborn (PPHN), characterized by respiratory distress and labile hypoxemia, occurs when the normal cardiopulmonary transition from fetal to neonatal life is disrupted.[1] It is reported in about 0.2% of term newborns and 2% to 8% of preterm infants.[2,3] Neonatal pulmonary hypertension (PH) can also complicate illness such as sepsis, meconium aspiration syndrome

Division of Neonatology, Department of Pediatrics, University of California, Davis, USA
[1] Present address. 2516 Stockton Boulevard, Sacramento, CA 95817, USA
* Corresponding author. 2516 Stockton Boulevard, Sacramento, CA 95817, USA.
E-mail address: estieren@ucdavis.edu

Clin Perinatol 51 (2024) 271–289
https://doi.org/10.1016/j.clp.2023.10.002   **perinatology.theclinics.com**

(MAS), respiratory distress syndrome (RDS), transient tachypnea of the newborn, bronchopulmonary dysplasia (BPD), and hypoxic-ischemic encephalopathy (HIE). The acute management of neonatal PH has advanced over the past few decades and now includes supplemental oxygen with gentle ventilation and lung recruitment strategies such as high-frequency ventilation and surfactant administration. There is an increased use of pulmonary vasodilators such an inhaled nitric oxide (iNO) in neonatal intensive care units, and extracorporeal membrane oxygenation (ECMO) is an option if these treatments are insufficient. Despite these therapeutic advances, PH is associated with significant long-term morbidities including adverse respiratory, cardiovascular, and neurodevelopmental (ND) outcomes. The extent and severity of these morbidities are determined by the underlying etiologies of PH, severity of hypoxemia, and the therapeutic interventions used. This review article aims to provide an overview of the comorbidities associated with neonatal PH and their impact on outcomes.

OUTCOMES

Outcomes among PPHN infants are classified based on gestation and need for ECMO.

Outcomes of Term Newborns with Pulmonary Hypertension Not Treated with Extracorporeal Membrane Oxygenation

Term neonates with PH are at risk of ND impairment (NDI) due to hypoxemic respiratory failure (HRF) and the underlying etiology of PH, and as an effect of therapeutic interventions including prolonged mechanical ventilation, exposure to hyperoxia, hypocapnia, acidosis, and ECMO (**Fig. 1**).[4] ND effects that are reported after neonatal PH include delay in cognitive or motor performance, cerebral palsy (CP), and sensorineural hearing

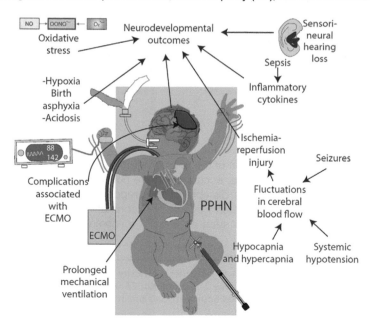

Fig. 1. Factors influencing neurodevelopmental outcomes in persistent pulmonary hypertension of the newborn (PPHN) in term infants. ECMO, extracorporeal membrane oxygenation. (Copyright Satyan Lakshminrusimha.)

loss (SNHL).[5] ND follow-up of newborns with PH from sites in the United States and Canada involved in the Neonatal Research Network at 18 to 24 months conducted by Konduri and colleagues demonstrated that approximately 25% had NDI (defined as the presence of any of the following: moderate or severe CP, Bayley Mental Developmental Index [MDI] < 70, Bayley Psychomotor Developmental Index [PDI] < 70, blindness, or permanent hearing impairment requiring amplification) with no difference based on iNO exposure.[4] Interestingly, ND outcomes were not different between the 24 infants who received ECMO (MDI, 85.8 ± 23.9; PDI, 92.8 ± 15.3) compared with 211 infants who did not receive ECMO support (MDI, 84.5 ± 20 [P = .66]; PDI, 91 ± 18.5 [P = .68]). In this study, moderate to severe CP, defined as abnormal muscle tone in at least one extremity and abnormal control of movement and posture that interfered with age-appropriate motor functioning, was observed in 3.8% of newborns with PH.[4] Furthermore, the use of muscle relaxants or postnatal steroids were not independent risk factors for NDI. Three other major trials have evaluated the effect of iNO and found no additional benefit of iNO in improving ND outcomes after neonatal PH.[5–7] In several studies, hearing impairment was found to be a common issue in patients with neonatal PH, notably even in infants with less severe illness. SNHL as a late outcome of neonatal PH is progressive and is thought to be associated with hyperventilation, longer duration of mechanical ventilation, hypocapnia, acidosis, and prolonged exposure to furosemide in neonates with PH (**Fig. 2**).[8] Relatively fewer studies have demonstrated longer term outcomes at school age. Eriksen and colleagues looked at cohort of children at age 5 to 11 years and found that those who had neonatal PH were more likely than age-matched controls to require remedial education.[9] In another cohort of 109 neonates, researchers reported Full-Scale Intelligence Quotient (IQ) less than 70 in 9.2%, IQ from 70 to 84 in 7.4%, and SNHL in 6.4%, with no difference between iNO-exposed versus nonexposed infants.[9]

In addition to NDI, short-term respiratory morbidities and feeding problems were observed in 24% after neonatal PH in a cohort of 109 neonates followed up at school

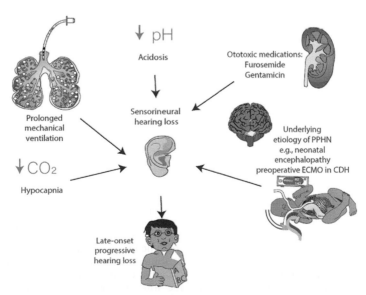

Fig. 2. Pathogenesis of sensorineural hearing loss in PPHN. CDH, congenital diaphragmatic hernia, ECMO, extracorporeal membrane oxygenation. (Copyright Satyan Lakshminrusimha.)

age by Rosenberg and colleagues.[9] Another cohort of neonates with PH demonstrated higher use of bronchodilator therapy at 5 to 11 years after birth.[10] In recent years, newer pulmonary vasodilator therapies, such as sildenafil, bosentan, and epoprostenol, have become more widely used in the neonatal population, and further studies are warranted to evaluate the impact of these new therapies on cardiorespiratory and ND outcomes after neonatal PH.

In contrast to reversible causes of neonatal PH such as MAS and pneumonia, pulmonary hypoplasia (secondary to congenital diaphragmatic hernia [CDH] or renal anomalies) and inherited causes of neonatal PH (such as *TBX4* gene mutations and deletions) are associated with worse outcomes. *TBX4* mutations and 17q23 deletions are often associated with either early neonatal-onset or late-onset PH and NDI, along with skeletal and other anomalies.[11]

Outcomes of Term Newborns with Pulmonary Hypertension Treated with Extracorporeal Membrane Oxygenation

For newborns with PH and HRF that do not improve with conventional medical management but have reversible cardiopulmonary disease, ECMO or extracorporeal life support may be indicated.[12] The availability of ECMO as a treatment option has improved survival and outcomes for HRF that is secondary to reversible etiologies such as MAS, HIE, RDS, and sepsis with overall survival rates of 73% to 85% with lower survival rates in CDH and sepsis.[13–15] Studies have reported worse ND outcomes among term neonates with PH that were treated with ECMO. However, it is challenging to define the extent to which the NDI is caused by the underlying cardiorespiratory instability due to the primary etiology of PH warranting escalation toward ECMO versus a direct complication from the utilization of ECMO (due to disruption of the cerebral circulation) (see **Figs. 1** and **3**).[16] Based on data from the UK Collaborative ECMO Trial, the underlying disease process and cardiorespiratory instability

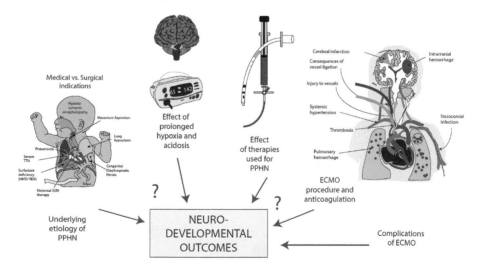

Fig. 3. Controversial contribution of extracorporeal membrane oxygenation (ECMO) to neurodevelopmental outcomes. The individual contribution of underlying etiology of pulmonary hypertension (such as congenital diaphragmatic hernia [CDH]), hypoxia, hypoperfusion, acidosis, impact of therapeutic interventions, and complications from ECMO are difficult to determine and separate out from effects of ECMO itself. (Copyright Satyan Lakshminrusimha.)

were thought to be the primary driver of NDI.[12] Additional factors implicated in intra-cranial injury after ECMO include hypoxemia, acidosis, hypercarbia, anticoagulant use, vasomotor shock, volume expansion, blood pressure fluctuations, increased cerebral blood volume, loss of autoregulation, reactive hyperperfusion, hemodilution, rupture of cerebral arterioles from exposure to high blood flow pressures, reduced pulsatility with venoarterial ECMO, and abnormal venous drainage from venovenous ECMO.[17,18]

The incidence of cerebral injury after ECMO is reported as 5% to 12% overall with severe hypoxia, with low birth weight and sepsis being risk factors.[19] Although there was a concern for lateralization of lesions after unilateral carotid artery ligation, there was no lateralization of lesions on neuroimaging in two large series.[19,20] Abnormalities on neuroimaging (**Fig. 4**) vary from mild (widened interhemispheric fissure, mild ventricular dilation, small extra-axial hemorrhages) to severe (generalized cortical atrophy, diffuse periventricular leukomalacia, parenchymal hemorrhages, parenchymal infarcts).[19] In a prospectively followed cohort of 152 neonates treated with ECMO, severity of findings on neonatal neuroimaging was inversely associated with IQ scores, pre-academic skills, and neuromotor function at age 5 year. The incidence of ND disability was 57% in those with severe lesions on imaging, 33% in those with moderate lesions, 13% in those with mild lesions, and 10% among those with no lesion on neuroimaging.[19] In another elegant study by Rais-Bahrami and colleagues that compared ND outcomes between 76 neonates who were treated with ECMO and 20 neonates who were critically ill but did not meet criteria for ECMO ("near-miss ECMO"), there was no difference in risk of cognitive and adaptive outcomes or school failure at 5 years, although a significant number (37%) in each group was at risk of school failure.[21] This finding was corroborated by Glass and colleagues who showed major disability in 17% (including 11% with intellectual disability) of ECMO-treated infants, school failure in 49% of ECMO-treated infants (compared with 22% in healthy controls), and normal yet lower mean full scale, verbal, and performance IQ compared with healthy controls (96 vs 115, $P < .001$).[22]

A prospective cohort study from the Netherlands conducted by Schiller and colleagues between 1996 and 2006 included 278 infants who were treated with ECMO within the first 28 days after birth and ultimately included 178 infants in whom MDI was evaluated at 2 years and IQ was evaluated at 8 years, respectively.[23] In this cohort, intelligence was stable and average across development at 2, 5, and 8 years of age. About 37% of ECMO-treated children needed extra help at school at 8 years of age despite average intelligence and 7% attended special education and had lower

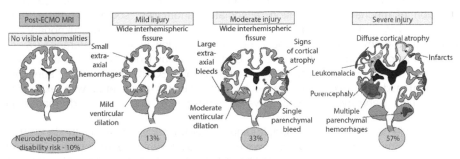

Fig. 4. Abnormalities in neuroimaging following ECMO (extracorporeal membrane oxygenation) for neonatal pulmonary hypertension. The severity of abnormalities are shown in the yellow rectangular boxes. The incidence of neurodevelopmental impairment is shown in pink oval/circles. (Copyright Satyan Lakshminrusimha.)

intelligence from age 2 onward. Children with CDH had lower scores for IQ and selective attention when compared with those with MAS and other diagnoses.[23] Eight-year follow-up after neonatal ECMO from a nationwide sample of 138 children from the United States showed normal range IQ (99.9, standard deviation 17.7).[24] However, the investigators observed a higher need for special education (39%), slower working speed and less accuracy, normal eye-hand coordination, more somatic and attention behavior issues per caregiver report, and more somatic, social, thought, and aggression problems per teacher report compared with normative data.[24] In a recent retrospective cohort study by Kim and colleagues that included 191 neonates who underwent ECMO for HRF between 2006 and 2016, survival to discharge was 71% with higher survival of 82% in those with medical indications for ECMO, such as MAS, and 60% for surgical indications such as CDH.[25] The investigators reported higher incidence of motor delays at 24 months in surgical indications compared with 15% in medical indications. In summary, neonatal respiratory ECMO is associated with abnormalities in neuroimaging and neurodevelopment that are worse in CDH when compared with medical indications for ECMO. It is possible that the outcomes are influenced more by the underlying etiology of HRF rather than ECMO itself.

Outcomes of Congenital Diaphragmatic Hernia with Pulmonary Hypertension with or Without Extracorporeal Membrane Oxygenation Support

Over the past few decades, the management of CDH has moved away from urgent surgery, hyperventilation, and zealous ventilation strategies[26] toward the use of protocolized management guidelines and gentle ventilation strategies (avoiding volutrauma and barotrauma), focus on management of PH, and delayed surgery after optimizing hemodynamic status. Despite advances in medical and surgical management, the mortality in CDH remained unchanged at approximately 30%, and survival after ECMO remains 40% to 50%.[27,28] A large retrospective study from CDH study group, an international collaborative body with a focus on studying and improving outcomes of CDH that included 5203 newborns with CDH showed a decrease in overall mortality over time between 1995 and 2020 comparing five eras of 5 years each.[29] In addition, there was a decrease in observed-to-expected mortality and risk-adjusted mortality over time, despite no difference in birth weight and repair rate. As expected, the timing of repair was later in the 2015 to 2020 era compared with the 1995 to 2000 era. Both right and left ventricular dysfunction occurring early in newborns with CDH are associated with ECMO and death.[30,31] Preoperative ECMO was associated with higher incidence of SNHL when compared with postoperative ECMO (see **Fig. 2**).[32] The etiology of NDI after neonatal PH in CDH is complex and is related to disease severity, duration of mechanical ventilation, associated anomalies, socioeconomic status, gestational age, and the use of iNO and ECMO.[33,34] In a study from the Pulmonary Hypoplasia Program database by Antiel and colleagues, low head circumference trajectory and longer Neonatal Intensive Care Unit (NICU) stay were associated with lower cognitive scores.[35] In another study comparing non-ECMO treated CDH survivors with matched controls, perioperative hypocapnia was associated with executive dysfunction, behavior problems, lowered intelligence, and poor performance in mathematics.[36]

In a single-center prospective longitudinal follow-up study from the Netherlands that included 52 newborns with CDH who were followed up with echocardiograms at 6 and 12 months of age, CDH infants with PH had a longer duration of mechanical ventilation (median [IQR] 77 days [49–181] vs 8 days [5–15], $P = .02$) and longer length of hospital stay (331 days [198–407] vs 33 days [16–59]) compared with CDH without PH.[37] Out of 37 newborns with CDH and PH, four infants (11%) had persistence of PH at 6 or

12 months after birth and required supplemental oxygen therapy, sildenafil, bosentan, diuretics, and tube feeding at 6 months.[37] PH is associated with worse cognitive outcomes and neuromuscular hypotonicity in CDH survivors.[33]

In a recent retrospective study of 193 CDH patients (32 treated with ECMO) who were followed for approximately 4 years following CDH repair, long-term survival rate was 96.4%, and seven (3.6%) patients died approximately 21 months after discharge, most commonly due to respiratory failure.[38] Asthma (23.6%), diminished exercise tolerance (29.5%), gastroesophageal reflux disease (21.8%), NDI (28.6%), attention-deficit/hyperactivity disorder (ADHD) (7.3%), hearing loss (2.1%), and autism (1.6%) were observed on long-term follow-up (**Fig. 5**).[38] A similar study that included 41 CDH survivors between 2004 and 2007 from Philadelphia showed borderline or delayed motor, cognitive, and psychomotor outcomes with ECMO use.[39] However, in another study by Sheikh and colleagues, mild versus severe CDH (based on prenatal risk factors: lung-to-head ratio, observed-to-expected total fetal lung volume) and use of ECMO were not associated with worse quality of life (QOL) in physical or psychosocial functioning.[40] This finding was corroborated in a chart review and phone survey-based study by Morsberger and colleagues evaluating children with a history of CDH at 5.8 ± 2.2 years in which defect side, patch versus primary repair, prenatal diagnosis, use of ECMO, or recurrence did not affect current neurocognitive functioning or QOL scores.[41] In a recent systematic review that included 2624 children from 13 studies with isolated CDH without other genetic defects, four studies reported

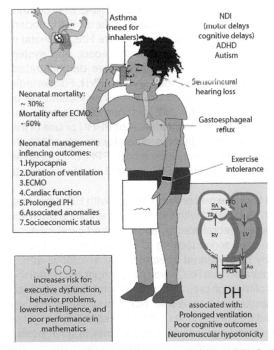

Fig. 5. Long-term outcomes in congenital diaphragmatic hernia (CDH). Pulmonary hypoplasia can lead to airway reactivity with asthma like symptoms and exercise intolerance. Gastroesophageal reflux, attention-deficit hyperactivity disorder (ADHD), autism, motor, and cognitive delays are common in children operated for CDH in the neonatal period. Negative outcomes associated with persistent pulmonary hypertension (PH) and hypocapnia are shown. (Copyright Satyan Lakshminrusimha.)

NDI in 16% of children that was mainly attributable to motor delays and in part to cognitive dysfunction and hearing loss.[42] However, they did not specifically evaluate the effect of PH or use of ECMO. Although studies that compared venovenous and venoarterial ECMO did not show any difference in severe neurologic complications, these studies are limited by potential selection bias and inability to control for disease severity.[43] In addition to risk of NDI, long-term ventilation, poor somatic growth, and poor ventilation–perfusion matching have been reported.[44,45] The standardization of multidisciplinary follow-up care is crucial for timely identification and management of long-term outcomes after CDH.[46]

Outcomes of Term Newborns with Hypoxic-Ischemic Encephalopathy and Pulmonary Hypertension

HIE is a serious neonatal condition that despite advances in neonatal care continues to contribute to long-term NDI and even death in the most severe cases. The brain injury associated with HIE is attributed to perinatal oxygen deprivation and reduced cerebral blood flow.[47] The standard of care for HIE is therapeutic hypothermia (TH) to decrease reperfusion injury.[47] Despite this, up to 30% of survivors with moderate to severe HIE have significant NDI.[48]

Moderate to severe HIE is often associated with neonatal PH. Several retrospective studies have demonstrated that approximately one-quarter of all infants undergoing TH for HIE are also diagnosed with neonatal PH by clinical or echocardiographic criteria.[48–50] The effects of hypoxia and acidosis on pulmonary vascular resistance (PVR), cardiac dysfunction, and co-occurrence of MAS may contribute to the neonatal PH in infants with HIE.[51] Among a cohort of infants with moderate or severe HIE, neonatal PH was more common with more severe HIE, perinatal metabolic acidosis, MAS, pulmonary hemorrhage, culture proven sepsis, and systemic hypotension.[49] Several studies, including in neonatal lambs, have demonstrated that hypothermia causes pulmonary vasoconstriction and elevated PVR. Furthermore, infants undergoing TH can require increased inspired oxygen as an indicator of increased PVR.[52,53] Initial trials that evaluated TH for HIE did not demonstrate that hypothermia to 33.5°C resulted in an increase in the incidence of PPHN or use of iNO.[48,54,55] However, in infants with preexisting HRF or increased risk for elevated PVR, the pulmonary vasoconstriction associated with TH may exacerbate PPHN.[51] Observational data suggest that the combination of HIE, PPHN, MAS, and TH may be associated with poor respiratory outcomes.[50]

PPHN could lead to worse outcomes in infants with HIE. Impaired systemic oxygenation and ventilation associated with PPHN could enhance brain injury in the setting of systemic hypotension, cerebral edema, and impaired cerebral autoregulation that can accompany HIE. A case series looking at regional cerebral oxygenation saturation (RSO$_2$) measured by near-infrared spectroscopy in infants with coexisting HIE and neonatal PH demonstrated that RSO$_2$ was most impacted by episodes of desaturation accompanied by splitting of pre- and post-ductal saturations suggestive of PH.[56] Whether these changes lead to worse ND outcomes is less clear.[57] There have been case series that demonstrate PH, and more specifically right ventricular dysfunction at 24 hours postnatal age, predisposes infants to have brain injury identified on MRI.[58,59] Conversely, other studies have failed to demonstrate this association.[50,60] The largest cohort of infants with HIE and PPHN was studied retrospectively from the TH arms of three randomized controlled trials (RCTs).[57] In this group of 280 infants with moderate or severe HIE, 67 (24%) had neonatal PH defined by clinical or echocardiographic evidence. In this group of patients, there was no difference in the primary outcome of death or moderate to severe disability after adjustment for the severity of encephalopathy, center, and specific RCT. Interestingly, in a subgroup analysis, infants with moderate HIE were more likely to have death or moderate/severe disability if they had PH (39 vs 20%; adjusted OR [95%CI] 2.58 [1.20–5.5]). Although there is need for further study, our current understanding suggests that careful management of neonatal PH in infants with HIE may help to optimize their ND outcomes.

Outcomes of Preterm Newborns with Early Pulmonary Hypertension

Most research regarding outcomes in this patient population has focused on mortality and/or the development of chronic respiratory conditions, including BPD. Several studies have highlighted the association between early PH and increased mortality rates in this population. In a prospective analysis of preterm patients less than 28 weeks birth gestational age who underwent screening echocardiogram at 10 to 14 days of life, researchers found that the evidence of PH (present in 8% of the cohort) was associated with moderate to severe BPD or death.[61] In a small single-center observational cohort study of infants born at 22 to 28 weeks gestation, echocardiographic evidence of PH at 72 to 96 hours of life, which was present in 55% of the cohort and inversely related to gestational age, was associated with the combined outcome of death or BPD, independent of birth gestational age, and duration of ventilatory support.[62] The infants in this study had serial echocardiograms over the first 14 days of life. Eighty-one percent of the patients with evidence of moderate to severe PH at 72 to 96 hours of life had PH that persisted beyond 96 hours, and for 38% of these infants, signs of moderate to severe PH were still present at day 14. All of the infants with echocardiographic evidence of moderate to severe PH on day 14 died or developed BPD. In a single-center retrospective cohort study of preterm infants with birth weight less than 1500 g, Berenz and colleagues found that echocardiographic evidence of PH between 72 hours and 14 days of age predicted death before hospital discharge.[63] In this study, echocardiograms were obtained for clinical indications rather than for screening or research purposes, and therefore, the patients included in the cohort likely had more severe illness or clinical instability compared with non-included patients. However, the statistical model for predicting mortality did control for gestational age, antenatal steroid exposure, 5-minute Apgar score, sepsis, necrotizing enterocolitis (NEC), and severe intraventricular hemorrhage (sIVH). In a case-control study comparing preterm patients with echocardiographic or clinical evidence of PH in the first 2 weeks of life to those without early PH, researchers found that early PH was associated with BPD and the combined outcome of BPD or death.[64] However, a longer duration of mechanical ventilation in the PH group may have mediated this relationship. Early PH was also associated with an increased use of inotropes and sIVH in this study and therefore could simply be an indicator of increased illness severity.

Contrasting results were reported in a study that used more stringent clinical and echocardiographic criteria to define PH. Seth and colleagues found that early PH was not associated with increased mortality in preterm infants less than 34 weeks (mean gestational age of 27 weeks).[64] However, most of the PH diagnoses in this study were based on echocardiogram findings within the first 12 to 24 hours of life and therefore could be consistent with normal postnatal transitional physiology. In agreement with this hypothesis, in a retrospective analysis of preterm infants (mean gestational age 27.7 weeks) treated with iNO for PH, Baczynski and colleagues found that PH during the first 3 days of life was associated with a higher response rate to iNO, lower mortality, and higher rate of survival without long-term disability at 18 months of age when compared with PH diagnosed after 3 days.[65] This suggests that early PH in preterm infants, especially when associated with preterm, premature rupture of membranes, oligohydramnios, or pulmonary hypoplasia might reflect a relative deficiency in endogenous nitric oxide synthesis during the neonatal transition period. In another single-center retrospective study, Kaluarachchi and colleagues found no difference in the combined outcome of severe BPD or death between patients with and without echocardiographic evidence of PH between 5 and 14 days of age.[66] The mean gestational age of subjects in this study was lower at 25.3 weeks, and the finding of PH was also associated with earlier timing of echocardiogram in this study.

Arjaans and colleagues also found that infants with early PH had echocardiograms performed earlier than those without PH. However, in this single-center prospective cohort study, echocardiographic evidence of early PH within day 3 to 10 of life among preterm infants born at 24 to 30 weeks gestational age was associated with an increased risk of mortality.[67] In this study, researchers defined distinct PH phenotypes based on echocardiogram findings to determine the differential impact on survival. Specifically, echocardiographic evidence of systemic or suprasystemic PVR with right-to-left or bidirectional shunting across a patent ductus arteriosus (PDA) or patent foramen ovale, which was present in 11.5% of the study cohort, was associated with increased mortality before 36 weeks postmenstrual age (PMA). Survival rate at 15 months was 46% for these infants. Subjects with echocardiographic evidence of PH and either left-to-right shunting (with low or normal PVR) or qualitative indicators of PH in the absence of a shunt were not at an increased risk of mortality before 36 weeks PMA. However, after adjusting for birth gestational age and age at the time of echocardiogram, PH with left-to-right shunting was associated with the combined outcome of death or BPD.

Some studies have focused specifically on respiratory outcomes of survivors. In one prospective study that included more than 200 preterm infants who underwent screening echocardiograms on day of life 7, evidence of early pulmonary vascular disease (which was present in 37% of survivors) was associated with higher rate of BPD at 36 weeks.[68] Survivors with early pulmonary vascular disease had threefold increased odds of developing late respiratory illness during the first 2 years of life compared with infants without early PH. When combined with mechanical ventilation at 7 days, the odds increased to eightfold. Of the patients who had signs of pulmonary vascular disease at 7 days of age and survived to 36 weeks, 75% had long-term respiratory comorbidities, such as asthma, bronchiolitis, or hospitalization for respiratory problem during the first 2 years of life. Interestingly, the presence of early PH had a prognostic value similar to that of severe BPD at 36 weeks in predicting late adverse respiratory outcomes, and adding BPD status to a model that included early PH and other perinatal factors did not appreciably improve its prognostic value. Berenz and colleagues found that early PH (within day 3–14 of life) was associated with moderate to severe BPD and need for mechanical ventilation at 36 weeks corrected gestational age after controlling for gestational age, race/ethnicity, PDA treatment, sepsis, and NEC.[63]

There is limited information regarding the role of early PH in preterm infants in predicting ND outcomes. In a large Japanese multicenter retrospective cohort of newborns less than 28 weeks gestational age, researchers found that PH diagnosed in the perinatal period was an independent predictor of visual impairment at 3 years of age, even after adjusting for severe (Stage 3 or greater) retinopathy of prematurity.[3] Among patients who developed BPD in this cohort, a history of early PH was associated with a lower cognitive score on developmental testing administered at 3-year follow-up visit and with lower body weight and head circumference at 3 years of age.

If exposure to iNO is considered a surrogate marker of PH, there are studies from Neonatal Research Network (NICHD) and the Pediatrix Data Warehouse that suggest high incidence of mortality and morbidity. Chandrasekharan and colleagues reported outcomes of 7639 extremely low birth weight infants born at ≤ 26 weeks gestation.[69] Early HRF (defined as the need for $FiO_2 ≥ 0.6$ on day 1 or 3) was associated with a mortality of 51.3% and moderate-to-severe NDI of 41.2% among survivors at 18 to 26 months. Although the precise incidence of PH was not determined, it is likely that many infants with early HRF may have had signs of PH on echocardiography. Exposure to iNO did not significantly influence mortality or morbidity in this population (**Fig. 6**). Ellsworth and colleagues described short-term outcomes of preterm infants (22–29 weeks gestation with a birth weight of ≥ 400g) with pulmonary hypoplasia and PPHN.[70] Mortality was approximately a third lower in this population with iNO exposure although this difference did not reach statistical significance in propensity matching (HR 0.67 [0.45–1.01]). Seventy one percent of infants exposed to iNO had BPD and 6% of them had PVL. Long-term outcomes are not available from this cohort.

Outcomes of Preterm Newborns with Bronchopulmonary Dysplasia and Pulmonary Hypertension

PH is a well-recognized complication of BPD and is associated with increased mortality in this group.[71] In a 2017 meta-analysis that included 384 subjects with BPD from three studies, in-hospital mortality ranged from 6% to 38% for patients with BPD-associated PH (BPD-PH), and subjects with BPD-PH had approximately five times greater odds of predischarge mortality compared with subjects with BPD alone.[72–75] A subsequent meta-analysis of studies that included patients with and without BPD reported an estimated in-hospital mortality rate of 16% for patients with BPD-PH and an estimated cumulative mortality rate of 40% at 2-year follow-up.[73,76–83] In a large multicenter retrospective cohort, Lagatta and colleagues found that among patients with a diagnosis of severe BPD, PH was associated with an adjusted threefold higher odds of in-hospital mortality compared with those without PH; however, among those who survived the NICU admission, there was no difference in mortality between the groups at 1 year corrected age.[84] Similarly, Arjaans and colleagues found that although the mortality rate for patients with BPD-PH was very high before 6 months corrected age, mortality beyond that time point was very low and nearly all survivors had resolution of PH by 2.5 years.[85]

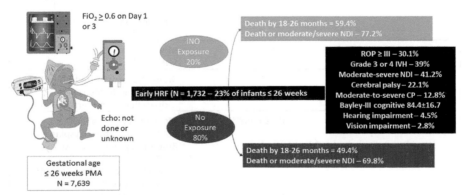

Fig. 6. Graphic abstract of Chandrasekharan and colleagues[69] Pediatrics on outcomes of early hypoxic respiratory failure (HRF) in extremely preterm neonates. There is no difference in clinical outcomes between those infants exposed to inhaled nitric oxide (iNO) versus those that were not exposed. Long-term outcomes are shown in the black box. (Copyright Satyan Lakshminrusimha)

Several studies report on late cardiopulmonary outcomes of BPD patients with and without associated PH. Mourani and colleagues investigated whether PH was associated with adverse late respiratory outcomes during the first 2 years life.[68] In this study, screening echocardiograms were performed on preterm infants at 7 days and

Table 1
Pulmonary hypertension outcome

PH Setting	Age at Follow-Up	Outcome
Term PPHN (excluding CDH)	18–24 mo[4]	NDI (25%)
		Moderate to severe CP (3.8%)
		SNHL
	School age[9,10]	Intellectual disability (9.2%)
		SNHL (6.4%)
		Short-term respiratory and feeding problems (24%)
		Higher use of bronchodilators
Term PPHN/HRF with ECMO	24 mo[25]	Mortality (15%–29%)
		Cerebral injury (5%–12%)[19]
		NDI (10%–57%)
		Motor delays (15%)
	School age[21–24]	Intellectual disability (11%)
		School failure (49%)
		Need for special education (7%–39%)
CDH		Mortality (30%–50%)[27,28]
		NDI (16%–29%)[38,42]
		ADHD (7.3%)
		Autism (1.6%)
		SNHL (2.1%)
		Cognitive impairment
		Motor impairment
		Executive dysfunction and behavior problems[36]
		Asthma (23.6%)
		Diminished exercise tolerance (29.5%)
		Gastroesophageal reflux disease (21.8%)
CDH with ECMO		Mortality (~50%)
		SNHL
PPHN with HIE		Brain injury identified on MRI[58]
		Death or moderate/severe disability (in moderate HIE)[57]
Preterm PPHN	18–26 mo[69]	Mortality (51%–54%)[63,67]
		Bronchopulmonary dysplasia
		Respiratory illness in first 2 y (75%)[68]
		Hospitalization in first 6 mo of life
		Moderate to severe NDI (41.2%)
	3 y[3]	Visual impairment
		Lower cognitive scores
BPD-PH	18–24 mo[87]	Mortality (6%–40%)[72,76]
		Cognitive delay (45%)
	3 y[88]	Developmental delay

36 weeks corrected age. Information regarding respiratory symptoms, respiratory support, and health care utilization was obtained via caregiver report in 6-month intervals for the first 2 years of life. They found that PH at 36 weeks did not increase the likelihood of late respiratory comorbidities, and even BPD status was not as useful in predicting late respiratory outcomes as a model that included day 7 echocardiogram findings and other early perinatal factors. In a retrospective study of patients who were referred to a BPD outpatient follow-up clinic, researchers found that PH that persisted beyond 2 months of age did not increase the risk of post-discharge respiratory outcomes, such as ER visits, hospital admissions, and respiratory symptoms, during the first 2 years of life.[86] However, this cohort represents a group that was engaging in close follow-up in BPD specialty clinic, and many eligible patients were excluded from analysis due to incomplete medical records, including echo reports. In a larger, more representative cohort of patients with severe BPD, infants with BPD-PH were more likely to have hospital readmissions and hospitalizations requiring mechanical ventilation before 1 year PMA.[84]

Although many researchers have published on ND outcomes of preterm infants with BPD, research looking into the specific contribution of PH in this population is limited. Choi and colleagues performed a retrospective chart review of patients with moderate to severe BPD who had no history of sIVH, PVL, or HIE and had returned for ND follow-up assessments at 18 to 24 months corrected age.[87] They found that subjects with BPD-PH had significantly lower scores in the language, cognitive, and motor domains of the Bayley Scales of Infant and Toddler Development, Third Edition (BSID-III). The prevalence of cognitive delay (BSID-III score <85 in the cognitive domain) was 45% in the BPD-PH group, which was significantly higher compared with BPD alone (9.8%). When the analysis was restricted to only subjects with severe BPD, there were no differences between groups for language and motor scores, but cognitive scores remained significantly lower in the PH group. A limitation of this study is the high risk of selection bias due to the retrospective study design. Only 48% of the eligible subjects had ND follow-up at 18 to 24 months corrected age, and clinical or ND characteristics of the subjects could have influenced the likelihood of attending a follow-up visit for ND assessment. Nakanishi and colleagues conducted a single-center retrospective cohort of preterm infants born at less than 28 weeks gestational age, in which 82% of eligible subjects completed follow-up ND assessments at 3 years of age.[88] They found that subjects with BPD-PH were more likely to have a developmental quotient (DQ) in the significantly delayed range compared with BPD alone. Multiple regression analysis revealed that periventricular leukomalacia (PVL) and BPD-PH were independently associated with developmental delay at age 3 year. When restricted only to severe BPD, those with PH still had significantly higher odds of having a DQ score in the significantly delayed range. There were no differences in the incidence of CP between the BPD and BPD-PH groups.

SUMMARY

Neonatal PH is associated with increased mortality and significant long-term morbidities, including NDI (**Table 1**). Term newborns with PH are at risk for NDI and SNHL. The use of iNO in this population reduces the need for ECMO but has little impact on mortality or ND outcomes. Although the use of ECMO for neonatal PH is associated with improved survival, the extent to which NDI is caused by the underlying disease or ECMO itself remains unclear. Despite improvements in the management of PH in neonates with CDH, mortality rates remain high at approximately 30%. ND outcomes after neonatal PH due to CDH are influenced by various factors, including disease severity, duration of mechanical ventilation, associated anomalies, and the use of ECMO. In preterm infants, PH can occur early in the postnatal course and both chronologic and gestational age at the time of diagnosis influence outcomes. Among patients who develop BPD, the presence of late-onset PH is associated with significantly higher mortality, particularly within the first year following PH diagnosis. Further research is needed to better understand the factors contributing to these outcomes and to develop strategies to improve long-term prognosis in infants with PH.

Best Practice Box

- Close neurodevelopmental follow-up including hearing assessment is important for neonates diagnosed with persistent pulmonary hypertension of newborn (PPHN) that require mechanical ventilation, inhaled nitric oxide, or extracorporeal membrane oxygenation.

- Infants with congenital diaphragmatic hernia are at high risk of neurodevelopmental impairment, nutritional difficulties, and pulmonary function test abnormalities and need close monitoring.

- Preterm infants who develop bronchopulmonary dysplasia with pulmonary hypertension are at risk of other comorbidities and require multidisciplinary follow-up.

- Optimal ventilator management to minimize fluctuations in $PaCO_2$ is critical to improve neurodevelopmental outcomes in PPHN.

FUNDING

S. Lakshminrusimha received HD072929 from NICHD. D. Sankaran received funding from the UC Davis Department of Pediatrics Children's Miracle Network and the American Academy of Pediatrics-Neonatal Resuscitation Program. The funding agencies did not have any role in the design of this manuscript. The authors have no financial relationships relevant to this article to disclose.

DISCLOSURE

The authors have no conflicts of interest to disclose.

REFERENCES

1. Lakshminrusimha S, Keszler M. Persistent pulmonary hypertension of the newborn. NeoReviews 2015;16(12):e680–92.
2. Sankaran D, Lakshminrusimha S. Pulmonary hypertension in the newborn- etiology and pathogenesis. Semin Fetal Neonatal Med 2022;27(4):101381.
3. Nakanishi H, Suenaga H, Uchiyama A, et al. Persistent pulmonary hypertension of the newborn in extremely preterm infants: a Japanese cohort study. Arch Dis Child Fetal Neonatal Ed 2018;103(6):F554–61.
4. Konduri GG, Vohr B, Robertson C, et al. Early inhaled nitric oxide therapy for term and near-term newborn infants with hypoxic respiratory failure: neurodevelopmental follow-up. J Pediatr 2007;150(3):235–40.e1.
5. Lipkin PH, Davidson D, Spivak L, et al. Neurodevelopmental and medical outcomes of persistent pulmonary hypertension in term newborns treated with nitric oxide. J Pediatr 2002;140(3):306–10.
6. Clark RH, Huckaby JL, Kueser TJ, et al. Low-dose nitric oxide therapy for persistent pulmonary hypertension: 1-year follow-up. J Perinatol 2003;23(4):300–3.

7. Group NINOS. Inhaled nitric oxide in term and near-term infants: neurodevelopmental follow-up of the neonatal inhaled nitric oxide study group (NINOS). J Pediatr 2000;136(5):611–7.

8. Hendricks-Munoz KD, Walton JP. Hearing loss in infants with persistent fetal circulation. Pediatrics 1988;81(5):650–6.

9. Rosenberg AA, Lee NR, Vaver KN, et al. School-age outcomes of newborns treated for persistent pulmonary hypertension. J Perinatol 2010;30(2):127–34.

10. Eriksen V, Nielsen LH, Klokker M, et al. Follow-up of 5- to 11-year-old children treated for persistent pulmonary hypertension of the newborn. Acta Paediatr 2009;98(2):304–9.

11. Galambos C, Mullen MP, Shieh JT, et al. Phenotype characterisation of TBX4 mutation and deletion carriers with neonatal and paediatric pulmonary hypertension. Eur Respir 2019;54(2). https://doi.org/10.1183/13993003.01965-2018.

12. Bennett CC, Johnson A, Field DJ, et al, UK Collaborative ECMO Trial Group. UK collaborative randomised trial of neonatal extracorporeal membrane oxygenation: follow-up to age 4 years. Lancet 2001;357(9262):1094–6.

13. Bahrami KR, Van Meurs KP. ECMO for neonatal respiratory failure. Semin Perinatol 2005;29(1):15–23.

14. Amodeo I, Di Nardo M, Raffaeli G, et al. Neonatal respiratory and cardiac ECMO in Europe. Eur J Pediatr 2021;180(6):1675–92.

15. Rycus P, Stead C. Extracorporeal life support organization registry report 2022. Journal of Cardiac Critical Care TSS 2022;6(02):100–2.

16. McNally H, Bennett CC, Elbourne D, et al. United Kingdom collaborative randomized trial of neonatal extracorporeal membrane oxygenation: follow-up to age 7 years. Pediatrics 2006;117(5):e845–54.

17. Short BL, Walker LK, Bender KS, et al. Impairment of cerebral autoregulation during extracorporeal membrane oxygenation in newborn lambs. Pediatr Res 1993; 33(3):289–94.

18. Hunter CJ, Blood AB, Bishai JM, et al. Cerebral blood flow and oxygenation during venoarterial and venovenous extracorporeal membrane oxygenation in the newborn lamb. Pediatr Crit Care Med 2004;5(5).

19. Bulas D, Glass P. Neonatal ECMO: neuroimaging and neurodevelopmental outcome. Semin Perinatol 2005;29(1):58–65.

20. Adolph V, Ekelund C, Smith C, et al. Developmental outcome of neonates treated with extracorporeal membrane oxygenation. J Pediatr Surg 1990;25(1):43–6.

21. Rais-Bahrami K, Wagner AE, Coffman C, et al. Neurodevelopmental outcome in ECMO vs near-miss ECMO patients at 5 years of age. Clin Pediatr (Phila) 2000;39(3):145–52.

22. Glass P, Wagner AE, Papero PH, et al. Neurodevelopmental status at age five years of neonates treated with extracorporeal membrane oxygenation. J Pediatr 1995;127(3):447–57.

23. Schiller RM, Madderom MJ, Reuser JJ, et al. Neuropsychological follow-up after neonatal ECMO. Pediatrics 2016;138(5). https://doi.org/10.1542/peds.2016-1313.

24. Madderom MJ, Reuser JJCM, Utens EMWJ, et al. Neurodevelopmental, educational and behavioral outcome at 8 years after neonatal ECMO: a nationwide multicenter study. Intensive Care Med 2013;39(9):1584–93.

25. Kim F, Bernbaum J, Connelly J, et al. Survival and developmental outcomes of neonates treated with extracorporeal membrane oxygenation: a 10-year single-center experience. J Pediatr 2021;229:134–40.e3.

26. Langham MR Jr, Kays DW, Beierle EA, et al. Twenty years of progress in congenital diaphragmatic hernia at the University of Florida. Am Surg 2003;69(1):45–52.

27. Tennant PWG, Pearce MS, Bythell M, et al. 20-year survival of children born with congenital anomalies: a population-based study. Lancet 2010;375(9715):649–56.

28. Guner YS, Delaplain PT, Zhang L, et al. Trends in mortality and risk characteristics of congenital diaphragmatic hernia treated with extracorporeal membrane oxygenation. Am Soc Artif Intern Organs J 2019;65(5):509.

29. Gupta VS, Harting MT, Lally PA, et al. Mortality in congenital diaphragmatic hernia: a multicenter registry study of over 5000 patients over 25 years. Ann Surg 2023;277(3):520–7.

30. Patel N, Massolo AC, Kipfmueller F. Congenital diaphragmatic hernia-associated cardiac dysfunction. Semin Perinatol 2020;44(1):151168.

31. Le LS, Kinsella JP, Gien J, et al. Failure to normalize biventricular function is associated with extracorporeal membrane oxygenation use in neonates with congenital diaphragmatic hernia. J Pediatr 2023;260:113490.

32. Rasheed A, Tindall S, Cueny DL, et al. Neurodevelopmental outcome after congenital diaphragmatic hernia: extracorporeal membrane oxygenation before and after surgery. J Pediatr Surg 2001;36(4):539–44.

33. Danzer E, Hoffman C, D'Agostino JA, et al. Neurodevelopmental outcomes at 5years of age in congenital diaphragmatic hernia. J Pediatr Surg 2017;52(3):437–43.

34. Benjamin JR, Gustafson KE, Smith PB, et al. Perinatal factors associated with poor neurocognitive outcome in early school age congenital diaphragmatic hernia survivors. J Pediatr Surg 2013;48(4):730–7.

35. Antiel RM, Lin N, Licht DJ, et al. Growth trajectory and neurodevelopmental outcome in infants with congenital diaphragmatic hernia. J Pediatr Surg 2017;52(12):1944–8.

36. Frisk V, Jakobson LS, Unger S, et al. Long-term neurodevelopmental outcomes of congenital diaphragmatic hernia survivors not treated with extracorporeal membrane oxygenation. J Pediatr Surg 2011;46(7):1309–18.

37. Kraemer US, Leeuwen L, Krasemann TB, et al. Characteristics of infants with congenital diaphragmatic hernia who need follow-up of pulmonary hypertension. Pediatr Crit Care Med 2018;19(5):e219–26.

38. Gerall CD, Stewart LA, Price J, et al. Long-term outcomes of congenital diaphragmatic hernia: a single institution experience. J Pediatr Surg 2022;57(4):563–9.

39. Danzer E, Gerdes M, Bernbaum J, et al. Neurodevelopmental outcome of infants with congenital diaphragmatic hernia prospectively enrolled in an interdisciplinary follow-up program. J Pediatr Surg 2010;45(9):1759–66.

40. Sheikh F, Akinkuotu A, Clark SJ, et al. Assessment of quality of life outcomes using the pediatric quality of life inventory survey in prenatally diagnosed congenital diaphragmatic hernia patients. J Pediatr Surg 2016;51(4):545–8.

41. Morsberger JL, Short HL, Baxter KJ, et al. Parent reported long-term quality of life outcomes in children after congenital diaphragmatic hernia repair. J Pediatr Surg 2019;54(4):645–50.

42. Van der Veeken L, Vergote S, Kunpalin Y, et al. Neurodevelopmental outcomes in children with isolated congenital diaphragmatic hernia: a systematic review and meta-analysis. Prenat Diagn 2022;42(3):318–29.

43. Yu PT, Jen HC, Rice-Townsend S, et al. The role of ECMO in the management of congenital diaphragmatic hernia. Semin Perinatol 2020;44(1):151166.

44. Spoel M, van der Cammen-van Zijp MHM, Hop WCJ, et al. Lung function in young adults with congenital diaphragmatic hernia; a longitudinal evaluation. Pediatr Pulmonol 2013;48(2):130–7.
45. Pal K, Gupta DK. Serial perfusion study depicts pulmonary vascular growth in the survivors of non-extracorporeal membrane oxygenation-treated congenital diaphragmatic hernia. Neonatology 2010;98(3):254–9.
46. Snoek KG, Capolupo I, Braguglia A, et al. Neurodevelopmental outcome in high-risk congenital diaphragmatic hernia patients: an appeal for international standardization. Neonatology 2015;109(1):14–21.
47. Bonifacio SL, Hutson S. The term newborn: evaluation for hypoxic-ischemic encephalopathy. Clin Perinatol 2021;48(3):681–95.
48. Jacobs SE, Berg M, Hunt R, et al. Cooling for newborns with hypoxic ischaemic encephalopathy. Cochrane Database Syst Rev 2013;2013(1):CD003311.
49. Lakshminrusimha S, Shankaran S, Laptook A, et al. Pulmonary hypertension associated with hypoxic-ischemic encephalopathy-antecedent characteristics and comorbidities. J Pediatr 2018;196:45–51 e3.
50. Joanna RGV, Lopriore E, Te Pas AB, et al. Persistent pulmonary hypertension in neonates with perinatal asphyxia and therapeutic hypothermia: a frequent and perilous combination. J Matern Fetal Neonatal Med 2022;35(25):4969–75.
51. Singh Y, Lakshminrusimha S. Pathophysiology and management of persistent pulmonary hypertension of the newborn. Clin Perinatol 2021;48(3):595–618.
52. Thoresen M, Whitelaw A. Cardiovascular changes during mild therapeutic hypothermia and rewarming in infants with hypoxic-ischemic encephalopathy. Pediatrics 2000;106(1 Pt 1):92–9.
53. Toubas PL, Hof RP, Heymann MA, et al. Effects of hypothermia and rewarming on the neonatal circulation. Arch Fr Pediatr 1978;35(10 Suppl):84–92.
54. Shankaran S, Laptook AR, Ehrenkranz RA, et al. Whole-body hypothermia for neonates with hypoxic-ischemic encephalopathy. N Engl J Med 2005;353(15): 1574–84.
55. Jacobs S, Hunt R, Tarnow-Mordi W, et al. Cooling for newborns with hypoxic ischaemic encephalopathy. Cochrane Database Syst Rev 2003;4:CD003311.
56. Gagnon MH, Wintermark P. Effect of persistent pulmonary hypertension on brain oxygenation in asphyxiated term newborns treated with hypothermia. J Matern Fetal Neonatal Med 2016;29(13):2049–55.
57. Agarwal P, Shankaran S, Laptook AR, et al. Outcomes of infants with hypoxic ischemic encephalopathy and persistent pulmonary hypertension of the newborn: results from three NICHD studies. J Perinatol 2021;41(3):502–11.
58. More KS, Sakhuja P, Giesinger RE, et al. Cardiovascular associations with abnormal brain magnetic resonance imaging in neonates with hypoxic ischemic encephalopathy undergoing therapeutic hypothermia and rewarming. Am J Perinatol 2018;35(10):979–89.
59. Giesinger RE, El Shahed AI, Castaldo MP, et al. Impaired right ventricular performance is associated with adverse outcome after hypoxic ischemic encephalopathy. Am J Respir Crit Care Med 2019;200(10):1294–305.
60. Yum SK, Seo YM, Kwun Y, et al. Therapeutic hypothermia in infants with hypoxic-ischemic encephalopathy and reversible persistent pulmonary hypertension: short-term hospital outcomes. J Matern Fetal Neonatal Med 2018;31(23): 3108–14.
61. Mirza H, Ziegler J, Ford S, et al. Pulmonary hypertension in preterm infants: prevalence and association with bronchopulmonary dysplasia. J Pediatr 2014;165(5): 909–14.e1.

62. Mirza H, Garcia JA, Crawford E, et al. Natural history of postnatal cardiopulmonary adaptation in infants born extremely preterm and risk for death or bronchopulmonary dysplasia. J Pediatr 2018;198:187–93.e1.

63. Berenz A, Vergales JE, Swanson JR, et al. Evidence of early pulmonary hypertension is associated with increased mortality in very low birth weight infants. Am J Perinatol 2017;34(8):801–7.

64. Seth SA, Soraisham AS, Harabor A. Risk factors and outcomes of early pulmonary hypertension in preterm infants. J Matern Fetal Neonatal Med 2018; 31(23):3147–52.

65. Baczynski M, Ginty S, Weisz DE, et al. Short-term and long-term outcomes of preterm neonates with acute severe pulmonary hypertension following rescue treatment with inhaled nitric oxide. Arch Dis Child Fetal Neonatal Ed 2017;102(6): F508–14.

66. Kaluarachchi DC, Woo KM, Colaizy TT. Role of early pulmonary hypertension as a risk factor for late pulmonary hypertension in extremely preterm infants. Am J Perinatol 2018;35(2):120–6.

67. Arjaans S, Fries MWF, Schoots MH, et al. Clinical significance of early pulmonary hypertension in preterm infants. J Pediatr 2022;251:74–81.e3.

68. Mourani PM, Mandell EW, Meier M, et al. Early pulmonary vascular disease in preterm infants is associated with late respiratory outcomes in childhood. Am J Respir Crit Care Med 2019;199(8):1020–7.

69. Chandrasekharan P, Lakshminrusimha S, Chowdhury D, et al. Early hypoxic respiratory failure in extreme prematurity: mortality and neurodevelopmental outcomes. Pediatrics 2020;146(4). https://doi.org/10.1542/peds.2019-3318.

70. Ellsworth KR, Ellsworth MA, Weaver AL, et al. Association of early inhaled nitric oxide with the survival of preterm neonates with pulmonary hypoplasia. JAMA Pediatr 2018;172(7):e180761.

71. Hilgendorff A, Apitz C, Bonnet D, et al. Pulmonary hypertension associated with acute or chronic lung diseases in the preterm and term neonate and infant. the european paediatric pulmonary vascular disease network, endorsed by ISHLT and DGPK. Heart 2016;102(Suppl 2):ii49–56.

72. Al-Ghanem G, Shah P, Thomas S, et al. Bronchopulmonary dysplasia and pulmonary hypertension: a meta-analysis. J Perinatol 2017;37(4):414–9.

73. Bhat R, Salas AA, Foster C, et al. Prospective analysis of pulmonary hypertension in extremely low birth weight infants. Pediatrics 2012;129(3):e682–9.

74. Choi EK, Jung YH, Kim HS, et al. The impact of atrial left-to-right shunt on pulmonary hypertension in preterm infants with moderate or severe bronchopulmonary dysplasia. Pediatr Neonatol 2015;56(5):317–23.

75. Slaughter JL, Pakrashi T, Jones DE, et al. Echocardiographic detection of pulmonary hypertension in extremely low birth weight infants with bronchopulmonary dysplasia requiring prolonged positive pressure ventilation. J Perinatol 2011; 31(10):635–40.

76. Arjaans S, Zwart EAH, Ploegstra M-J, et al. Identification of gaps in the current knowledge on pulmonary hypertension in extremely preterm infants: a systematic review and meta-analysis. Paediatr Perinat Epidemiol 2018;32(3):258–67.

77. Mourani PM, Sontag MK, Younoszai A, et al. Early pulmonary vascular disease in preterm infants at risk for bronchopulmonary dysplasia. Am J Respir Crit Care Med 2015;191(1):87–95.

78. Weismann CG, Asnes JD, Bazzy-Asaad A, et al. Pulmonary hypertension in preterm infants: results of a prospective screening program. J Perinatol 2017/5 2017; 37(5):572–7.

79. Khemani E, McElhinney DB, Rhein L, et al. Pulmonary artery hypertension in formerly premature infants with bronchopulmonary dysplasia: clinical features and outcomes in the surfactant era. Pediatrics 2007;120(6):1260–9.
80. del Cerro MJ, Sabaté Rotés A, Cartón A, et al. Pulmonary hypertension in bronchopulmonary dysplasia: clinical findings, cardiovascular anomalies and outcomes. Pediatr Pulmonol 2014;49(1):49–59.
81. Cuna A, Kandasamy J, Sims B. B-type natriuretic peptide and mortality in extremely low birth weight infants with pulmonary hypertension: a retrospective cohort analysis. BMC Pediatr 2014;14:68.
82. Aswani R, Hayman L, Nichols G, et al. Oxygen requirement as a screening tool for the detection of late pulmonary hypertension in extremely low birth weight infants. Cardiol Young 2016;26(3):521–7.
83. Waruingi W, Mhanna MJ. Pulmonary hypertension in extremely low birth weight infants: characteristics and outcomes. World J Pediatr 2014;10(1):46–52.
84. Lagatta JM, Hysinger EB, Zaniletti I, et al. The impact of pulmonary hypertension in preterm infants with severe bronchopulmonary dysplasia through 1 year. J Pediatr 2018;203:218–24.e3.
85. Arjaans S, Haarman MG, Roofthooft MTR, et al. Fate of pulmonary hypertension associated with bronchopulmonary dysplasia beyond 36 weeks postmenstrual age. Arch Dis Child Fetal Neonatal Ed 2021;106(1):45–50.
86. Stuart BD, Sekar P, Coulson JD, et al. Health-care utilization and respiratory morbidities in preterm infants with pulmonary hypertension. J Perinatol 2013;33(7): 543–7.
87. Choi EK, Shin SH, Kim E-K, et al. Developmental outcomes of preterm infants with bronchopulmonary dysplasia-associated pulmonary hypertension at 18-24 months of corrected age. BMC Pediatr 2019;19(1):26.
88. Nakanishi H, Uchiyama A, Kusuda S. Impact of pulmonary hypertension on neurodevelopmental outcome in preterm infants with bronchopulmonary dysplasia: a cohort study. J Perinatol 2016;36(10):890–6.